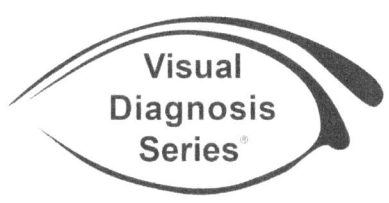

www.visualdxseries.com

Visual Stimuli Review for the Emergency Medicine Board Examinations

Gil Z. Shlamovitz, MD

Copyright © 2014 Gil Shlamovitz, MD

All rights reserved.

DISCLAIMER

1) This publication is intended for medical professionals and **contains graphic medical images**.

2) While the authors and publisher of this work did their best to verify that this work represents acceptable diagnostic and therapeutic standards at the time of publication, neither the authors nor the publisher nor any other party who has been involved in the preparation or publication of this work warrants that the information contained herein is in every respect accurate or complete, and they do not accept responsibility or legal liability for any errors or omissions in this work or for the results obtained from the use of the information contained in this work.

3) Readers are encouraged to verify the information contained herein with other sources. Nonmedical professionals who read this work are encouraged to seek the advice of a physician and not to use any of the diagnostic or therapeutic recommendations that may be included herein.

4) The authors and publisher are not affiliated with the USMLE®, NBME®, FSMB®, or ECFMG® organizations.

PREFACE

Visual stimuli and clinical vignettes are frequently used in medical, nursing, and other allied health examinations. The learner's ability to correctly answer multiple questions is often dependent on his or her initial correct diagnosis of a visual case.

In this publication, which is a part of the Visual Diagnosis Series®, we will review classic clinical vignettes and visual stimuli of disease processes that are commonly asked about on the Emergency Medicine in-service, written and oral board examinations. Each case will include a brief review of the findings seen in the visual stimuli as well as multiple- choice questions that will highlight important clinical aspects of the medical condition.

I hope this publication will appeal to a wide range of readers and assist medical professionals in improving their diagnostic skills and exam scores.

Gil Shlamovitz, MD

TABLE OF CONTENTS

CASE #1:	WEAKNESS AND SYNCOPE	1
CASE #2:	ABDOMINAL DISCOMFORT	4
CASE #3:	VAGINAL BLEEDING AND PELVIC PAIN	7
CASE #4:	LEG PAIN	11
CASE #5:	SHOULDER PAIN	14
CASE #6:	BURNING PAIN	18
CASE #7:	WEAKNESS AND SKIN DISCOLORATION	21
CASE #8:	PALPITATIONS	25
CASE #9:	CHEST PAIN	28
CASE #10:	SWOLLEN TONGUE	31
CASE #11:	CHEST AND BACK PAIN	34
CASE #12:	PAINFUL ULCER	38
CASE #13:	RLQ PAIN	41
CASE #14:	SEVERE LEG PAIN	44
CASE #15:	ABDOMINAL DISTENTION	48
CASE #16:	FEVER AND NIGHT SWEATS	52
CASE #17:	PENILE RASH	55
CASE #18:	PAINFUL LUMP	58
CASE #19:	HEADACHE	61
CASE #20:	SKIN LESION	64
CASE #21:	FACIAL WEAKNESS	68
CASE #22:	BACK PAIN	71
CASE #23:	BREAST LUMP	75

CASE #24:	LEG PAIN	79
CASE #25:	NECK PAIN	82
CASE #26:	WEAKNESS	86
CASE #27:	SKIN LUMPS	89
CASE #28:	DRY COUGH	92
CASE #29:	SHORTNESS OF BREATH	95
CASE #30:	NAUSEA AND VOMITING	98
CASE #31:	LEG SWELLING	101
CASE #32:	CONFUSION AND QUADRIPLEGIA	104
CASE #33:	PAINLESS ULCER	107
CASE #34:	PAINFUL ULCER	110
CASE #35:	RASH & FEVER	113
CASE #36:	EPIGASTRIC PAIN	117
CASE #37:	FINGER SWELLING	121
CASE #38:	DOUBLE VISION	125
CASE #39:	VOMITING	129
CASE #40:	WATERY DIARRHEA	132
CASE #41:	PAINFUL SORE	136
CASE #42:	WRIST PAIN	139
CASE #43:	LEG PAIN	142
CASE #44:	SMALL BUMPS	145
CASE #45:	RED EYE	148
CASE #46:	ITCHY RASH	151
CASE #47:	EYE PAIN	155

CASE #48:	PAINFUL EYE	158
CASE #49:	BARKING COUGH	161
CASE #50:	DYSPNEA	165
CASE #51:	WEAKNESS	169
CASE #52:	TOOTHACHE	172
CASE #53:	ITCHY RASH	175
CASE #54:	RASH	178
CASE #55:	LLQ PAIN	181
CASE #56:	SHORTNESS OF BREATH	184
CASE #57:	LEG PAIN	187
CASE #58:	SEIZURES AND VISION LOSS	191
CASE #59:	UNRESPONSIVENESS	194
CASE #60:	ELBOW PAIN	197
CASE #61:	ABDOMINAL PAIN	200
CASE #62:	SORE THROAT	203
CASE #63:	RASH	206
CASE #64:	ALTERED MENTAL STATUS	209
CASE #65:	RESPIRATORY DISTRESS	212
CASE #66:	NECK SWELLING	215
CASE #67:	FACIAL WEAKNESS	219
CASE #68:	COUGH	223
CASE #69:	FINGER PAIN	226
CASE #70:	RASH	229
CASE #71:	SWOLLEN HAND	232

CASE #72:	FINGER PAIN	235
CASE #73:	EPIGASTRIC PAIN	239
CASE #74:	FINGER PAIN	242
CASE #75:	FACIAL RASH	246
CASE #76:	POOR FEEDING	249
CASE #77:	FOOT PAIN	252
CASE #78:	PAINFUL SCROTUM	255
CASE #79:	EPIGASTRIC PAIN	258
CASE #80:	FOOT PAIN	262
CASE #81:	FINGER PAIN	266
CASE #82:	EYE PAIN	269
CASE #83:	FOOT PAIN	272
CASE #84:	RASH AND FEVER	275
CASE #85:	HEMATURIA	279
CASE #86:	PAINFUL LUMP	282
CASE #87:	GROIN SWELLING	285
CASE #88:	RASH	288
CASE #89:	SHORTNESS OF BREATH	292
CASE #90:	HIP PAIN	296
CASE #91:	VISION LOSS	301
CASE #92:	ABDOMINAL PAIN	304
CASE #93:	PAINFUL LESIONS	308
CASE #94:	NECK PAIN	311
CASE #95:	WEAKNESS	315

CASE #96:	EYE PAIN	318
CASE #97:	WEAKNESS	321
CASE #98:	LLQ PAIN	324
CASE #99:	BLEEDING GUMS	327
CASE #100:	SHORTNESS OF BREATH	331
CASE #101:	RASH AND WEIGHT LOSS	335
CASE #102:	PAINFUL LUMP	338
CASE #103:	ABDOMINAL PAIN	341
CASE #104:	GROIN PAIN	345
CASE #105:	ITCHY SCALP	348
CASE #106:	EPIGASTRIC PAIN	351
CASE #107:	KNEE PAIN	354
CASE #108:	ABDOMINAL PAIN	357
CASE #109:	SORE THROAT	360
CASE #110:	PRODUCTIVE COUGH	363
CASE #111:	RASH AND FEVER	367
CASE #112:	FEVER AND WEIGHT LOSS	370
CASE #113:	FEVER AND MUSCLE ACHES	373
CASE #114:	BREAST PAIN	376
CASE #115:	EARACHE	379
CASE #116:	FEVER	382
CASE #117:	FEVER AND FATIGUE	385
CASE #118:	AGITATION	388
CASE #119:	FACE PAIN	391

CASE #120:	SWOLLEN EYE	394
CASE #121:	SEIZURES	397
CASE #122:	ELBOW SWELLING	401
CASE #123:	UMBILICAL DISCHARGE	404
CASE #124:	EYE PAIN	407
CASE #125:	TESTICULAR PAIN	410
CASE #126:	ALTERED MENTAL STATUS	413
CASE #127:	KNEE PAIN	416
CASE #128:	BACK PAIN	420
CASE #129:	BACK PAIN	423
CASE #130:	SHOULDER PAIN	427
CASE #131:	EARACHE	430
CASE #132:	PELVIC PAIN	433
CASE #133:	EPIGASTRIC PAIN	437
CASE #134:	DIFFICULTY URINATING	441
CASE #135:	FINGER PAIN	444
CASE #136:	SHORTNESS OF BREATH	447
CASE #137:	FEVER AND CONFUSION	451
CASE #138:	PAINFUL RASH	455
CASE #139:	SHORTNESS OF BREATH	458
CASE #140:	EYE SWELLING	463
CASE #141:	SORE THROAT	466
CASE #142:	PELVIC PAIN	469
CASE #143:	DRAINING LUMP	472

CASE #144:	DIFFICULTY SLEEPING	475
CASE #145:	ITCHY RASH	479
CASE #146:	ITCHY RASH	483
CASE #147:	DOUBLE VISION	486
CASE #148:	EARACHE	490
CASE #149:	SKIN DISCOLORATION	494
CASE #150:	KNEE PAIN	499
CASE #151:	ANAL PAIN	502
CASE #152:	ITCHY RASH	505
CASE #153:	SHORTNESS OF BREATH	508
CASE #154:	SHORTNESS OF BREATH	511
CASE #155:	RASH AND FEVER	515
CASE #156:	HEADACHE	518
CASE #157:	VOMITING	521
CASE #158:	ITCHY RASH	524
CASE #159:	LEG PAIN	528
CASE #160:	JOINT PAIN	532
CASE #161:	PAINFUL RASH	535
CASE #162:	PAINFUL FINGERS	538
CASE #163:	CONSTIPATION	541
CASE #164:	WRIST PAIN	544
CASE #165:	ALTERED MENTAL STATUS	547
CASE #166:	CHEST PAIN	550
CASE #167:	RIGHT-SIDED WEAKNESS	553

CASE #168:	VISION LOSS	556
CASE #169:	SHORTNESS OF BREATH	559
CASE #170:	COUGH	562
CASE #171:	PAINFUL RASH	566
CASE #172:	TESTICULAR PAIN	569
CASE #173:	SORE THROAT	573
CASE #174:	WHITE TONGUE	577
CASE #175:	NECK PAIN	580
CASE #176:	ITCHY RASH	583
CASE #177:	RASH	586
CASE #178:	SORE THROAT	589
CASE #179:	CONFUSION	592
CASE #180:	RASH AND FEVER	596
CASE #181:	DYSURIA	599

CASE #1: WEAKNESS AND SYNCOPE

CASE

A 72-year-old female with a past medical history of hypertension and diabetes presents to the emergency department after an episode of syncope in bed, complaining of generalized weakness. She reports fatigue and dizziness over the previous two days and denies any recent medication changes. She denies having chest pain or dyspnea. She is awake, alert, and oriented; her heart rate is 40/min, and her blood pressure is 110/70. An EKG is performed.

QUESTIONS

1. What is the likely diagnosis?
    a. 1st Degree Atrioventricular Block
    b. Mobitz I 2nd Degree Atrioventricular Block
    c. Mobitz II 2nd Degree Atrioventricular Block
    d. 3rd Degree Atrioventricular Block

2. What artery supplies the AV node in most patients?
   a. Circumflex Artery
   b. Left Anterior Descending
   c. Left Marginal Artery
   d. Right Coronary Artery

3. What is the likely cause of her condition?
   a. Congenital
   b. Ischemic
   c. Lyme Disease
   d. Sarcoidosis

4. Which of the following treatments is recommended for this patient?
   a. Atropine 1 mg IV
   b. Ceftriaxone 1 gr IV
   c. Dopamine 5 mcg/kg/min IV
   d. Pacemaker Implantation

ANSWERS

1. d
2. d
3. b
4. d

VISUAL STIMULUS REVIEW

The EKG tracing shows there is no relationship between the rhythm of P waves and the rhythm of QRS complexes. The frequency of P waves is higher than the frequency of QRS complexes.

REFERENCES

- Epstein AE, Dimarco JP, Ellenbogen KA, et al. ACC/AHA/HRS 2008 guidelines for Device-Based Therapy of Cardiac Rhythm Abnormalities: executive summary. Heart Rhythm. Jun 2008;5(6):934-55.

CASE #2: ABDOMINAL DISCOMFORT

CASE

A 67-year-old male patient with a history of hypertension, smoking, and obesity is referred for an abdominal ultrasound for vague abdominal discomfort that he had for the past four months. The patient denies any pain at this time; his blood pressure is 160/90 mmHg, and his heart rate is 72/min. An ultrasound image, obtained at the midline and 5 cm above his umbilicus, is shown below.

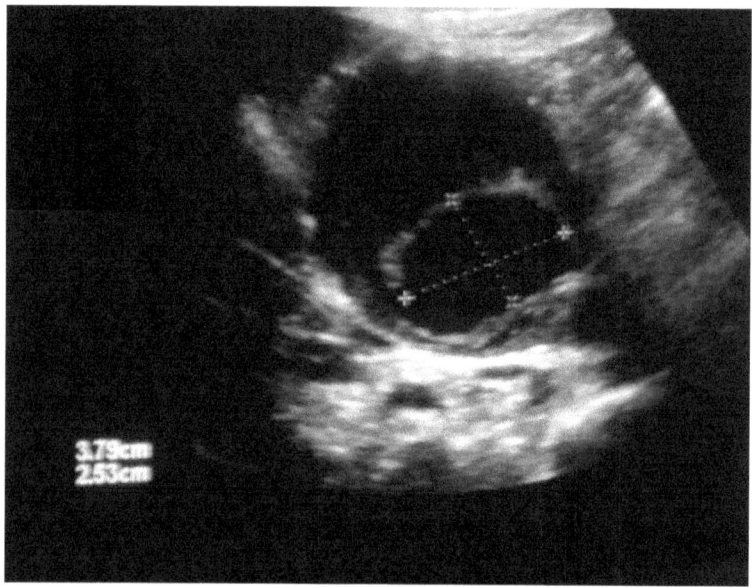

QUESTIONS

5. What is the likely diagnosis?
    a. Abdominal Aortic Aneurism
    b. Atherosclerotic Aortic Disease
    c. Retroperitoneal Hematoma
    d. Ruptured Abdominal Aortic Aneurism

6. What distance is measured in the image?
    a. Clot Burden
    b. Cyst Diameter
    c. False Lumen
    d. True Lumen

7. The patient arrives to your office shortly after the ultrasound exam, and he is asymptomatic. How will you manage this patient?
    a. Immediate referral for CT Angiogram of his thoracic and abdominal aorta.
    b. Initiate Coumadin therapy.
    c. Initiate Esmolol and Nitroprusside IV drips and transfer the patient emergently to the emergency department.
    d. Referral for repeat ultrasound in six months.
    e. Urgent referral to a vascular surgeon.

ANSWERS

5. a

6. d

7. e

VISUAL STIMULUS REVIEW

The ultrasound image demonstrates a large (~7 cm) abdominal aortic aneurism, with a mural thrombus and a "true lumen" of 2.09 cm.

REFERENCES

- Guirguis-Blake J, Wolff TA. Screening for abdominal aortic aneurism. Am Fam Physician. 2005 Jun 1;71(11):2154-5.

CASE #3: VAGINAL BLEEDING AND PELVIC PAIN

CASE

A 19-year-old African-American female patient, who is P1G0 with an estimated gestational age of 30 weeks, presents to the emergency department complaining of waves of vaginal bleeding and pelvic pain for last three hours. She reports that she bumped her abdomen against a table a week ago but had no pain and felt the baby moving normally until a few hours ago. On physical examination, she has a heart rate of 124/min, blood pressure of 100/60, and a tender and hard uterus on palpation. Fetal heart tones are 100/min. A bedside transabdominal ultrasound is obtained.

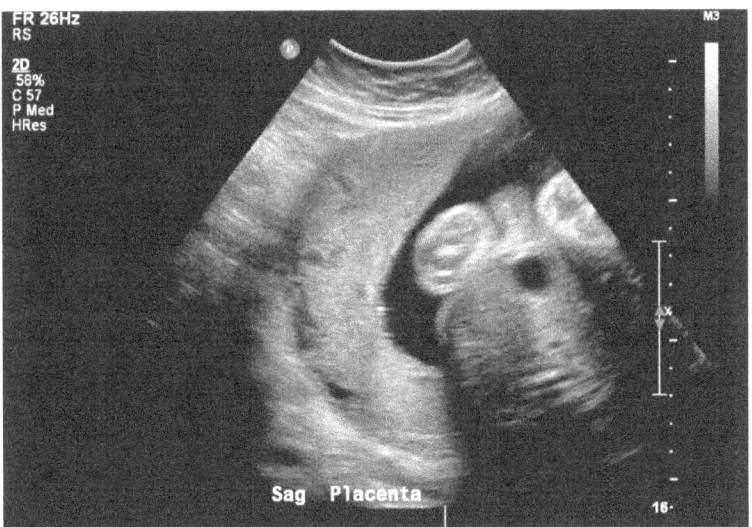

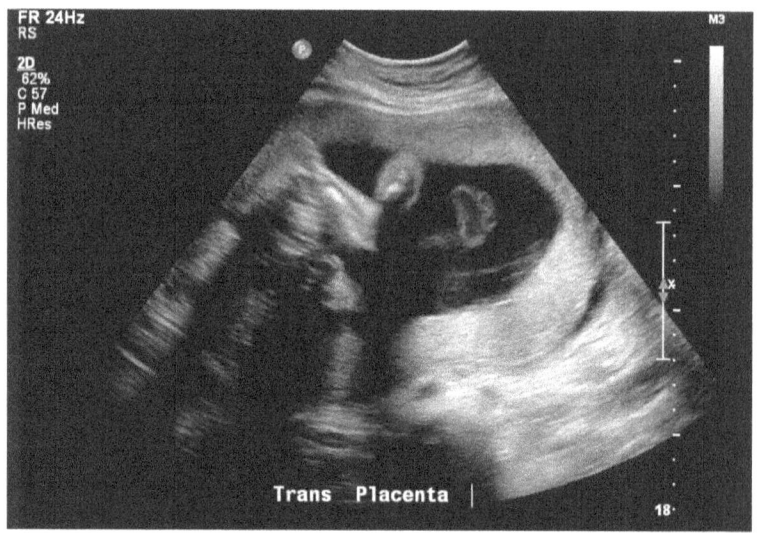

QUESTIONS

8. What is the likely diagnosis?
    a. Abruptio Placenta
    b. Ectopic Pregnancy
    c. Labor with Bloody Show
    d. Placenta Previa
    e. Preeclampsia

9. How would you treat this patient?
    a. Emergent Maternal and Fetal OB Consult
    b. Magnesium Sulfate 4 g IV
    c. Pitocin IV and Emergent Vaginal Delivery
    d. Stat Cesarean Section

10. How should you position the patient?
    a. Counter Trendelenburg
    b. Flexed hips and flexed knees while supine

c. Left Lateral Decubitus
   d. Right Lateral Decubitus
   e. Trendelenburg
11. Which of the following statements is true?
   a. Maternal hypertension does not increase the risk of this condition.
   b. Absence of vaginal bleeding does not exclude the diagnosis.
   c. Normal ultrasound evaluation and normal fetal monitoring excludes the diagnosis.
   d. Normal fibrinogen levels exclude the diagnosis and are reassuring.

ANSWERS

8. a

9. d

10. c

11. b

VISUAL STIMULUS REVIEW

The ultrasound image shows hypodense retroplacental fluid collection. In the acute phase, retroplacental hemorrhage is usually hyperechoic, or even isoechoic, compared with the placenta.

REFERENCES

- Oyelese Y, Ananth CV. Placental abruption. Obstet Gynecol. 2006 Oct;108(4):1005-16.

CASE #4: LEG PAIN

CASE

A 30-year-old male patient with no significant past medical history presents to the ED complaining of pain and swelling of his right lower leg, where he thinks he had a spider bite. On examination, he is afebrile, and his vital signs are all within normal limits. He has a large ill-defined erythematous and edematous plaque on his right medial calf with a 5 cm centrally ulcerated fluctuating mass at its superior pole. The area is warm and fairly tender to the touch.

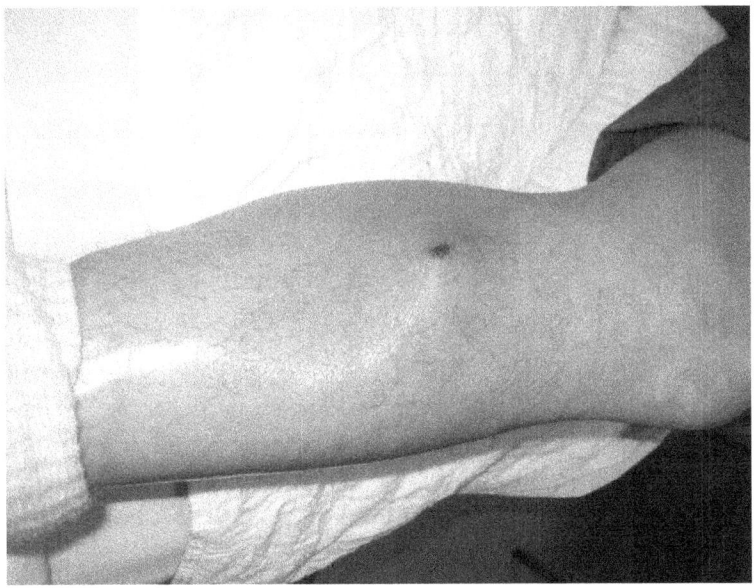

QUESTIONS

12. What is the likely diagnosis?
    a. Abscess
    b. Brown Recluse Spider Bite
    c. Cellulitis
    d. Necrotizing Fasciitis

13. What is the likely cause of this condition?
    a. Anthrax
    b. Brown Recluse Spider Toxins
    c. Methicillin Resistant Staphylococcus Aureus
    d. Streptococcus Pyogenous

14. Which of the following statement is correct?
    a. Brown Recluse Spider (BRS) envenomation usually causes severe initial pain and rarely goes unnoticed.
    b. Most BRS bites will not heal without aggressive surgical treatment.
    c. Drainage alone is usually curative for uncomplicated abscesses measuring less than 5 cm in diameter.
    d. Methicillin Sensitive Staph Aureus (MSSA) is responsible for the majority of skin and soft tissue infections seen in the United States.

ANSWERS

12. a
13. c
14. c

VISUAL STIMULUS REVIEW

The image shows erythematous skin with central black ulceration. The ulcer seems to be the roof of a soft tissue mass, likely an abscess.

REFERENCES

- Breen JO. Skin and soft tissue infections in Immunocompetent patients. Am Fam Physician. 2010 Apr 1;81(7):893-9.
- Dryden MS. Complicated skin and soft tissue infection. J Antimicrob Chemother. 2010 Nov;65 Suppl 3:iii35-44.

CASE #5: SHOULDER PAIN

CASE

A right-handed 20-year-old man presents to the emergency department an hour after he fell on his left shoulder during a soccer game. He has limited range of motion of his left shoulder because of pain but has a normal distal neurovascular exam. A shoulder radiograph is obtained.

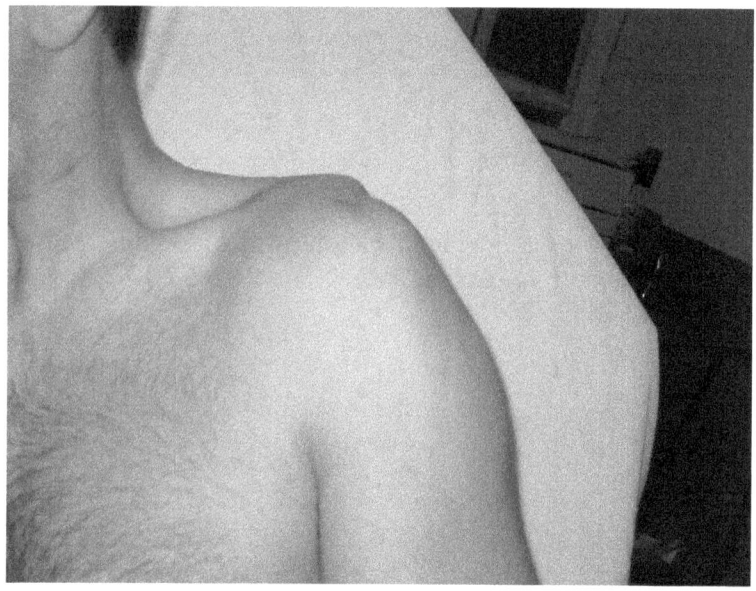

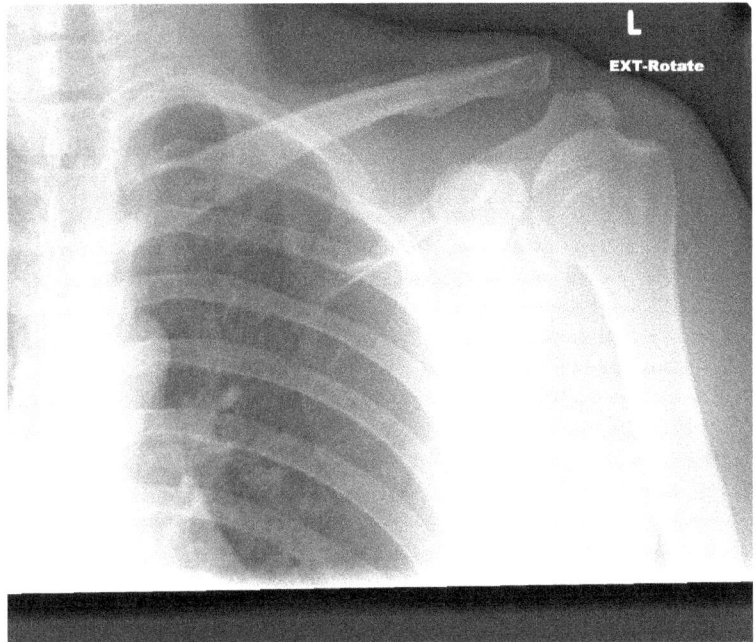

QUESTIONS

15. What is the likely diagnosis?

    a. Acromioclavicular Joint Separation

    b. Clavicular Fracture

    c. Shoulder Dislocation

    d. Shoulder Subluxation

16. Which of the following statements is true?

    a. Heavy lifting and contact sports should be avoided for one to two weeks.

    b. Immediate reduction under moderate sedation is indicated.

    c. Range-of-motion training should be recommended to start at least six weeks after the initial injury.

d. Use of a sling for two weeks or until symptoms improve is recommended.

17. Which of the following statements is true?

    a. This type of injury is common in nonactive elderly patients.

    b. This type of injury most often occurs as a result of a fall on an outstretched arm.

    c. Sagging of the acromion in relation to the clavicle is highly suggestive of a ligamentous disruption of the AC joint.

    d. Immediate operative repair should be recommended to this patient.

ANSWERS

15. a
16. d
17. c

VISUAL STIMULUS REVIEW

The clinical image shows sagging of the acromion in relation to the clavicle.

The radiograph shows that the humerus head is positioned within the glenoid fossa. There is also subluxation of the acromioclavicular space of less than 1 cm with normal coracoclavicular space.

REFERENCES

- Willimon SC, Gaskill TR, Millett PJ. Acromioclavicular joint injuries: anatomy, diagnosis, and treatment. Phys Sportsmed. 2011 Feb;39(1):116-22.

CASE #6: BURNING PAIN

CASE

A 20-year-old male student presents to the ED with severe bilateral upper extremity pain. He was working in a chemistry laboratory when an unknown solution spilled on both his forearms. He immediately washed his hands with a large volume of running water. He complained of severe pain and progression of the skin marks despite washing the substance off.

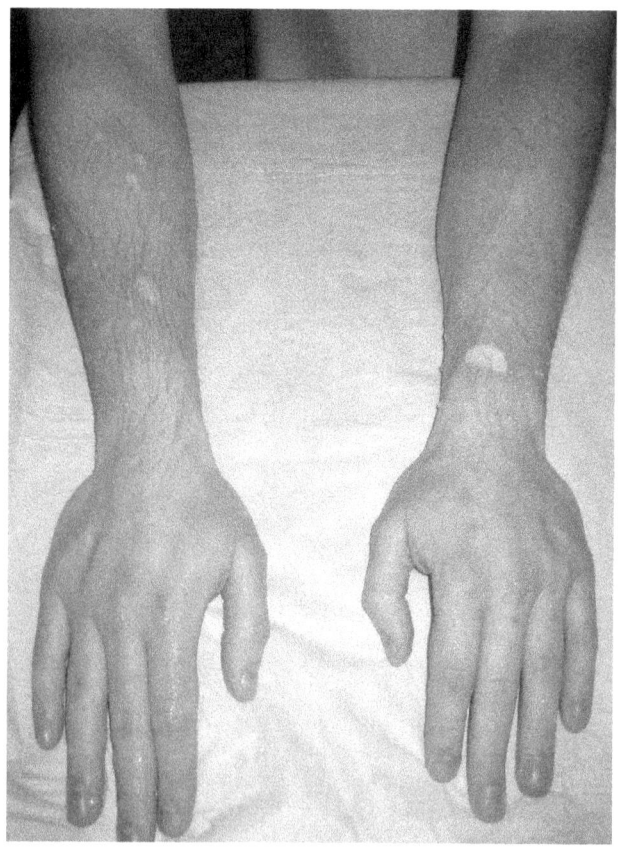

QUESTIONS

18. What is the likely diagnosis?
    a. Acute Bleach Burn
    b. Alkaline Burn
    c. Hydrofluoric Acid Burn
    d. Severe Contact Dermatitis

19. What is the recommended first line treatment for this condition?
    a. Continuous Water Irrigation
    b. Immersion in Milk of Magnesia
    c. Intravenous Steroids and Antihistamines
    d. Topical Application of Calcium Gluconate

20. Which of the following statements is true?
    a. Calcium chloride subcutaneous injections are indicated in refractory cases.
    b. Systemic exposure is an indication for cardiac monitoring and immediate intravenous therapy.
    c. Opioids analgesics should be avoided in order to allow close monitoring of patient's response to therapy.
    d. Serum sodium levels should be closely monitored and are a sensitive marker of disease severity.

ANSWERS

18. c
19. d
20. b

VISUAL STIMULUS REVIEW

The image shows white burn marks with surrounding erythema.

REFERENCES

- Stuke LE, Arnoldo BD, Hunt JL, Purdue GF. Hydrofluoric acid burns: a 15-year experience. J Burn Care Res. Nov-Dec 2008;29(6):893-6.
- Hatzifotis M, Williams A, Muller M, Pegg S. Hydrofluoric acid burns. Burns. 2004 Mar;30(2):156-9.

CASE #7: WEAKNESS AND SKIN DISCOLORATION

CASE

A 32-year-old woman presents to her family doctor complaining of generalized weakness for six months. She has no past medical history and is not taking any medications. She also reports darkening of her skin, especially her palmar skin creases, as well as painless brownish spots over her inner lips. A detailed review of systems reveals progressive fatigue, generalized weakness, and weight loss. Her vital signs are a temperature of 99.7F (37.6C), heart rate of 68/min, blood pressure of 110/60 mmHg, respiratory rate of 11/min, and pulse oximetry of 99%. Her physical examination reveals absence of axillary and pubic hair.

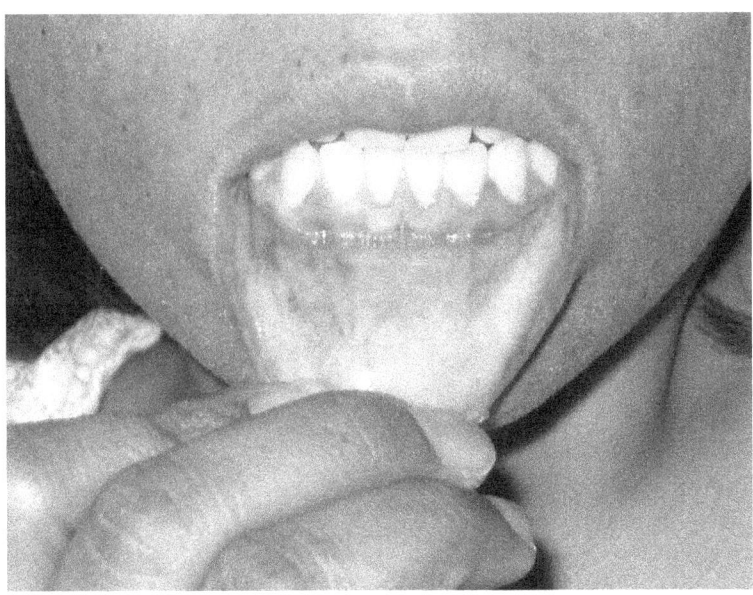

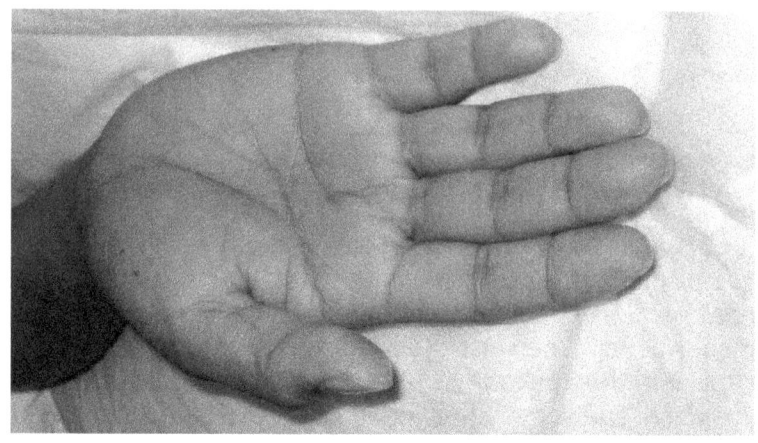

QUESTIONS

21. What is the likely diagnosis?

    a. Addison's Disease

    b. Sarcoidosis

    c. Systemic Lupus Erythematosus

    d. Bilateral Adrenal Infarcts

22. What is the most common cause of this condition?

    a. Amyloidosis

    b. Autoimmune (Idiopathic)

    c. Hemorrhagic Necrosis

    d. Malignant (Lymphoma)

    e. Tuberculosis

23. Once confirmed, what is the most appropriate therapy for this patient?

    a. Hydrocortisone 100 mg IV Push

    b. Prednisone 40 mg PO Daily

    c. Prednisone 40 mg PO + Fludrocortisone 0.1 mg PO Daily

d. IVIG 60 g IV

e. Methotrexate 7.5 mg PO Once Weekly

24. Which of the following medications may cause this condition?

    a. Acetaminophen

    b. Amiodarone

    c. Ketoconazole

    d. Sulfamethoxazole

ANSWERS

21. a
22. b
23. c
24. c

VISUAL STIMULUS REVIEW

The images show generalized hyperpigmentation, including the palmar creases, the dentogingival margins, and the mucosal surface of lips.

REFERENCES

- Betterle C, Morlin L. Autoimmune Addison's disease. Endocr Dev. 2011;20:161-72.

CASE #8: PALPITATIONS

CASE

A 60-year-old woman presents to her family doctor's office complaining of intermittent palpitations and generalized fatigue for the last four days. On the morning of her presentation, the palpitations got worse, and she also experienced shortness of breath with minimal activity. She has a history of hypertension and hyperlipidemia and is compliant with her current medical therapy (Aspirin, Simvastatin, and Hydrochlorothiazide). The patient's vital signs are a heart rate of 140/min, blood pressure of 130/96 mmHg, respiratory rate of 20/min, and O_2Sat of 99%. On physical examination, she is in mild distress, with elevated jugular pressure at 6 cm, bilateral rales over lower and middle fields, and irregularly irregular rapid heart sounds.

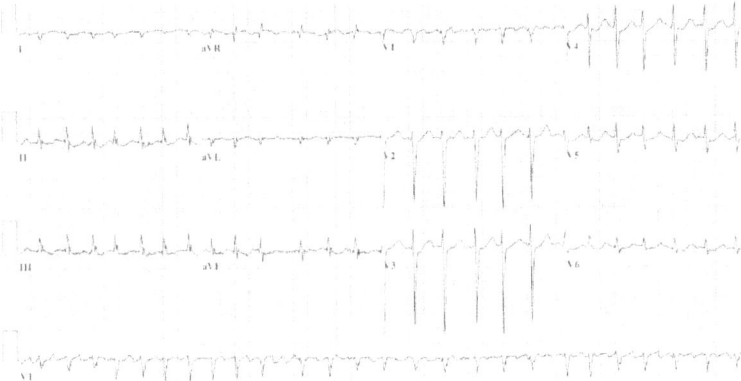

QUESTIONS

25. What is the likely diagnosis?
    a. Atrial Fibrillation
    b. Atrial Flutter
    c. Multifocal Atrial Tachycardia
    d. Normal Sinus Rhythm

26. Which of the following is the most common cause of this condition?
    a. Alcohol and Drug Abuse
    b. Atrial Ischemia
    c. Inflammatory Conduction System Disease
    d. Valvular Heart Disease
    e. Ventricular Ischemia

27. What treatment would you initiate first?
    a. Anticoagulation
    b. Electrical Cardioversion
    c. Pharmaceutical Rhythm Control
    d. Rate Control

ANSWERS

25. a
26. e
27. d

VISUAL STIMULUS REVIEW

The EKG tracing shows irregularly irregular narrow complex tachycardia with visible fibrillation waves.

REFERENCES

- Gutierrez C, Blanchard DG. Atrial fibrillation: diagnosis and treatment. Am Fam Physician. 2011 Jan 1;83(1):61-8.

CASE #9: CHEST PAIN

CASE

A 40-year-old man with no past medical history presents to the emergency department complaining of severe chest pressure that started about 45 minutes ago. He is anxious and diaphoretic. He reports some nausea and dyspnea. His vital signs are a heart rate of 80/min, blood pressure of 150/80 mmHg, respiratory rate of 16/min, and O_2Sat of 99%. He has a normal heart and lung examination and has some tenderness to palpation over his left chest wall that did worsen his pain. An EKG is performed.

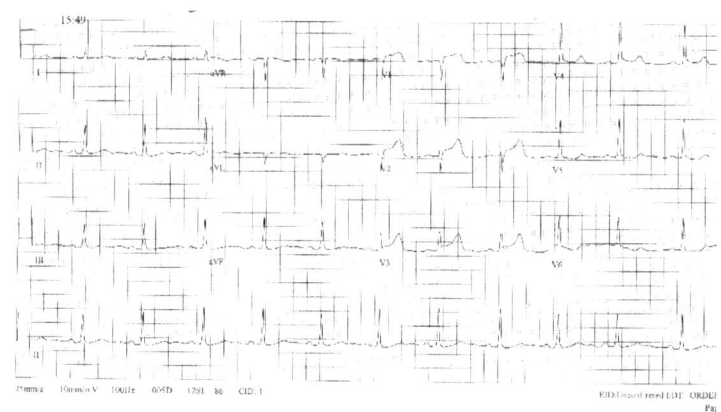

QUESTIONS

28. What is the likely diagnosis?

    a. Aortic Dissection
    b. Endocarditis
    c. Musculoskeletal Pain
    d. Myocardial Infarction
    e. Myocarditis

29. What medication would you order at this time?
    a. Aspirin 324 mg PO
    b. Enoxaparin 80 mg SC
    c. Ibuprofen 600 mg PO
    d. Metoprolol 50 mg PO
    e. Tenecteplase (TNKase) 35 mg IV
30. A point of care Troponin-I test is performed and is within normal limits. The patient is still having chest pressure, and a repeat EKG looks the same. What should be your next course of action?
    a. Discharge the patient.
    b. Hospitalize the patient for serial EKGs and cardiac enzyme measurements.
    c. Order an emergent treadmill stress testing.
    d. Send the patient to the cath lab.

ANSWERS

28. d

29. a

30. e

VISUAL STIMULUS REVIEW

The EKG tracing shows >2 mm ST segment elevations in V1, V2, and V3 suggestive of an anteroseptal myocardial infarction.

REFERENCES

- Anderson JL, Adams CD, Antman EM, Bridges CR, Califf RM, et al. ACC/AHA 2007 guidelines for the management of patients with unstable angina/non-ST-Elevation myocardial infarction: a report of the American College of Cardiology/American Heart Association Task Force on Practice Guidelines (Writing Committee to Revise the 2002 Guidelines for the Management of Patients With Unstable Angina/Non-ST-Elevation Myocardial Infarction) developed in collaboration with the American College of Emergency Physicians, the Society for Cardiovascular Angiography and Interventions, and the Society of Thoracic Surgeons endorsed by the American Association of Cardiovascular and Pulmonary Rehabilitation and the Society for Academic Emergency Medicine. J Am Coll Cardiol. Aug 14 2007;50(7):e1-e157.

CASE #10: SWOLLEN TONGUE

CASE

A 30-year-old male presents to the emergency department complaining of progressive tongue swelling for the last two hours. He has a past medical history of hypertension and diabetes and is taking Metformin, Glipizide, Lisinopril, and Metoprolol. He denies any known allergies or history of similar episodes. There is no recent change to his medication regimen. He denies any recent illness, sore throat, pruritus, or dyspnea. He is in no acute distress, and his vital signs are all within normal limits.

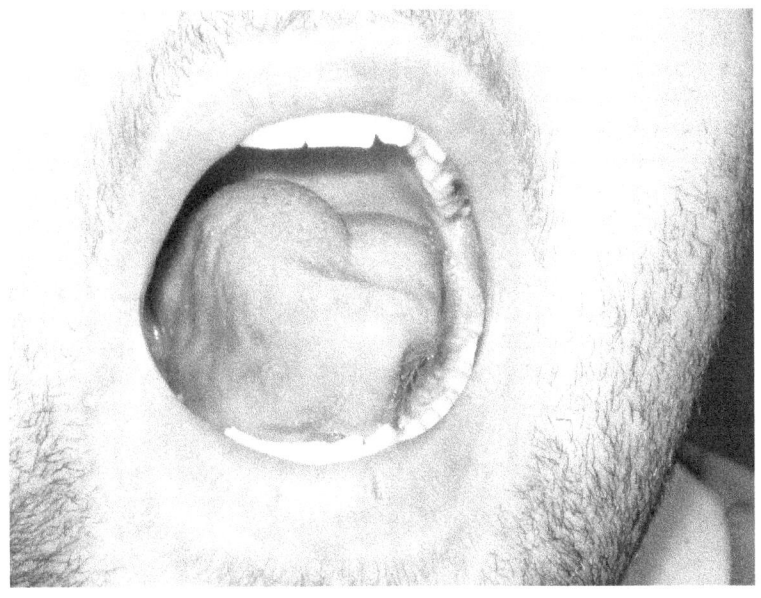

QUESTIONS

31. What is the likely diagnosis?

    a. Anaphylaxis

    b. Angioedema

c. Ludwig's Angina

   d. Urticaria

32. What is the likely cause of this condition in this patient?

   a. Allergic Reaction

   b. Hereditary

   c. Idiopathic

   d. Glipizide

   e. Lisinopril

   f. Metformin

33. What is the likely mechanism responsible for this presentation?

   a. Bradykinin Mediated

   b. Histamine Mediated

   c. IgE Mediated

   d. IgG Mediated

34. The patient starts drooling and points toward his throat and is having a hard time speaking. What should be your next course of action while you set up for an emergent surgical airway placement?

   a. Epinephrine 1 mg IM

   b. Epinephrine 1 mg IV

   c. Fiberoptic Nasotracheal Intubation

   d. Icatibant 30 mg IV

   e. Orotracheal Intubation

ANSWERS

31. b
32. e
33. a
34. c

VISUAL STIMULUS REVIEW

The image shows a normal mouth opening and markedly swollen tongue. The floor of the mouth does not appear to be elevated, and the patient is not drooling.

REFERENCES

- Kanani A, Schellenberg R, Warrington R. Urticaria and angioedema. Allergy Asthma Clin Immunol. 2011 Nov 10;7 Suppl 1:S9.
- Caballero T, Baeza ML, Cabañas R. Consensus statement on the diagnosis, management, and treatment of angioedema mediated by bradykinin. Part II. Treatment, follow-up, and special situations. J Investig Allergol Clin Immunol. 2011;21(6):422-41.

CASE #11: CHEST AND BACK PAIN

CASE

A 52-year-old man presents to the emergency department complaining of severe chest pain that radiates to his back that started 60 minutes ago. The pain is described as sharp and severe and moves down to his left flank. The patient appears to be in severe distress. His heart rate is 104/min, blood pressure of 200/105 mmHg, respiratory rate of 16/min, and O₂Sat of 97%. On examination he is diaphoretic. He has clear bilateral breath sounds and a diastolic murmur. His left radial pulse is weaker on the left than on his right.

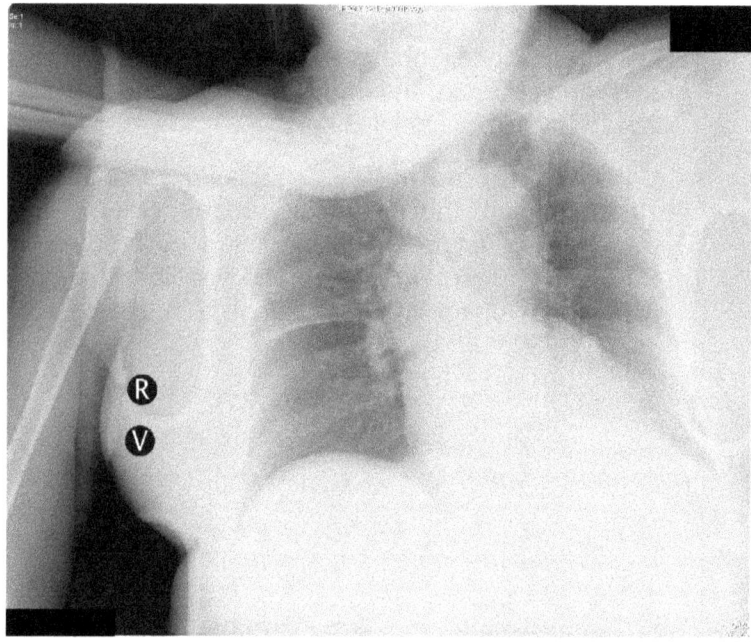

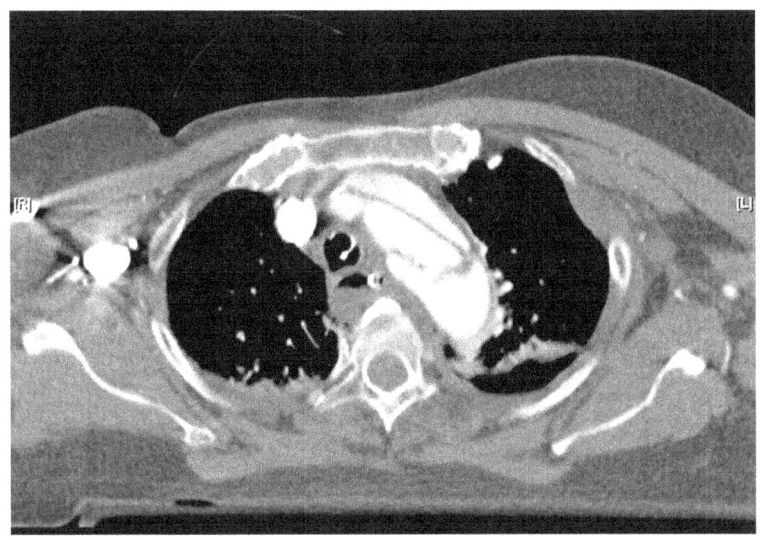

QUESTIONS

35. What is the likely diagnosis?

   a. Aortic Dissection

   b. Aortic Rupture

   c. Myocardial Infarction

   d. Pulmonary Embolism

   e. Renal Colic

36. What medication would you give to this patient first?

   a. Aspirin 324 mg PO

   b. Esmolol 80 mg IV bolus than 150 mcg/kg/min IV

   c. Heparin 5000 Units IV than 1000 Units/hr IV

   d. Nitroglycerin 0.4 mg SL x1 than 200 mcg/min IV

   e. Nitroprusside 0.25 mcg/kg/min IV

37. The patient is complaining of ongoing severe pain. What medication would you use to help manage his pain?
    a. Acetaminophen 650 mg PO
    b. Ibuprofen 600 mg PO
    c. Ketorolac 60 mg IV
    d. Fentanyl 50 mcg IV
    e. Morphine 5 mg IV
    f. Nitroglycerin 200 mcg/min IV

38. Which of the following statements is true?
    a. This condition is less common in black than in white patients.
    b. This condition is more common in males than in females.
    c. Syphilis is a common cause of this condition.
    d. Patients with Marfan syndrome presents later in life than other patients who develop this condition.
    e. Surgical management will not offer this patient improved prognosis when compared with nonsurgical management because of the anatomic location of the pathology.

ANSWERS

35. a
36. b
37. d
38. b

VISUAL STIMULUS REVIEW

The chest radiograph demonstrates a widened mediastinum and loss of the normal aortic contour.

The chest CT angiogram shows an aortic flap that originates from the aortic arch.

REFERENCES

- Wittels K. Aortic emergencies. Emerg Med Clin North Am. 2011 Nov;29(4):789-800, vii.
- Patel PD, Arora RR. Pathophysiology, diagnosis, and management of aortic dissection. Ther Adv Cardiovasc Dis. Dec 2008;2(6):439-68.

CASE #12: PAINFUL ULCER

CASE

A 30-year-old man presents to his family doctor complaining of a painful mouth sore that started three days before his presentation. He recalls having similar episodes once or twice a year that last up to 10 days per episode. He has no past medical history and is not taking any medications. He denies fevers, arthralgias, rashes, abdominal pain, diarrhea, lesions in other locations, or any other complaints.

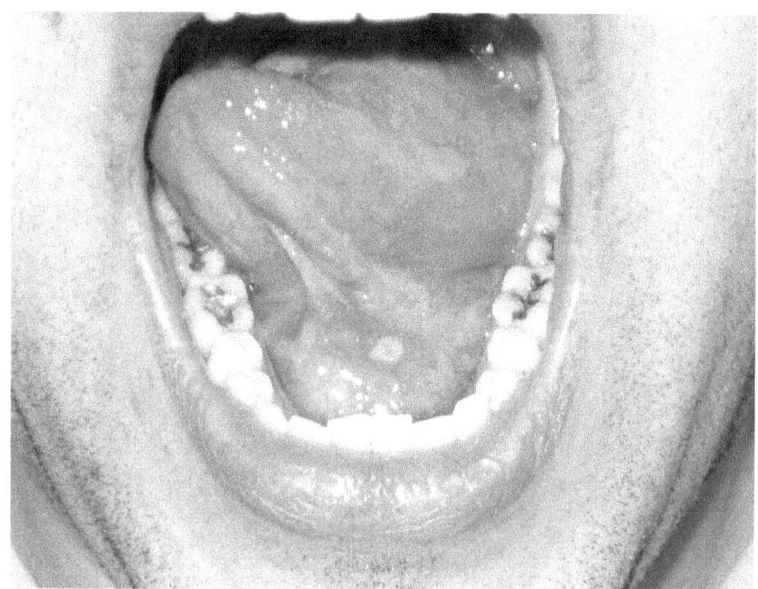

QUESTIONS

39. What is the likely diagnosis?

    a. Behçet Disease

    b. Herpangina

    c. Herpes Simplex

    d. Pemphigus Vulgaris

    e. Recurrent Aphthous Ulcer

    f. Squamous Cell Carcinoma

40. What is the likely cause?

    a. Herpes Simplex Type 1

    b. Idiopathic

    c. Iron Deficiency

    d. Tobacco

    e. Vitamin B12 Deficiency

41. Which of the following statements is true?

    a. Amlexanox is the recommended first line therapy.

    b. Biopsy is recommended in patients that experience more than two flare-ups a year.

    c. Topical or intralesional corticosteroids are the recommended first line therapy.

    d. Most lesions develop on the dorsal surface of the tongue.

ANSWERS

39. e

40. b

41. a

VISUAL STIMULUS REVIEW

The image demonstrates a single shallow ulcer over a nonkeratinized oral mucosa and is covered by a yellow exudate and surrounded by an erythematous halo.

REFERENCES

- Chattopadhyay A, Shetty KV. Recurrent aphthous stomatitis. Otolaryngol Clin North Am. 2011 Feb;44(1):79-88.

CASE #13: RLQ PAIN

CASE

A seven-year-old girl is brought to the emergency department by her parents and is complaining of diffuse abdominal pain for the last 12 hours that is localized to the right lower quadrants. She has no past medical history and is not taking any medications. She reports loss of appetite and nausea, and she vomited twice before arrival. She also had two very soft bowel movements. Her vital signs are temperature of 99.7F (37.6), heart rate of 100/min, blood pressure of 100/60, and respiratory rate of 16/min. On physical examination she has RLQ tenderness to palpation without guarding or rebound. An ultrasound of the RLQ was obtained.

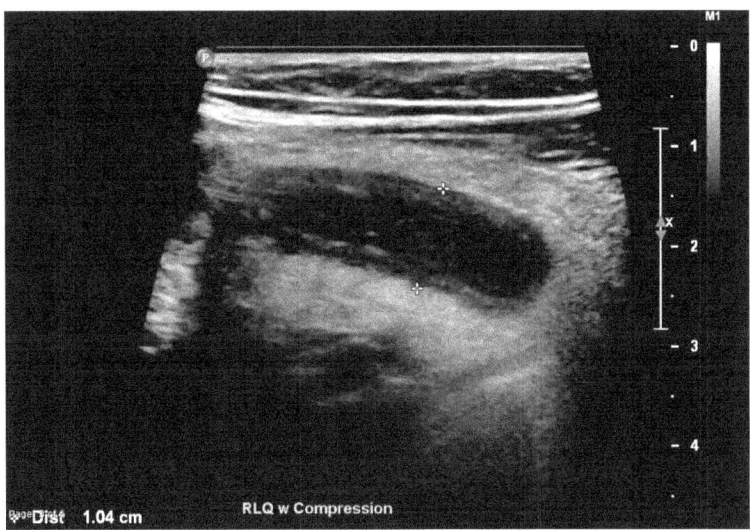

QUESTIONS

42. What is the likely diagnosis?
    a. Acute Appendicitis
    b. Gastroenteritis
    c. Intra-Abdominal Abscess
    d. Meckel's Diverticulum
    e. Ovarian Torsion
    f. Tubo Ovarian Abscess

43. What is the most common cause of this condition?
    a. Bacterial Overgrowth
    b. Bilirubin or Calcium Stones
    c. Congenital Malformation
    d. Fecal Stasis
    e. Luminal Lymphoid Hyperplasia
    f. Malignancy
    g. Sexually Transmitted Bacteria

44. What is the recommended first line treatment?
    a. CT Guided Drainage
    b. Intravenous Antibiotics
    c. Oral Antibiotics
    d. Surgery
    e. Ultrasound Guided Drainage

ANSWERS

42. a

43. e

44. d

VISUAL STIMULUS REVIEW

The ultrasound image shows a noncompressible tubular structure (1.04 cm in diameter) in the right lower quadrant, which is surrounded by a thin rim of fluid.

REFERENCES

- Pepper VK, Stanfill AB, Pearl RH. Diagnosis and management of pediatric appendicitis, intussusception, and Meckel diverticulum. Surg Clin North Am. 2012 Jun;92(3):505-26.

- Bundy DG, Byerley JS, Liles EA, Perrin EM, Katznelson J, Rice HE. Does this child have appendicitis? JAMA. 2007 Jul 25;298(4):438-51.

CASE #14: SEVERE LEG PAIN

CASE

A 64-year-old man presents to the emergency department complaining of sudden onset severe left lower leg pain that developed over the last six hours. He has a history of hypertension that is controlled on Metoprolol and Hydrochlorothiazide. He denies any history of chest pain or palpitations. He reports a history of progressively worsening left leg pain with exertion over the last two years that usually goes away within 10 minutes of rest. His vital signs are all within normal limits, and his EKG shows normal sinus rhythm of 72/min with no acute ST-T changes. On physical examination, his lung and heart sounds are normal, and he has strong bilateral inguinal pulses. His left popliteal, dorsalis pedis, and tibialis posterior pulses are not palpable. His left lower leg is swollen, cold to touch, and purple in color with delayed capillary refill (~10 sec) of the toes. He has decreased sensation to the foot and decreased big toe and foot dorsiflexion strength when compared with the right. On Doppler auscultation, a monophasic, very faint dorsalis pedis signal waveform is intermittently found.

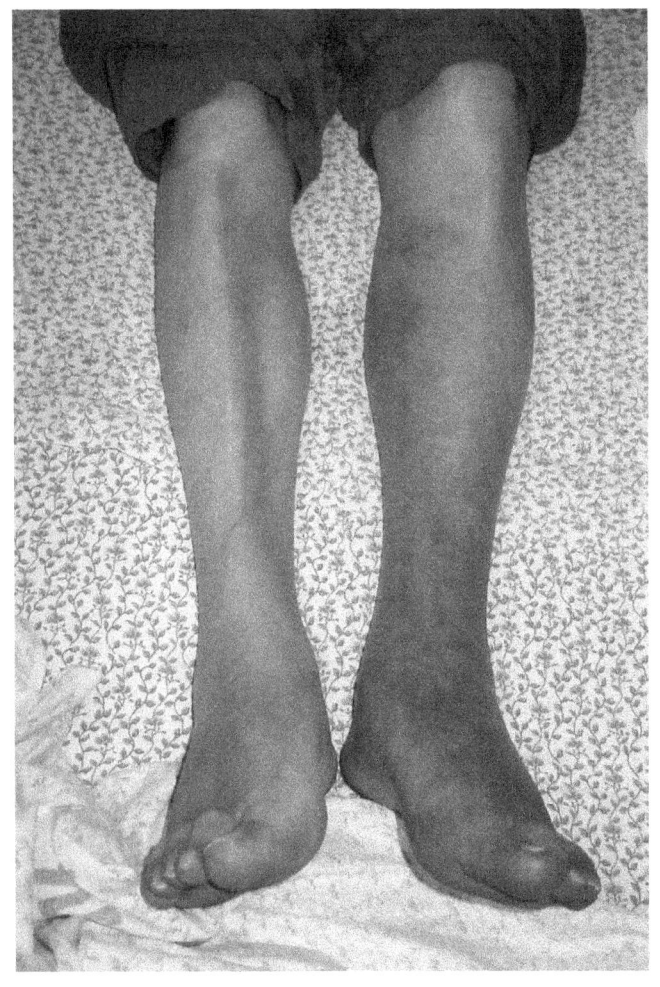

QUESTIONS

45. What is the likely diagnosis?
    a. Arterial Embolism
    b. Arterial Thrombosis
    c. Compartment Syndrome
    d. Deep Venous Thrombosis
    e. Septic Thrombophlebitis

46. What would you expect the left-sided Ankle to Brachial Index (ABI) to be in this patient?
    a. 0.3
    b. 0.8
    c. 1
    d. 1.5

47. What medication should be given to the patient at this time?
    a. Aspirin 324 mg PO
    b. Heparin 5000 units IV followed by 1000 units/hr IV
    c. Morphine 6 mg IV
    d. All of the above

48. What should be the next step in managing the patient?
    a. Alteplase 100 mg IV over 2 h
    b. Arteriogram
    c. CT Angiogram
    d. Doppler Duplex Arterial of the Left Leg
    e. Doppler Duplex Arterial of Both Legs
    f. Surgical Revascularization

ANSWERS

45. b

46. a

47. d

48. b

VISUAL STIMULUS REVIEW

The image shows a mildly swollen left lower leg with normal-colored skin to the proximal tibia. There does not seem to be a clear demarcation of skin discoloration.

REFERENCES

- Creager MA, Kaufman JA, Conte MS. Clinical practice. Acute limb ischemia. N Engl J Med. 2012 Jun 7;366(23):2198-206

- Costantini V, Lenti M. Treatment of acute occlusion of peripheral arteries. Thromb Res. 2002 Jun 1;106(6):V285-94.

- Henke PK. Approach to the patient with acute limb ischemia: diagnosis and therapeutic modalities, Cardiol Clin 20 (2002) 513–520.

CASE #15: ABDOMINAL DISTENTION

CASE

A 67-year-old woman presents to her family doctor complaining of abdominal distention and shortness of breath that developed over the last three months. She has a history of chronic alcoholism and is not on any medications. Her last visit to her doctor was three years ago. She denies having abdominal pain, nausea, fever, pruritus, or diarrhea. Her vital signs are temp 99.7F (37.6C), heart rate of 72/min, blood pressure of 90/58 mmHg, respiratory rate of 24/min, and O_2Sat of 91% on room air. Physical examination findings include scleral jaundice, decreased bilateral breath sounds, distended abdominal wall veins, and a distended and tense abdomen with no tenderness to palpation. A bedside ultrasound image tracing is shown below.

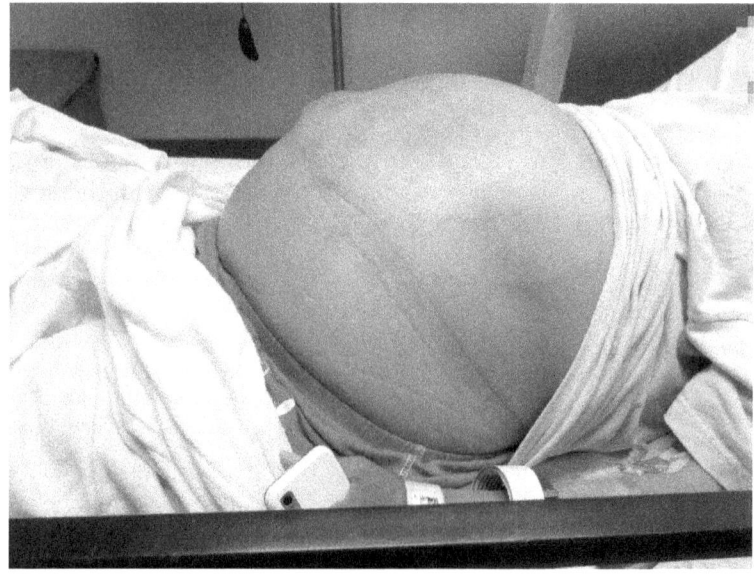

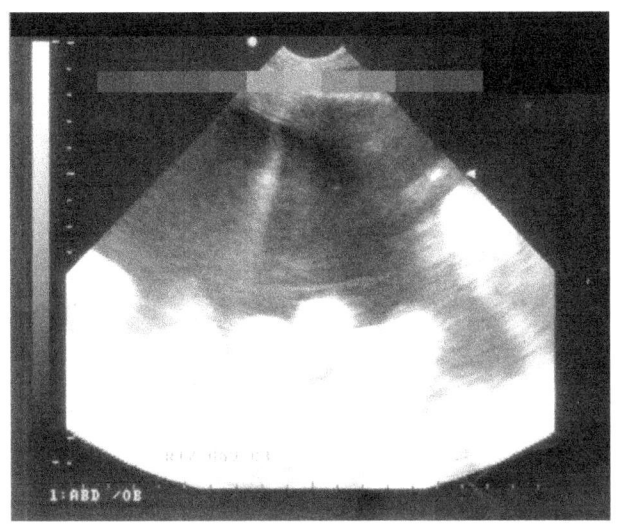

QUESTIONS

49. What is the likely diagnosis?

   a. Biliary Cancer

   b. Cirrhosis

   c. Congestive Heart Failure

   d. Hemoperitoneum

   e. Nephrotic Syndrome

   f. Spontaneous Bacterial Peritonitis

50. Which of the following statements is true?

   a. Most ascitic fluid is transparent and tinged red.

   b. Cytology smear of ascites samples is 98% sensitive for detection of malignant cells.

   c. SAAG (Serum Ascites Albumin Gradient) > 1.1 g/dl suggests portal hypertension etiology.

d. Ascites polymorphonuclear cell count greater than 50 cell/microliter is highly suggestive of bacterial peritonitis.

51. Which of the following statements is true?

   a. Transjugular Intrahepatic Portosystemic Shunt (TIPS) is indicated in all patients with recurrent ascites.

   b. Sodium restriction and diuretic therapy are effective in most patients with this condition.

   c. Removal of 2 L of fluid or more is considered large-volume paracentesis.

   d. Infusing patients with 5 g of albumin per each liter that is removed during paracentesis over 2 L is considered standard recommendation.

ANSWERS

49. b

50. c

51. b

VISUAL STIMULUS REVIEW

The image shows a markedly distended abdomen with visibly distended abdominal wall veins (caput medusa).

The ultrasound image shows large hypoechoic intraperitoneal fluid and free-floating loops of small bowel.

REFERENCES

- Starr SP, Raines D. Cirrhosis: diagnosis, management, and prevention. Am Fam Physician. 2011 Dec 15;84(12):1353-9.

CASE #16: FEVER AND NIGHT SWEATS

CASE

A 64-years-old man presents to his family doctor complaining of fever, shaking chills, and episodes of diaphoresis for the past week. He reports night sweats and fevers up to 104.9F (40.5C), headaches, arthralgias, dyspnea, abdominal pain, nausea, and vomiting. He denies any international travel or exposure to animals. He did visit a family member in Connecticut two weeks before the onset of symptoms, but he does not recall a tick bite or direct contact with deer.

His vital signs are temp 102F (38.9C), heart rate 104/min, respiratory rate of 26/min, and O_2Sat at 93% on room air. His physical examination is within normal limits—of note there is no heart murmur, no abdominal tenderness, no hepatomegaly, no jaundice, and no rash.

Serum chemistry demonstrates mildly elevated AST, ALT, Total Bilirubin, and Alkaline Phosphatase.

QUESTIONS

52. What is the likely diagnosis?
    a. Acute Leukemia
    b. Babesiosis
    c. Ehrlichiosis
    d. Lyme Disease
    e. Malaria
    f. Rocky Mountain Spotted Fever

53. Which of the following blood tests is likely to be elevated?
    a. Platelet Count
    b. Lactate Dehydrogenase
    c. Red Blood Cell Count
    d. Sodium
    e. White Blood Cell Count

54. Which of the following treatments is recommended?
    a. Atovaquone PO + Azithromycin IV
    b. Azithromycin IV
    c. Doxycycline IV
    d. Clindamycin IV
    e. Clindamycin IV + Atovaquone PO
    f. Quinine PO

ANSWERS

52. b

53. b

54. a

VISUAL STIMULUS REVIEW

The blood smear image demonstrates ring form parasites both inside as well as outside erythrocytes.

REFERENCES

- Vannier E, Gewurz BE, Krause PJ. Human babesiosis. Infect Dis Clin North Am. 2008 Sep;22(3):469-88, viii-ix.

CASE #17: PENILE RASH

CASE

A 27-year-old uncircumcised man presents to his family doctor's clinic complaining of burning and draining rash to his penis for four days. He has no past medical history and is not taking any medications. He denies dysuria, hematuria, or urethral discharge. He is sexually active with one long-term partner and always uses condoms. His vital signs are all within normal limits. His nongenital physical examination is normal, and his genital examination shows no urethral discharge and normal scrotal and testicular exam. His foreskin is not easily retractable, and the glans and distal foreskin show the following findings. The glans is tender to palpation.

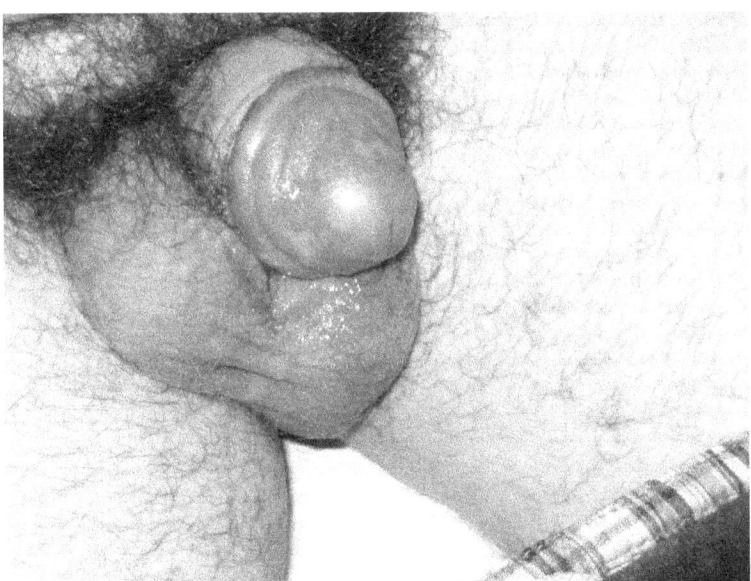

QUESTIONS

55. What is the likely diagnosis?
    a. Balanitis
    b. Balanoposthitis
    c. Penile Cancer
    d. Psoriasis
    e. Smegma Overproduction
    f. Urethritis

56. What is the most common cause of this condition?
    a. Anaerobic Bacteria
    b. Candida Albicans
    c. Chlamydia Trachomatis
    d. Neisseria Gonorrhea
    e. Treponema Pallidum
    f. Beta-Hemolytic Streptococci

57. What is the most common risk factor for this condition?
    a. Cirrhosis
    b. Congestive Heart Failure
    c. Diabetes
    d. Obesity

ANSWERS

55. b
56. b
57. c

VISUAL STIMULUS REVIEW

The image shows erythematous and swollen penile glans and distal foreskin with yellow discharge.

REFERENCES

- Lisboa C, Ferreira A, Resende C, Rodrigues AG. Infectious balanoposthitis: management, clinical and laboratory features. Int J Dermatol. 2009 Feb;48(2):121-4.
- Edwards S. Balanitis and balanoposthitis: a review. Genitourin Med. Jun 1996;72(3):155-9.

CASE #18: PAINFUL LUMP

CASE

A 23-year-old woman presents to her gynecologist complaining of severe pain to her vagina. She has no past medical history, and she is not taking any medications. She reports a painful and tender lump that developed over the last two days. She reports that sitting or walking makes the pain even worse. She denies history of same, fever, chills, or drainage. The patient's vital signs are normal, and on exam she has an extremely tender lump as shown below.

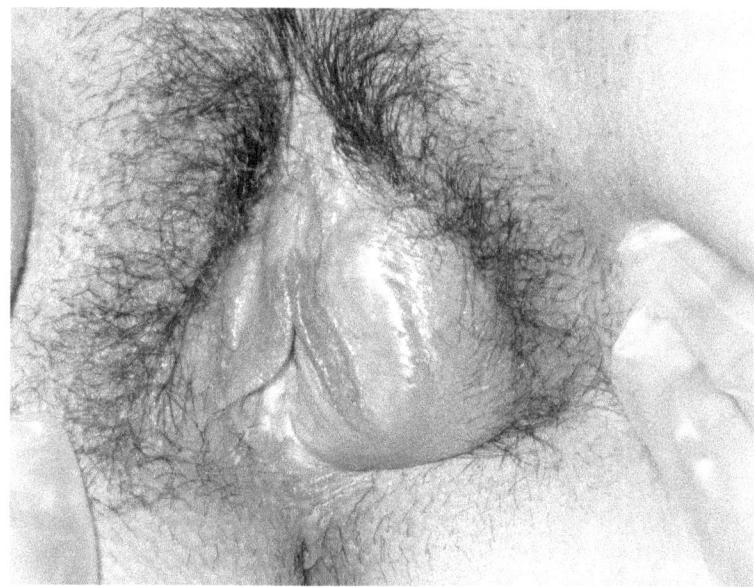

QUESTIONS

58. What is the likely diagnosis?
    a. Adenocarcinoma
    b. Bartholin Abscess
    c. Gartner Duct Cyst
    d. Lipoma
    e. Sebaceous Cyst
    f. Squamous Cell Carcinoma

59. What is the likely cause of this condition?
    a. Adipose Tissue Hypertrophy
    b. Chlamydia
    c. Neisseria Gonorrhea
    d. Malignancy
    e. Polymicrobial Infection
    f. Sebum Over Production

60. Which of the following treatments would you recommend for this patient?
    a. Ciprofloxacin 500 mg PO q12 hrs for seven days.
    b. Incision and drainage (I&D) alone.
    c. I&D and insertion of a Ward catheter.
    d. Twice daily sitz baths until spontaneous drainage.
    e. Wide excision with frozen section.

ANSWERS

58. b

59. e

60. c

VISUAL STIMULUS REVIEW

The image shows a large and erythematous mass in the vestibular area.

REFERENCES

- Wechter ME, Wu JM, Marzano D, Haefner H. Management of Bartholin duct cysts and abscesses: a systematic review. Obstet Gynecol Surv. 2009 Jun;64(6):395-404.

- Hill DA, Lense JJ. Office management of Bartholin gland cysts and abscesses. Am Fam Physician. 1998 Apr 1;57(7):1611-6, 1619-20.

CASE #19: HEADACHE

CASE

A 27-year-old male presents to the emergency department complaining of headache and vomiting two days status post motor vehicle accident, where his head collided with the windshield. He denies loss of consciousness, vertigo, or vision changes. The next day he noticed some drainage from his left ear. On examination, he is alert and oriented. He has no bruising to his face and no rhinorrhea. His face is symmetric with intact bilateral CN-V and CN-VII and no nystagmus. His hearing is grossly intact with Rinne test showing left ear bone conduction better than air conduction and Weber test that lateralizes to the left. The rest of his neurological exam is normal.

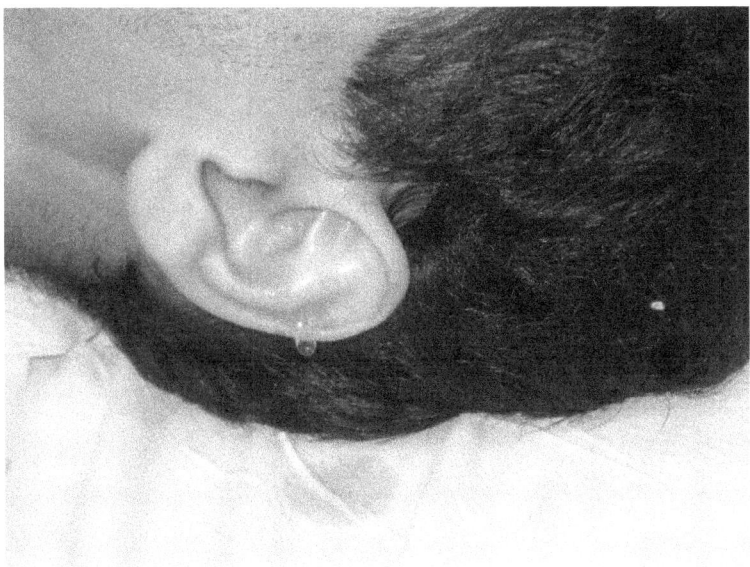

QUESTIONS

61. What is the likely diagnosis?
    a. Anterior Cranial Fossa Fracture
    b. Occipital Bone Fracture
    c. Perforated Tympanic Membrane
    d. Petrous Temporal Bone Fracture
62. The Rinne and Weber tests in this patient suggest?
    a. Conductive Hearing Loss
    b. Mixed Hearing Loss
    c. Normal Hearing
    d. Sensorineural Hearing Loss
63. Where would you expect to find bruising in this patient?
    a. Mastoid
    b. Nose Bridge
    c. Periorbital
    d. Scalp

ANSWERS

61. d
62. a
63. a

VISUAL STIMULUS REVIEW

The image shows clear otorrhea from the left ear.

REFERENCES

- Prosser JD, Vender JR, Solares CA. Traumatic cerebrospinal fluid leaks. Otolaryngol Clin North Am. 2011 Aug;44(4):857-73, vii.
- Samii M, Tatagiba M. Skull base trauma: diagnosis and management. Neurol Res. 2002 Mar;24(2):147-56.

CASE #20: SKIN LESION

CASE

A 40-year-old man presents to his family doctor complaining of a painless slowly growing lesion to his right upper chest that he noticed five weeks ago. He has no past medical history and is not taking any medications. He reports that the lesion bleeds when traumatized.

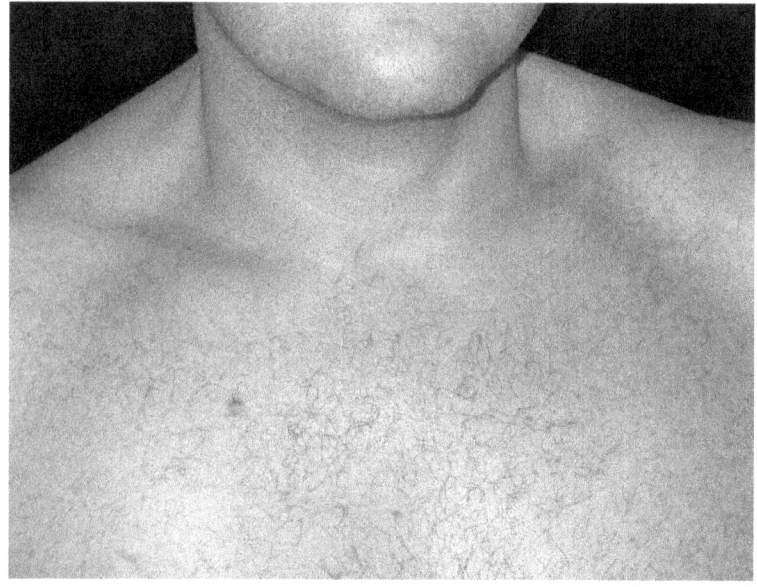

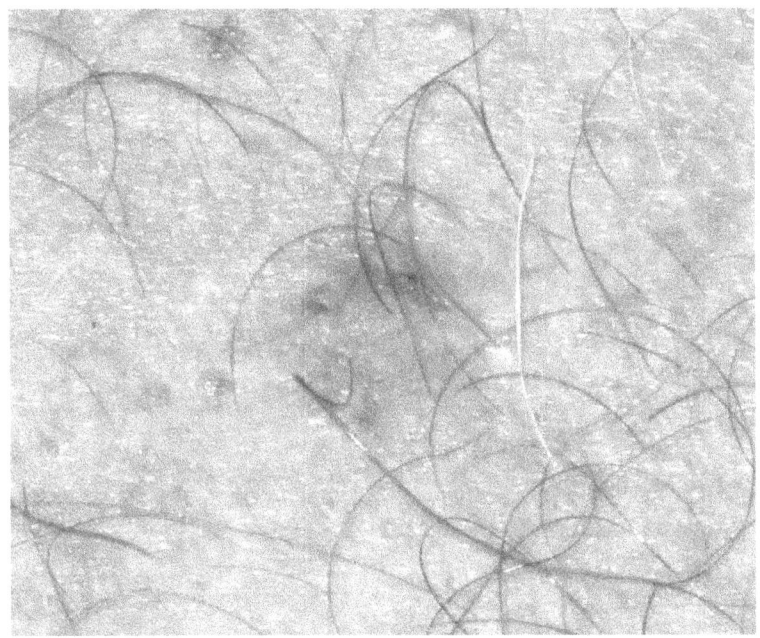

QUESTIONS

64. What is the likely diagnosis?

    a. Actinic Keratosis

    b. Angiofibroma

    c. Basal Cell Carcinoma

    d. Malignant Melanoma

    e. Squamous Cell Carcinoma

65. What should be the next step in diagnosing/treating this lesion?

    a. 5-fluorouracil 5% Topical BID x Six Weeks

    b. Mohs Micrographic Surgery

    c. Shave Biopsy

    d. Wide Excision

e. Wide Excision and Sentinel Lymph Node Biopsy

66. Which of the following statements is true?

   a. Dark-skinned individuals are rarely affected by this condition.

   b. This condition often metastasizes.

   c. This condition is fast growing.

   d. This condition is the most common cancer in humans.

ANSWERS

64. c

65. c

66. d

VISUAL STIMULUS REVIEW

The image shows a raised, mostly pink, and waxy lesion.

REFERENCES

- Kim RH, Armstrong AW. Nonmelanoma skin cancer. Dermatol Clin. 2012 Jan;30(1):125-39, ix. Epub 2011 Oct 21.
- Kwasniak LA, Garcia-Zuazaga J. Basal cell carcinoma: evidence-based medicine and review of treatment modalities. Int J Dermatol. 2011 Jun;50(6):645-58.

CASE #21: FACIAL WEAKNESS

CASE

A 40-year-old man presents to his family doctor complaining of facial weakness that started a day before his presentation. He reports that he woke up the day before and noticed some weakness that progressed over the last 24 hours. He has no medical history and is not taking any medications. He reports some pain behind his right ear and difficulty closing his right eye. He denies any headache, difficulty speaking or swallowing, or blurry vision. The patient is unable to close his right eye or raise his right eyebrow. The rest of his physical exam is unremarkable.

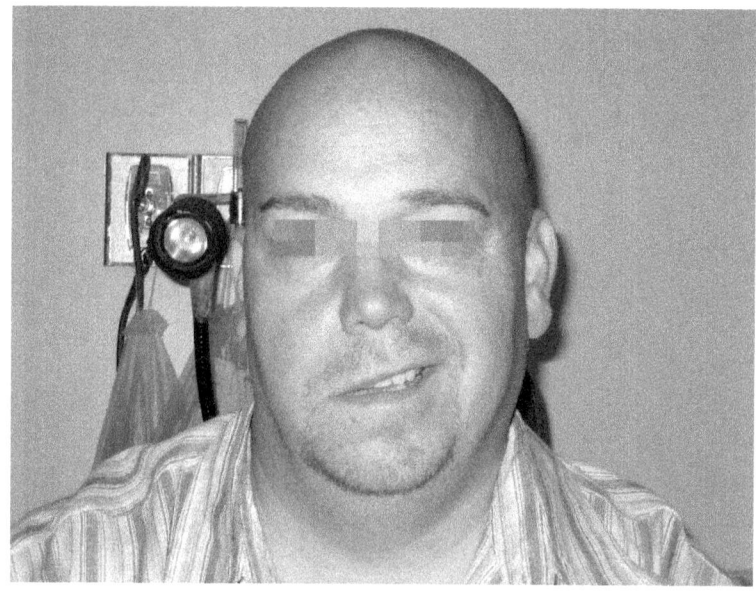

QUESTIONS

67. What is the likely diagnosis?
    a. Acute Stroke
    b. CN VI Palsy
    c. Central CN VII Palsy
    d. Peripheral CN VII Palsy
    e. Posterior Fossa Tumor

68. What is the most common cause of this condition?
    a. Borrelia Burgdorferi
    b. Cerebral Artery Thrombosis
    c. Glioblastoma
    d. Herpes Simplex Virus
    e. Idiopathic
    f. Meningioma

69. What is the recommended treatment for this patient?
    a. CT Brain with and without Contrast
    b. Doxycycline 100 mg PO q12 hrs x 21 Days
    c. Prednisone 60 mg PO Daily x Five Days
    d. Valacyclovir 1 g PO q8 hrs x Seven Days

ANSWERS

67. d
68. e
69. c

VISUAL STIMULUS REVIEW

The image shows paralysis of his right-sided facial muscles with flattening of his right-sided nasolabial folds and facial creases.

REFERENCES

- Tiemstra JD, Khatkhate N. Bell's palsy: diagnosis and management. Am Fam Physician. 2007 Oct 1;76(7):997-1002.

- Salinas RA, Alvarez G, Daly F, Ferreira J. Corticosteroids for Bell's palsy (idiopathic facial paralysis). Cochrane Database Syst Rev. 2010 Mar 17;(3):CD001942.

- Lockhart P, Daly F, Pitkethly M, Comerford N, Sullivan F. Antiviral treatment for Bell's palsy (idiopathic facial paralysis). Cochrane Database Syst Rev. 2009 Oct 7;(4):CD001869.

CASE #22: BACK PAIN

CASE

A 36-year-old man presents to the emergency department, complaining of severe back pain after a spider bite. The patient was in his house without his shirt on when he felt an insect bite to his right upper back. He describes gradual onset of severe back pain during the next two hours that did not respond to over-the-counter medications. The patient is ill-appearing, with diffuse diaphoresis, temperature of 99.7°F (37.6°C), pulse rate of 120 beats/min, respiration rate of 20 breaths/min, blood pressure of 200/110 mmHg, and O_2Sat of 99% on room air. Physical examination reveals a single bite mark in the center of a 4 cm erythematous and anhidrotic circle. The erythematous circle is surrounded by a 15 cm pale and oval halo that is hyperhidrotic. The hyperhidrotic halo leaves an impression on the sheet the patient is resting on.

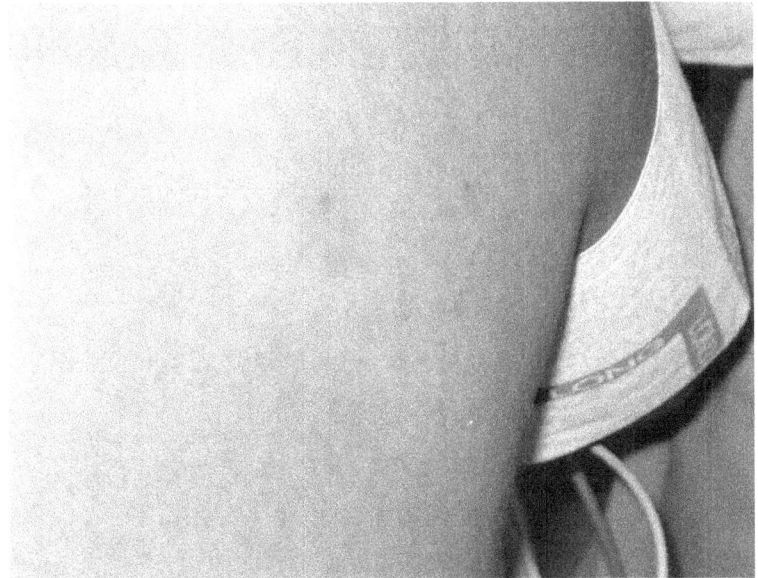

QUESTIONS

70. What is the likely diagnosis?
    a. Black Widow Spider Bite
    b. Brown Recluse Spider Bite
    c. Centipede Envenomation
    d. Scorpion Envenomation
71. What is the first line treatment for this condition?
    a. Antivenom
    b. Benzodiazepines and Opiates
    c. Calcium Gluconate 2 g IV
    d. Magnesium Sulfate 4 g IV

72. Which of the following statement regarding this condition is true?
    a. Diaphoresis is an uncommon sign.
    b. Most cases take two to three weeks to resolve.
    c. Nystagmus is a common finding.
    d. The onset of pain is usually gradual.

ANSWERS

70. a

71. b

72. d

VISUAL STIMULUS REVIEW

The image shows a small central fang mark in the center of an area of anhidrosis. The area of anhidrosis is surrounded by a peripheral hyper hidrotic halo.

REFERENCES

- Monte AA, Bucher-Bartelson B, Heard KJ. A US perspective of symptomatic Latrodectus species envenomation and treatment: a National Poison Data System review. Ann Pharmacother. 2011 Dec;45(12):1491-8.

- Shlamovitz GZ. Man with back pain. Black widow spider bite. Man with back pain. Ann Emerg Med. 2011 Nov;58(5):496, 500.

CASE #23: BREAST LUMP

CASE

A 63-year-old woman presents to a walk-in clinic complaining of a painless breast mass that has been growing for the past four years. She is not seeing doctors routinely, has no known medical history, and is not taking any medications. She denies any fevers, weight loss, or discharge from her nipples. Her vital signs are all within normal limits. Her physical examination is significant for hard, nonmobile and nontender left breast mass and enlarged, hard and nontender left axillary lymph nodes. An urgent mammogram is performed.

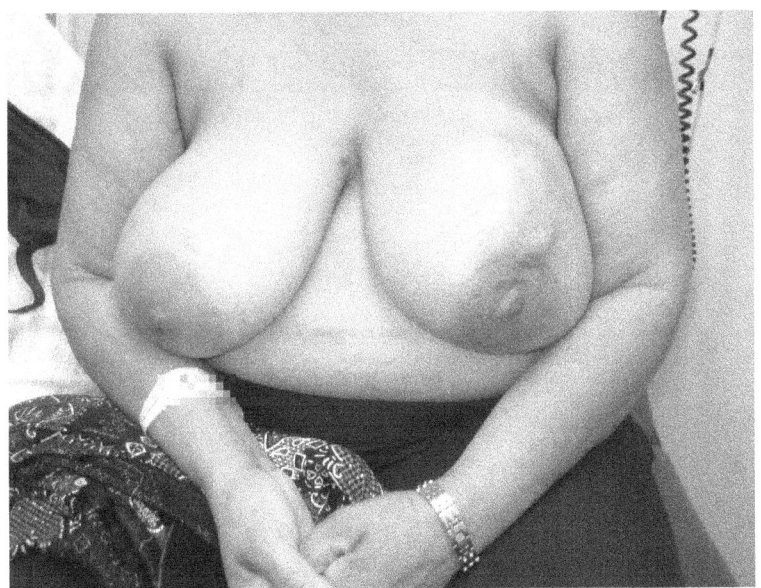

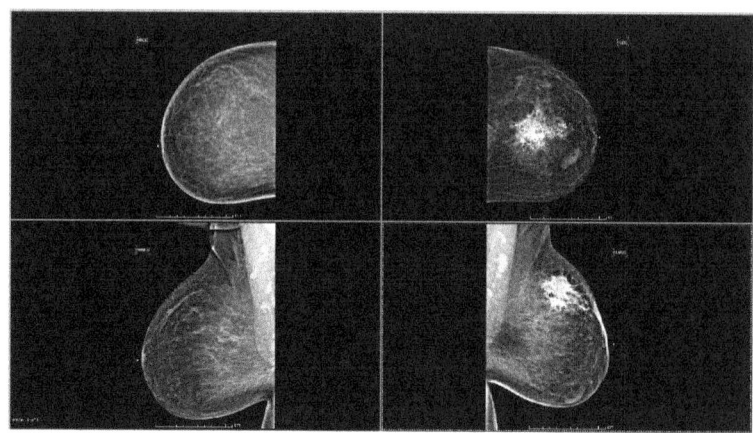

QUESTIONS

73. What is the likely diagnosis?

    a. Breast Abscess

    b. Breast Cancer

    c. Breast Fibroadenoma

    d. Inflammatory Mastitis

74. The most commonly diagnosed type of this condition is?

    a. Ductal Carcinoma in Situ

    b. Lobular Carcinoma in Situ

    c. Medullary Carcinoma

    d. Mucinous Adenoma

    e. Multiloculated Abscess

    f. Post Infectious

75. The next step in diagnosing/managing this patient would be?
    a. Antibiotic Trial
    b. Chemotherapy
    c. CT Chest Abdomen and Pelvis
    d. Needle Biopsy
    e. Radiation Therapy
    f. Surgical Excision

ANSWERS

73. b

74. a

75. d

VISUAL STIMULUS REVIEW

The image shows a large left breast mass with skin tethering and retracted nipple.

The mammogram images show normal right breast tissue, and the left breast images show spiculated and irregular calcifications.

REFERENCES

- Barnes NL, Ooi JL, Yarnold JR, Bundred NJ. Ductal carcinoma in situ of the breast. BMJ. 2012 Feb 29;344:e797.

- DeSantis C, Siegel R, Bandi P, Jemal A. Breast cancer statistics, 2011. CA Cancer J Clin. 2011 Nov-Dec;61(6):409-18.

CASE #24: LEG PAIN

CASE

A 27-year-old woman presents to the emergency department complaining of severe pain to her left calf as a result of hot grease that spilled on her leg an hour before her arrival. She denies any known past medical history and is not taking any medications. She has no other injuries. Her skin is very tender and blanches to palpation.

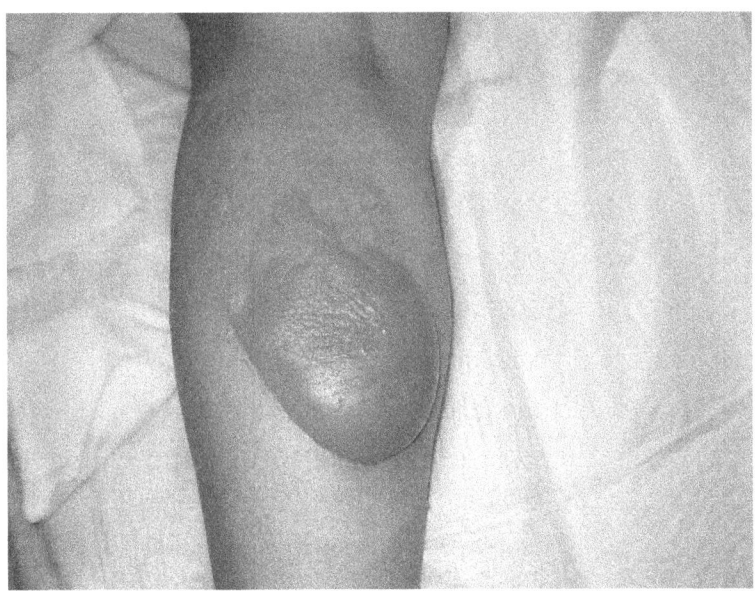

QUESTIONS

76. What is the likely diagnosis?

    a. Superficial 1st Degree Burn
    b. Superficial Partial 2nd Degree Burn
    c. Deep Partial 2nd Degree Burn
    d. Deep 3rd Degree Burn
    e. 4th Degree Burn

77. What is the estimated volume (using the parkland formula) of intravenous fluids to be given in the first 24 hours to a 50 kg patient with partial and full thickness burns over 40% of his total body surface area?

    a. 2,000 ml
    b. 4,000 ml
    c. 6,000 ml
    d. 8,000 ml
    e. 10,000 ml

78. Which of the following statement is true?

    a. Intact blisters should be debrided in order to promote wound healing.
    b. Major burns rarely cause systemic inflammatory response.
    c. Most burns have a central zone of hyperemia and a peripheral zone of coagulation.
    d. The depth of burn wounds evolves over time.

ANSWERS

76. b

77. d

78. d

VISUAL STIMULUS REVIEW

The image shows a large, intact, and moist blister and a surrounding erythema.

REFERENCES

- Endorf FW, Ahrenholz D. Burn management. Curr Opin Crit Care. 2011 Dec;17(6):601-5.
- Evers LH, Bhavsar D, Mailänder P. The biology of burn injury. Exp Dermatol. 2010 Sep;19(9):777-83.
- Pham TN, Gibran NS. Thermal and electrical injuries. Surg Clin North Am. 2007 Feb;87(1):185-206, vii-viii.

CASE #25: NECK PAIN

CASE

A 19-year-old man is brought to the emergency department by ambulance after a shallow pool diving accident. He had been drinking alcohol when he jumped head first into a shallow pool. He was able to get out of the pool on his own but complained of neck pain. He is awake and alert and is still complaining of neck pain but is unable to localize the exact location. On examination he has diffuse neck tenderness and no gross neurological deficit. A CT scan of his head is normal; images from his cervical spine CT are shown below.

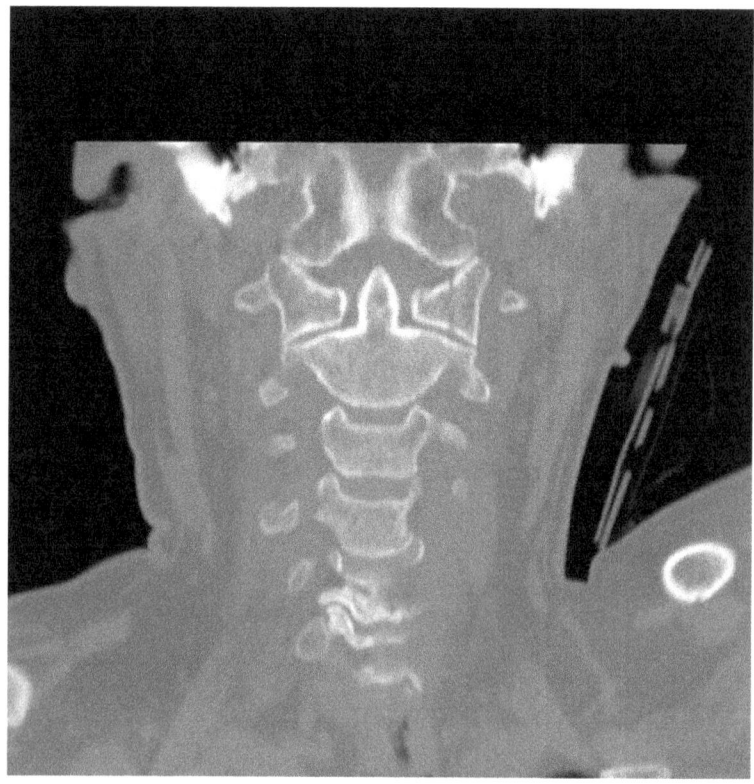

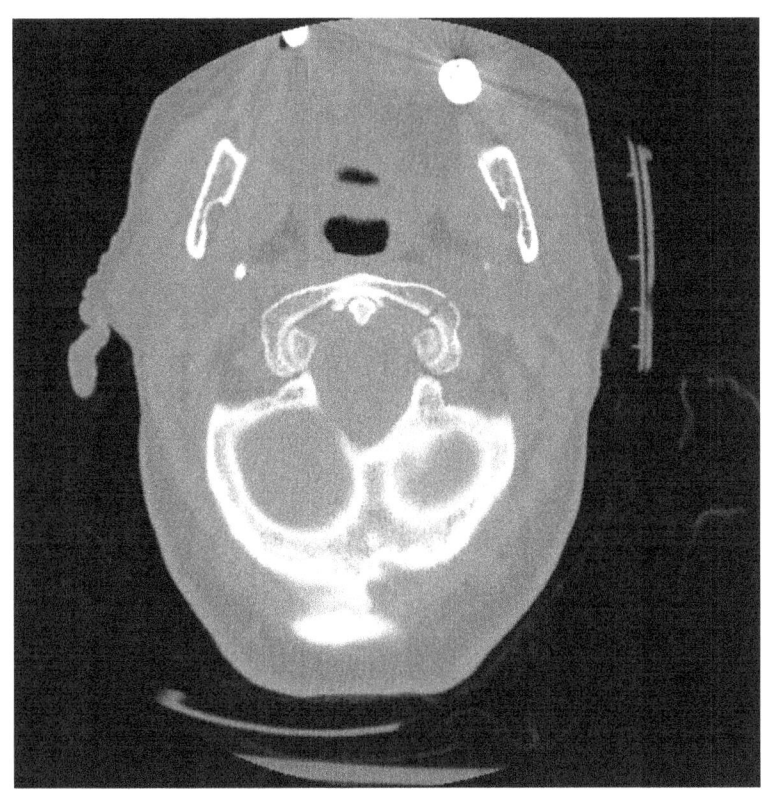

QUESTIONS

79. What is the likely diagnosis?

    a. C1 Fracture

    b. C2 Fracture

    c. Basilar Skull Fracture

    d. Hangman's Fracture

80. Spinal cord compression at the level of this injury is likely to cause which of the following?

    a. Ataxia

    b. Diplopia

    c. Hemiparesis

    d. Hemiplegia

    e. Phrenic Nerve Paralysis

81. What additional injury should you suspect if the patient starts complaining of dizziness and develops dysmetria?

    a. C2 Level Cord Compression

    b. C3 Level Cord Compression

    c. Hemorrhagic Stroke

    d. Vertebral Artery Dissection

ANSWERS

79. a

80. e

81. d

VISUAL STIMULUS REVIEW

The CT images demonstrate a nondisplaced linear fracture through the left anterior ring of C1 (Atlas).

REFERENCES

- Longo UG, Denaro L, Campi S, Maffulli N, Denaro V. Upper cervical spine injuries: indications and limits of the conservative management in Halo vest. A systematic review of efficacy and safety. Injury. 2010 Nov;41(11):1127-35.

CASE #26: WEAKNESS

CASE

A 67-year-old woman is brought to the emergency department for generalized muscle weakness and fatigue for two days. Her family reports a history of hypertension, coronary artery disease, and heart failure. The patient has normal vital signs and a nonfocal neurological exam.

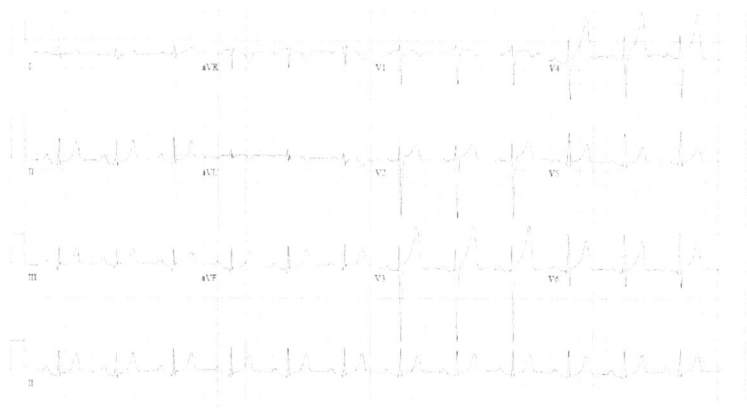

QUESTIONS

82. What is the likely diagnosis?
    a. Hypercalcemia
    b. Hyperkalemia
    c. Hyperphosphatemia
    d. Hypocalcemia
    e. Hypokalemia

83. Which of the following medications might cause this condition?
    a. Furosemide
    b. Metoprolol
    c. Spironolactone
    d. Valacyclovir

84. Which of the following treatment is considered an acceptable first line treatment for this condition?
    a. Calcium Chloride
    b. Calcium Gluconate
    c. Potassium Phosphate
    d. Insulin and Glucose
    e. a, b, or d
    f. a, b, c, or d

ANSWERS

82. b

83. c

84. e

VISUAL STIMULUS REVIEW

The electrocardiogram shows picked t waves.

REFERENCES

- Elliott MJ, Ronksley PE, Clase CM, Ahmed SB, Hemmelgarn BR. Management of patients with acute hyperkalemia. CMAJ. 2010 Oct 19;182(15):1631-5.
- Nyirenda MJ, Tang JI, Padfield PL, Seckl JR. Hyperkalaemia. BMJ. 2009 Oct 23;339:b4114.

CASE #27: SKIN LUMPS

CASE

A 15-year-old man presents to his pediatrician complaining of multiple skin nodules that increased in size over the last year. He has no other symptoms. On physical examination, he has axillary and inguinal freckles as well as eight pigmented flat skin lesions as seen in the image below. He has about 14 deep skin nodules over his trunk and extremities.

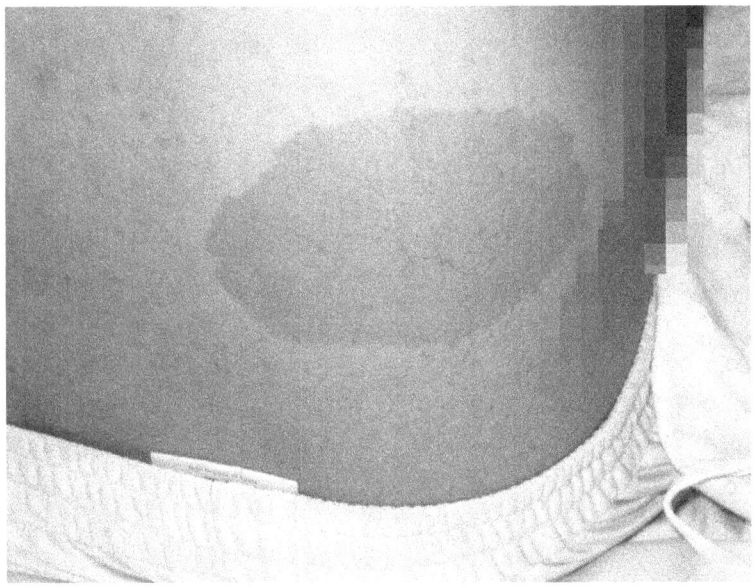

QUESTIONS

85. What is the likely diagnosis?
    a. Cystic Fibrosis
    b. Gaucher Disease
    c. Neurofibromatosis
    d. Tuberous Sclerosis

86. What is the name of the skin lesion?
    a. Acanthosis Nigricans
    b. Café Au Lait Spot
    c. Mongolian Spot
    d. Port Wine Stain

87. Which of the following is a common manifestation of this disease process?
    a. Colon Carcinoma
    b. Dysplastic Teratoma
    c. Malignant Melanoma
    d. Optic Nerve Glioma

ANSWERS

85. c

86. b

87. d

VISUAL STIMULUS REVIEW

The image shows a hyperpigmented patch.

REFERENCES

- Shah KN. The diagnostic and clinical significance of café-au-lait macules. Pediatr Clin North Am. 2010 Oct;57(5):1131-53.
- Ferner RE. The neurofibromatoses. Pract Neurol. 2010 Apr;10(2):82-93.

CASE #28: DRY COUGH

CASE

A 17-year-old man presents to his family doctor complaining of dyspnea on exertion and some dry cough progressively worsening over the last six months. He has no known medical history, is not taking any medications, and he denies fevers, sputum production, weight loss, pain, or travel outside of the USA. His lung examination reveals normal breath sounds and good symmetric bilateral air movement. A chest radiograph is ordered.

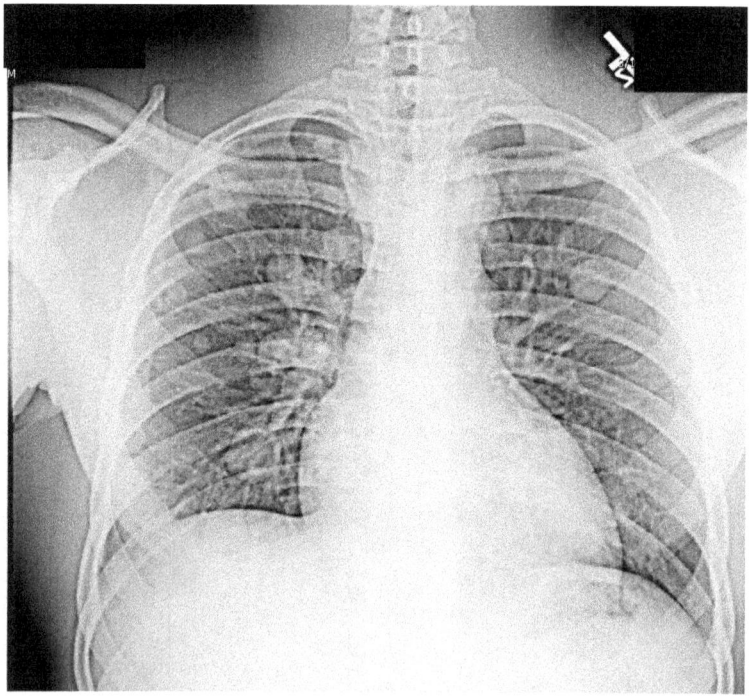

QUESTIONS

88. What is the likely diagnosis?
    a. Community Acquired Pneumonia (RUL)
    b. Diffuse Pulmonary TB Infection
    c. Lung Metastasis
    d. Pneumocystis Carinii Pneumonia

89. What is the main finding in this Image?
    a. Cannonball Lesions
    b. Diffuse Cavitary Lesions
    c. Patchy Infiltrates
    d. Peribronchial Cuffing

90. Which of the following conditions is a likely cause of this finding?
    a. Malignant Melanoma
    b. Mycobacteria Tuberculosis
    c. Staphylococcus Aureus
    d. Streptococcus Pneumonia
    e. Seminoma
    f. Tuberculosis

ANSWERS

88. c

89. a

90. e

VISUAL STIMULUS REVIEW

The chest radiograph shows multiple lung nodules in all lobes.

REFERENCES

- Dishop MK, Kuruvilla S. Primary and metastatic lung tumors in the pediatric population: a review and 25-year experience at a large children's hospital. Arch Pathol Lab Med. Jul 2008;132(7):1079-103.

CASE #29: SHORTNESS OF BREATH

CASE

A 65-year-old woman presents to her family doctor's office complaining of shortness of breath for two weeks. She has a known history of type 2 diabetes and hypertension. She is taking Aspirin, Hydrochlorothiazide, Metoprolol, and Glucophage with no recent change in medications. She reports progressively worsening dyspnea on minimal exertion and swelling to both her feet. A PA chest X-ray is obtained.

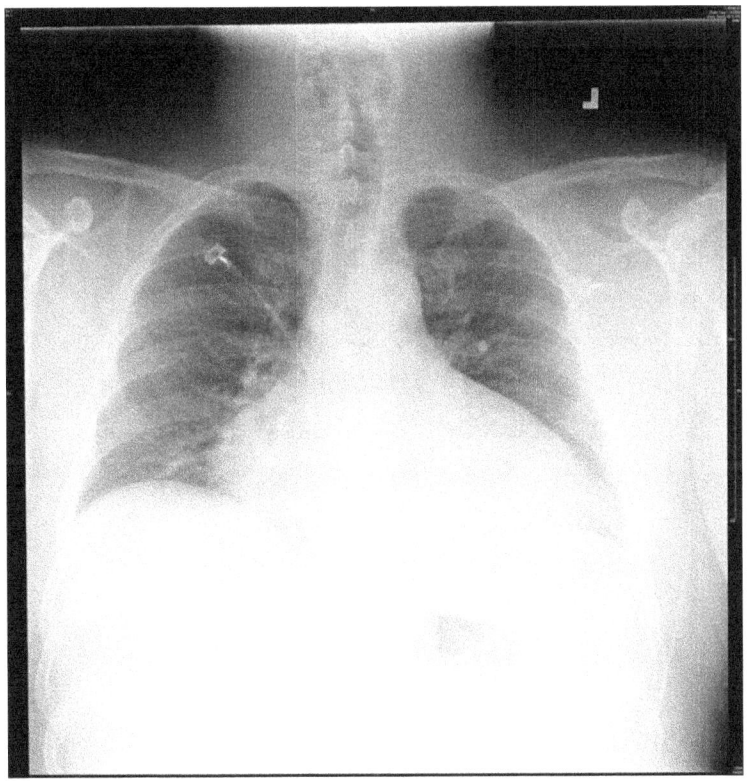

QUESTIONS

91. What is the likely diagnosis?

    a. Acute Renal Failure

    b. Congestive Heart Failure

    c. Chronic Obstructive Pulmonary Disease

    d. Pneumonia

92. Which of the following is a common complaint in patients with this condition?

    a. Decreased Urine Output

    b. Orthopnea

    c. Productive Cough

    d. Weight Loss

    e. Wheezing on Exertion

93. What is the likely cause of this condition in this patient?

    a. Amyloidosis

    b. Bacterial

    c. Carcinoid Syndrome

    d. Coronary Artery Disease

    e. Pulmonary Embolism

ANSWERS

91. b

92. b

93. d

VISUAL STIMULUS REVIEW

The image shows enlarged cardiac silhouette.

REFERENCES

- Onwuanyi A, Taylor M. Acute decompensated heart failure: pathophysiology and treatment. Am J Cardiol. Mar 26 2007;99(6B):25D-30D.

CASE #30: NAUSEA AND VOMITING

CASE

A 22-year-old man is brought to the emergency department by ambulance eight hours after ingesting eight cracked seeds of the plant pictured in the image below in an attempt to commit suicide. The patient is awake and alert but is having multiple episodes of vomiting and diarrhea.

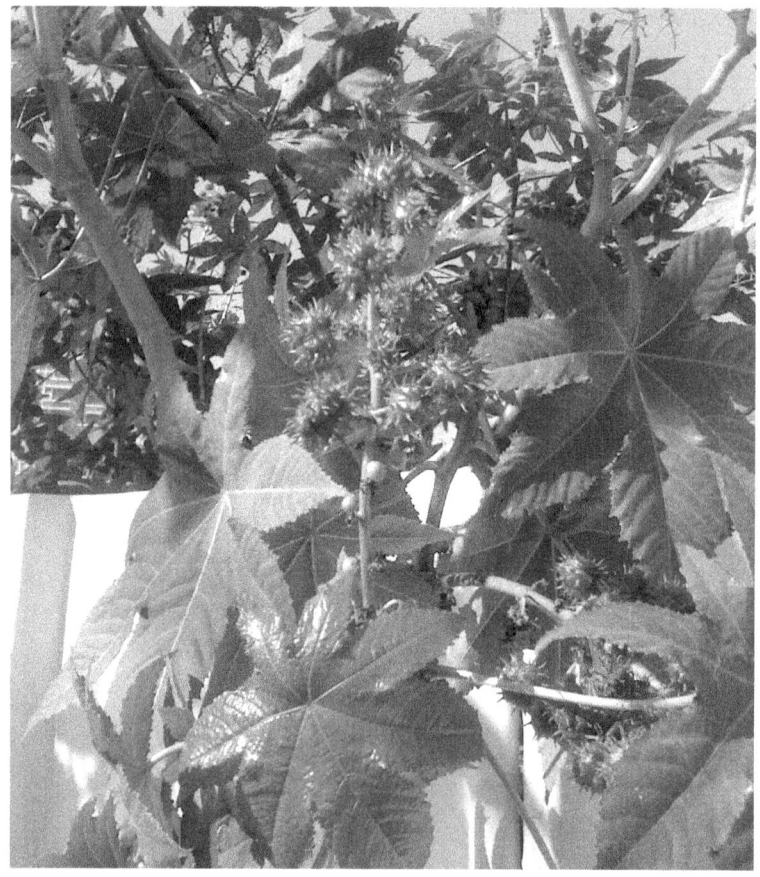

QUESTIONS

94. What is the likely diagnosis?
    a. Cyanide Toxicity
    b. Digitalis Toxicity
    c. Physostigmine Toxicity
    d. Ricin Toxicity

95. What is the name of the plant shown in the image?
    a. Agave Bean Plant
    b. Castor Bean Plant
    c. Foxglove Plant
    d. Jequirity Bean Plant
    e. Lima Bean Plant

96. What is the first line treatment for this condition?
    a. Atropine
    b. Digoxin Immune Fab
    c. Neostigmine
    d. Symptomatic and Supportive Care
    e. Whole Bowel Irrigation

ANSWERS

94. d

95. b

96. d

VISUAL STIMULUS REVIEW

The image shows castor bean plant and beans.

REFERENCES

- Lim H, Kim HJ, Cho YS. A case of ricin poisoning following ingestion of Korean castor bean. Emerg Med J. 2009 Apr;26(4):301-2.
- Audi J, Belson M, Patel M, Schier J, Osterloh J. Ricin poisoning: a comprehensive review. JAMA. 2005 Nov 9;294(18):2342-51.

CASE #31: LEG SWELLING

CASE

A 64-year-old woman presents to her doctor complaining of painful swelling to her left lower leg for the last three days. She has a medical history of diabetes and hypertension and three weeks prior underwent coronary artery bypass graft surgery with a vein that was harvested from her left lower leg. She has a temperature of 101.3F (38.5C), heart rate of 96/min, respirations 16/min, blood pressure of 163/75 mmHg, and O_2Sat of 99% on room air. Her left calf and foot are tender to palpation and warm both anteriorly (as shown) and posteriorly.

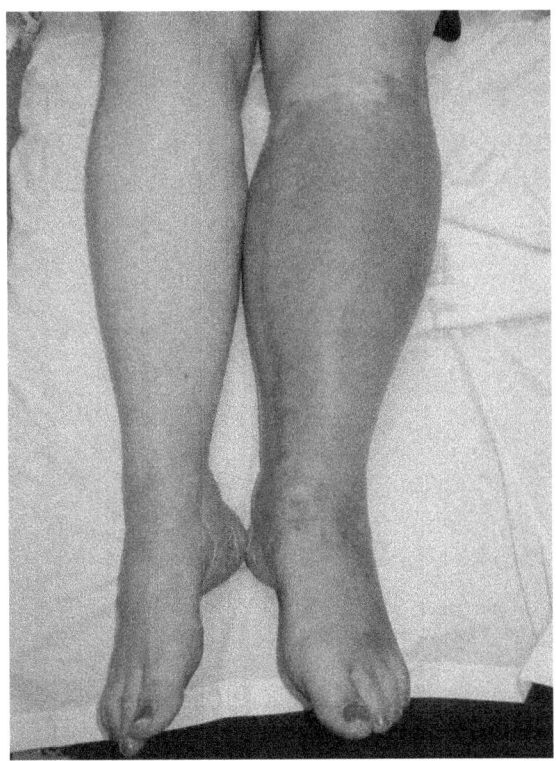

QUESTIONS

97. What is the likely diagnosis?

   a. Cellulitis

   b. Compartment Syndrome

   c. Deep Vein Thrombosis

   d. Necrotizing Fasciitis

   e. Osteomyelitis

98. What is the likely cause of this condition?

   a. Neisseria Meningitidis

   b. Pseudomonas Aeruginosa

   c. Staphylococcus Aureus

   d. Streptococcus Pyogenes

   e. Venous Thrombus

99. Which of the following medications should be used to treat this patient?

   a. Ciprofloxacin

   b. Enoxaparin

   c. Levofloxacin

   d. Penicillin G

   e. Vancomycin

ANSWERS

97. a

98. c

99. e

VISUAL STIMULUS REVIEW

The image shows swollen and erythematous left lower leg and foot with sharp proximal demarcation.

REFERENCES

- Bailey E, Kroshinsky D. Cellulitis: diagnosis and management. Dermatol Ther. 2011 Mar-Apr;24(2):229-39.
- May AK. Skin and soft tissue infections. Surg Clin North Am. 2009 Apr;89(2):403-20, viii.

CASE #32: CONFUSION AND QUADRIPLEGIA

CASE

A 65-year-old man with a history of consuming four glasses of wine daily and newly diagnosed hypertension is brought to the emergency department by ambulance as he was found to have had a seizure by a neighbor that checked on him. The patient has no other medical history, and the only history provided by the neighbor is that he started on a blood pressure pill three weeks ago and that the last time that he was seen at his baseline normal health was three days ago. The patient is confused and found to have serum sodium of 114 mEq/L. He is treated with hypertonic saline and admitted to the intensive care unit. The next morning he is awake and alert and feels much better; his serum sodium is 138 meq/L. He is discharged home on hospital day number three to return to the hospital two days later for severe confusion, horizontal gaze paralysis, and spastic quadriplegia. His gag reflex is absent, and he is endotracheally intubated for airway protection. An emergent MRI is obtained.

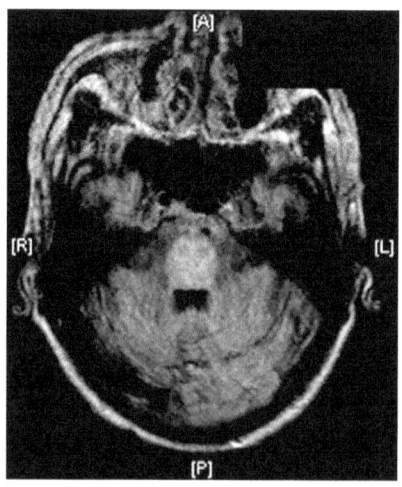

QUESTIONS

100. What is the likely diagnosis?
    a. Alcohol Withdrawal Encephalopathy
    b. Central Pontine Myelinolysis
    c. Delirium Tremens
    d. Herpes Encephalitis
    e. Ischemic Stroke

101. Which of the following is a known risk factor for development of this condition?
    a. Diabetes Mellitus
    b. Hypertension
    c. Immunocompromised State
    d. Malnutrition
    e. Recent Hospitalization

102. What medication is likely responsible for the patient's initial presentation to the emergency department?
    a. Clonidine
    b. Hydralazine
    c. Hydrochlorothiazide
    d. Lisinopril
    e. Metoprolol
    f. Nifedipine

ANSWERS

100. b

101. d

102. c

VISUAL STIMULUS REVIEW

The Axial FLAIR MRI image shows hyperintense signal to the pons.

REFERENCES

- Hurley RA, Filley CM, Taber KH. Central pontine myelinolysis: a metabolic disorder of myelin. J Neuropsychiatry Clin Neurosci. 2011 Fall;23(4):369-74.

- Martin RJ. Central pontine and extrapontine myelinolysis: the osmotic demyelination syndromes. J Neurol Neurosurg Psychiatry. 2004 Sep;75 Suppl 3:iii22-8.

CASE #33: PAINLESS ULCER

CASE

A 23-year-old man presents to his family doctor complaining of a painless ulcer to his penis for the last three days. He has no past medical history and is sexually active with multiple female partners. He reports that three weeks prior he did not use a condom. He reports a small "bump" that turned into an ulcer within a couple of days. His vital signs are within normal limits, and his physical examination shows no abnormalities other than his genital exam as shown below.

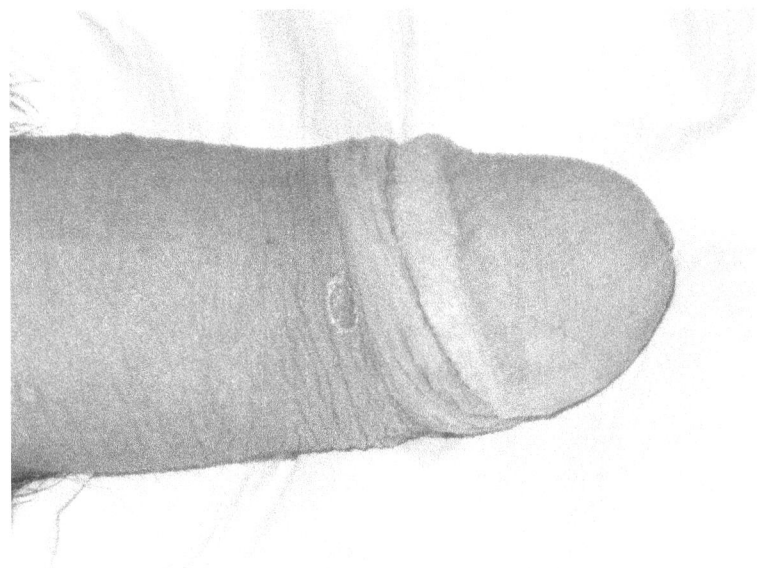

QUESTIONS

103. What is the likely diagnosis?
    a. Carcinoma
    b. Condyloma
    c. Lymphogranuloma Venereum
    d. Syphilis

104. What is the name of this skin lesion?
    a. Bubo
    b. Cancerous Ulcer
    c. Chancre
    d. Chancroid
    e. Genital Wart

105. What is the likely cause of this lesion?
    a. Chlamydia Trachomatis
    b. Haemophilus Ducreyi
    c. Herpes Simplex Virus
    d. Human Papilloma Virus
    e. Malignant Transformation
    f. Treponema Pallidum

106. What medication should you use to treat this condition?
    a. Acyclovir PO
    b. Ciprofloxacin PO
    c. Imiquimod Topical
    d. Levofloxacin PO
    e. Penicillin G IM

ANSWERS

103. d

104. c

105. f

106. e

VISUAL STIMULUS REVIEW

The image shows a small, dry ulcer with surrounding hard edge.

REFERENCES

- Roett MA, Mayor MT, Uduhiri KA. Diagnosis and management of genital ulcers. Am Fam Physician. 2012 Feb 1;85(3):254-62.
- Lee V, Kinghorn G. Syphilis: an update. Clin Med. 2008 Jun;8(3):330-3.
- Centers for Disease Control and Prevention. Sexually transmitted diseases treatment guidelines 2006. MMWR 2006;55(no. RR-11).

CASE #34: PAINFUL ULCER

CASE

A 23-year-old man presents to his family doctor complaining of a painful ulcer to his penis for the last three days. He has no past medical history and is sexually active with multiple female partners. He reports that two weeks prior he did not use a condom. He reports a small "bump" that released some pus and then turned into an ulcer within a couple of days. His vital signs are within normal limits, and his physical examination shows no abnormalities other than right inguinal tender lymphadenopathy and an abnormal genital exam as shown below.

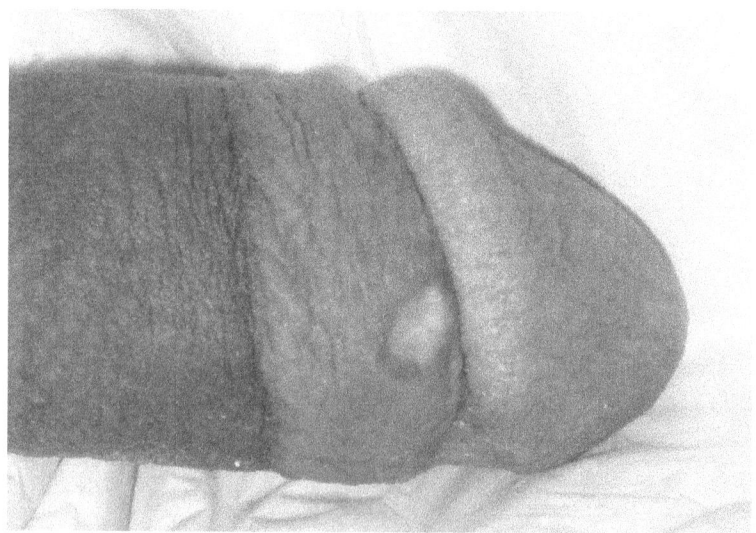

QUESTIONS

107. What is the likely diagnosis?
    a. Carcinoma
    b. Chancroid
    c. Condyloma
    d. Lymphogranuloma Venereum
    e. Syphilis

108. What is the name of this skin lesion?
    a. Bubo
    b. Cancerous Ulcer
    c. Chancre
    d. Chancroid
    e. Genital Wart

109. What is the likely cause of this lesion?
    a. Chlamydia Trachomatis
    b. Haemophilus Ducreyi
    c. Herpes Simplex Virus
    d. Human Papilloma Virus
    e. Malignant Transformation
    f. Treponema Pallidum

110. What medication should you use to treat this condition?
    a. Acyclovir PO
    b. Ceftriaxone IM
    c. Imiquimod Topical
    d. Penicillin G IM
    e. Trimethoprim - Sulphamethoxazole PO

ANSWERS

107. b

108. d

109. b

110. b

VISUAL STIMULUS REVIEW

The image shows an ulcer with a soft erythematous border and what appears to be a wet yellowish exudate covering its base.

REFERENCES

- Roett MA, Mayor MT, Uduhiri KA. Diagnosis and management of genital ulcers. Am Fam Physician. 2012 Feb 1;85(3):254-62.

- Centers for Disease Control and Prevention, National Center for HIV/AIDS, Viral Hepatitis, STD, and TB Prevention, Division of STD Prevention. Accessed 6/11/2012

CASE #35: RASH & FEVER

CASE

A 14-year-old boy presents to his pediatrician complaining of two days of pruritic rash that started on his face but since progressed to his torso and extremities. He is fully immunized and has no medical history. His vital signs are temp 102.5F (39.1C), heart rate 108/min, respiratory rate 17/min, blood pressure 110/60, and O_2Sat 99% on room air. He is well-appearing, and his physical exam is within normal limits excluding his skin and oropharynx exam.

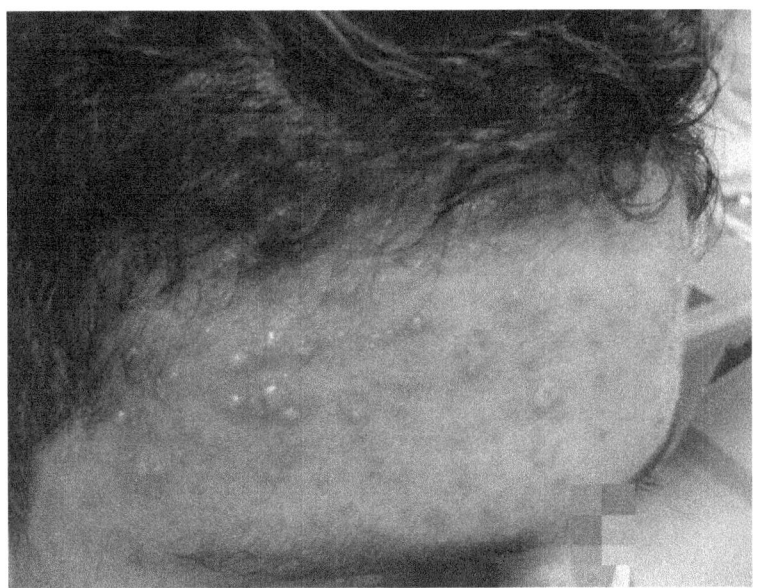

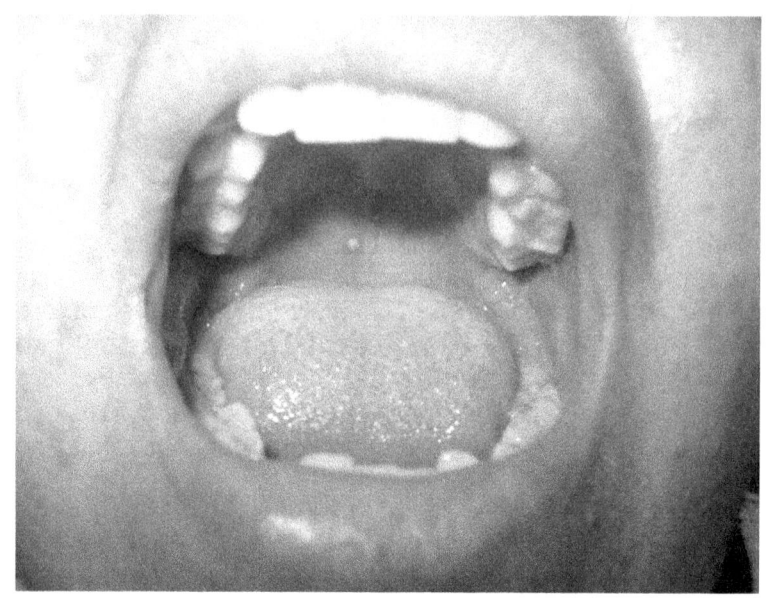

QUESTIONS

111. What is the likely diagnosis?
   a. Chickenpox
   b. Erythema Multiforme
   c. Herpes Simplex
   d. Measles
   e. Rubella
   f. Shingles

112. What is the likely causative organism?
   a. Herpes Simplex Virus
   b. Measles Virus
   c. Rubella Virus
   d. Varicella Virus

113. Which of the following is a concerning complication of this condition?

   a. Cataract
   b. Orchitis
   c. Pneumonitis
   d. Renal Failure

114. What is the recommended treatment for this patient?

   a. Acyclovir PO
   b. Amoxicillin PO
   c. Prednisone PO
   d. Symptomatic Care

ANSWERS

111. a

112. d

113. c

114. a

VISUAL STIMULUS REVIEW

The first image shows multiple lesions to the patient's forehead (macules, papules, vesicles, pustules, and umbilicated vesicles). The second image shows a pharyngeal vesicle on an erythematous base.

REFERENCES

- Tunbridge AJ, Breuer J, Jeffery KJ; Chickenpox in adults - clinical management. J Infect. 2008 Aug;57(2):95-102.
- National Center for Immunization and Respiratory Diseases (NCIRD), Division of Viral Diseases. Managing Persons at Risk for Severe Varicella; Accessed: 6/11/2012.

CASE #36: EPIGASTRIC PAIN

CASE

A 40-year-old woman presents to the emergency department complaining of six hours of right upper and epigastric pain with nausea and vomiting. She has no medical history and is taking no medications. She reports occasional epigastric pain after eating fatty foods over the last six months, which used to come and go over a couple of hours. This episode started while she was eating lunch but is more severe than her previous pains and has become constant. Her vital signs are temperature of 99.7F (37.6C), blood pressure 140/75 mmHg, heart rate 96/min, respirations 16/min, and O_2Sat of 99% on room air. On physical examination she has right upper quadrant and epigastric tenderness with guarding. An ultrasound is obtained.

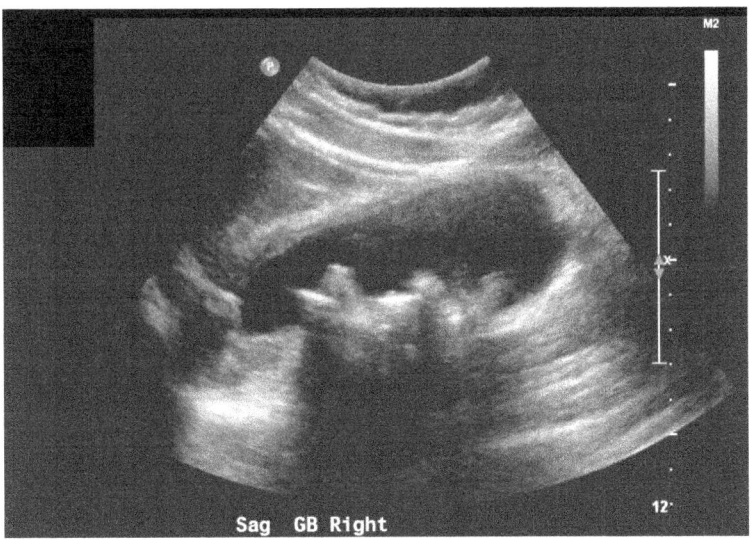

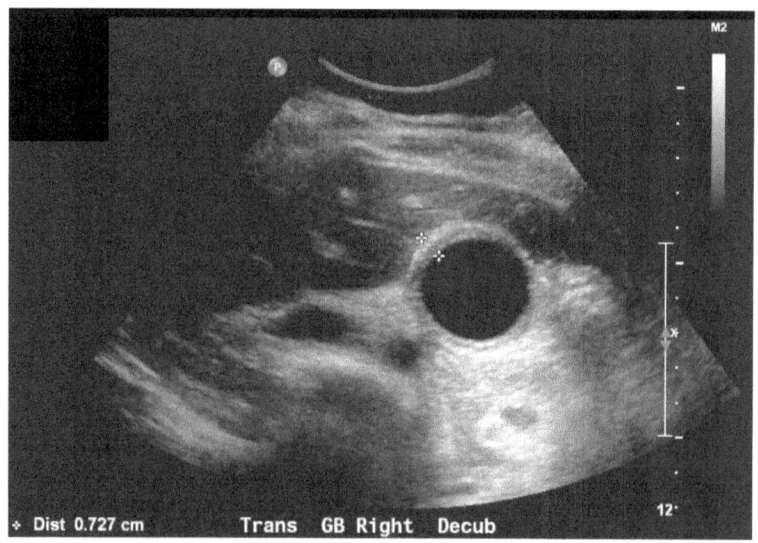

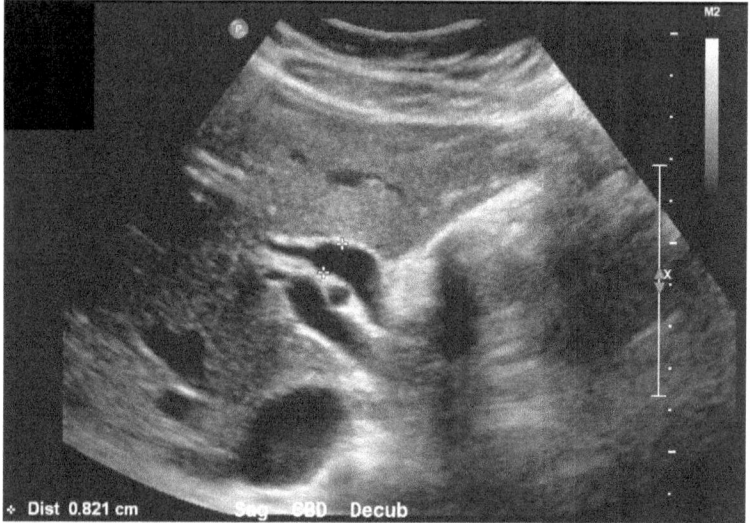

QUESTIONS

115. What is the likely diagnosis?
    a. Acute Pancreatitis
    b. Biliary Colic

c. Cholecystitis
   d. Choledocholithiasis
   e. Pancreatitis
   f. Renal Colic

116. Where is the likely site of obstruction?
   a. Common Bile Duct
   b. Cystic Duct
   c. Pancreatic Duct
   d. Right Hepatic Duct
   e. Right Ureter

117. In which of the following is this condition more common?
   a. Asians
   b. Children
   c. Chronic Alcoholics
   d. Females
   e. Malnourished People

118. What is the most sensitive finding/sign for the diagnosis of this condition?
   a. Elevated Alkaline Phosphatase
   b. Elevated Direct Bilirubin
   c. Elevated Indirect Bilirubin
   d. Elevated White Blood Cell count
   e. Murphy's Sign
   f. Right Upper Quadrant Rebound Tenderness

ANSWERS

115. c

116. b

117. d

118. e

VISUAL STIMULUS REVIEW

The first ultrasound image shows multiple gallstones. The second ultrasound image shows a thickened gallbladder wall of 0.7 cm. The third ultrasound image shows a mildly dilated common bile duct at 0.8 cm.

REFERENCES

- Elwood DR. Cholecystitis. Surg Clin North Am. 2008 Dec;88(6):1241-52, viii.
- Strasberg SM. Clinical practice. Acute calculous cholecystitis. N Engl J Med. 2008 Jun 26;358(26):2804-11.

CASE #37: FINGER SWELLING

CASE

A 27-year-old man presents to his doctor complaining of painless swelling to his fingertips that developed over the last year. He has no medical history and is taking no medications. He denies any shortness of breast, fevers, chills, abdominal pain, diarrhea, weight loss, joint pain, or any other symptoms. He is physically active and runs 20 miles a week with no decrease in his exercise tolerance. His physical exam is normal except for his distal fingers as shown below.

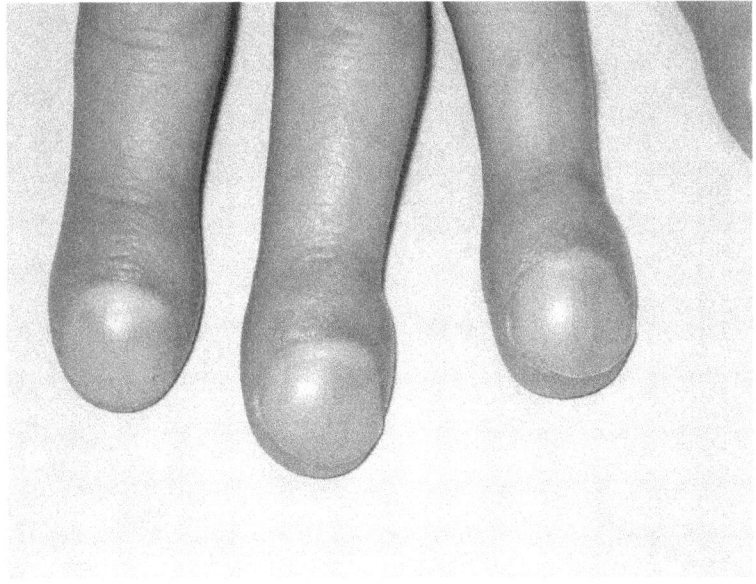

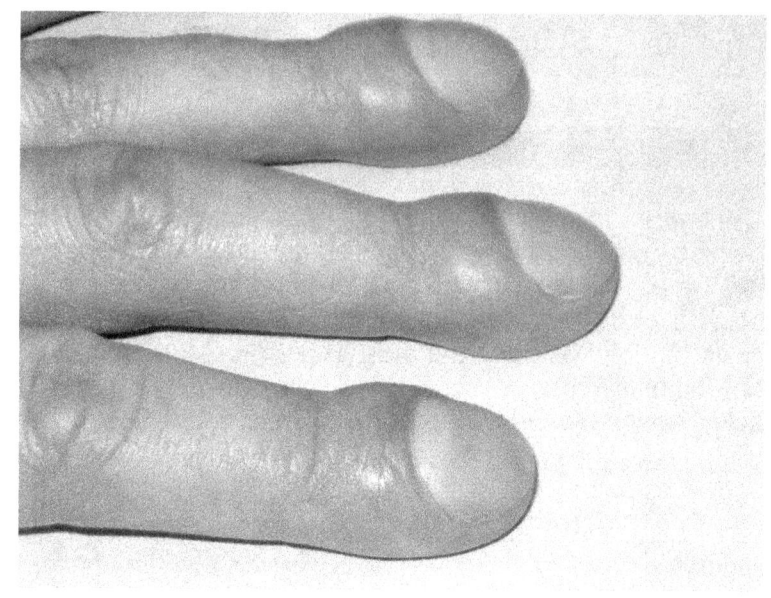

QUESTIONS

119. What is the likely diagnosis?
    a. Crohn's Disease
    b. Emphysema
    c. Endocarditis
    d. Hypertrophic Osteoarthropathy
    e. Tuberculosis

120. What is the name of the physical finding shown?
    a. Clubbing
    b. Koilonychia
    c. Leukonychia
    d. Schamroth Sign

121. What is the recommended treatment for this condition?
    a. 5-aminosalicylic Acid
    b. Intravenous Antibiotics for Six Weeks
    c. Lung Transplant
    d. Oral Antibiotic Treatment for Six Months
    e. Symptomatic Care

ANSWERS

119. d

120. a

121. e

VISUAL STIMULUS REVIEW

The images demonstrate bulbous fusiform enlargement of the distal portion of the digits with a proximal nail fold to nail plate (Lovibond) angle of more than 180 degrees.

REFERENCES

- Martinez-Lavin M, Vargas A, Rivera-Viñas M. Hypertrophic osteoarthropathy: a palindrome with a pathogenic connotation. Curr Opin Rheumatol. 2008 Jan;20(1):88-91.

- Spicknall KE, Zirwas MJ, English JC 3rd. Clubbing: an update on diagnosis, differential diagnosis, pathophysiology, and clinical relevance. J Am Acad Dermatol. 2005 Jun;52(6):1020-8.

CASE #38: DOUBLE VISION

CASE

A 65-year-old man presents to his family doctor complaining of two days of double vision where he sees double images side by side when he looks to the right. He has a history of hypertension and is taking Aspirin, Hydrochlorothiazide, and Lisinopril daily. He woke up a couple of days ago with this condition and decided to seek medical attention as it did not resolve. He denies any headache, hearing or vision loss, difficulty speaking or swallowing, unsteadiness, or any weakness. On physical exam he has normal pupillary exam and no nystagmus with a normal cranial nerve exam except as shown in the following images.

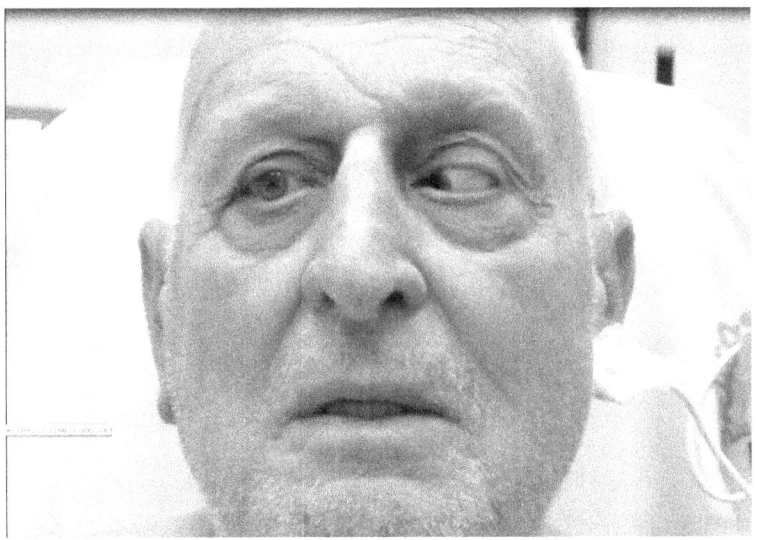

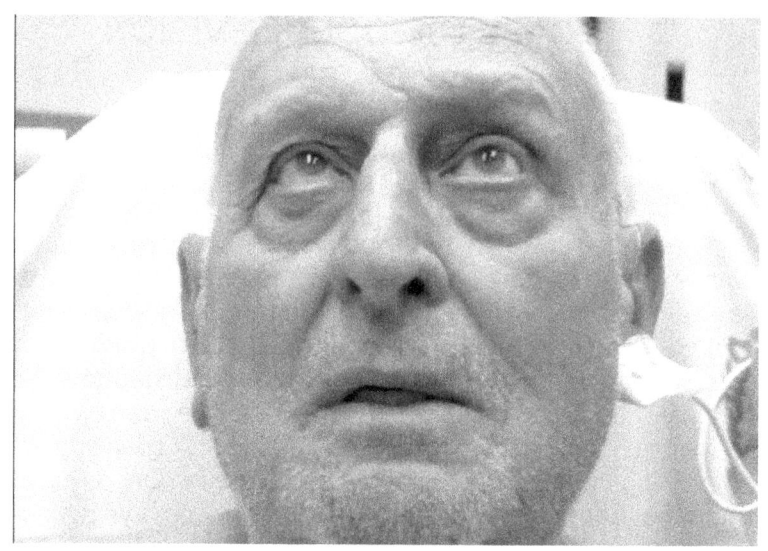

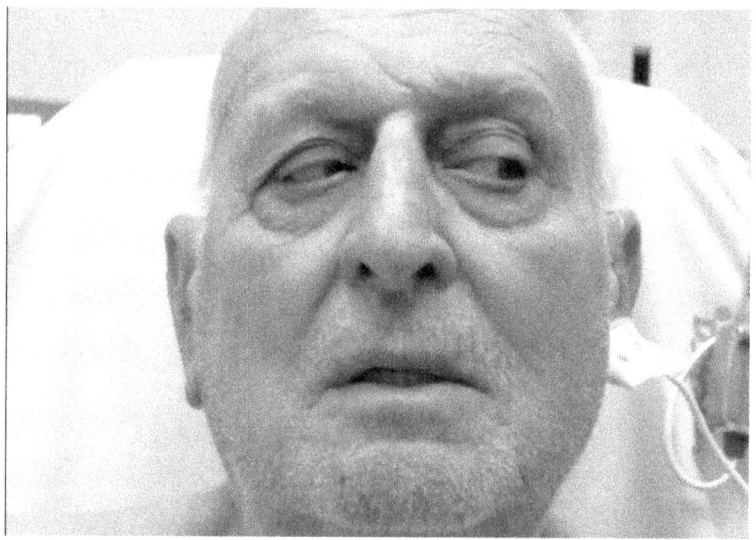

QUESTIONS

122. What is the clinical diagnosis?
   a. CN III Palsy
   b. CN IV Palsy

- c. CN V Palsy
- d. CN VI Palsy

123. What muscle is affected in this condition?
    - a. Inferior Rectus
    - b. Lateral Rectus
    - c. Levator Palpebrae
    - d. Medial Rectus
    - e. Superior Rectus

124. What is the likely cause of this condition in this patient?
    - a. Autoimmune
    - b. Hemorrhagic
    - c. Infectious
    - d. Ischemic
    - e. Malignant
    - f. Post-Infectious

125. What condition should be suspected in a patient with similar cranial nerves findings in the presence of nonfatigable nystagmus?
    - a. Myasthenia Gravis
    - b. Herpes Encephalitis
    - c. Pontine Glioma
    - d. Thalamic Ischemic Infarct
    - e. Vitamin B12 Deficiency

ANSWERS

122. d

123. b

124. d

125. c

VISUAL STIMULUS REVIEW

The images show right eye lateral rectus palsy as evident by the right eye not crossing the midline upon lateral gaze. There is no proptosis or ptosis, and the left and upper gazes appear to be intact.

REFERENCES

- Prasad S, Volpe NJ. Paralytic strabismus: third, fourth, and sixth nerve palsy. Neurol Clin. 2010 Aug;28(3):803-33.
- Brazis PW. Isolated palsies of cranial nerves III, IV, and VI. Brazis PW. Semin Neurol. 2009 Feb;29(1):14-28.

CASE #39: VOMITING

CASE

A 42-year-old woman presents to the emergency department complaining of two hours of vomiting and mild epigastric pain that started a couple of days ago. She has a history of mild rheumatoid arthritis for which she is taking over-the-counter medications that she uses almost daily. She denies alcohol use, fevers, chills, or shortness of breath. Her vital signs are temp 99.7F (37.4C), heart rate 106/min, blood pressure 95/60, respiratory rate of 16/min, and O$_2$Sat of 99% on room air. She appears to be in no distress, and her abdominal exam shows mild epigastric tenderness with no guarding or rebound.

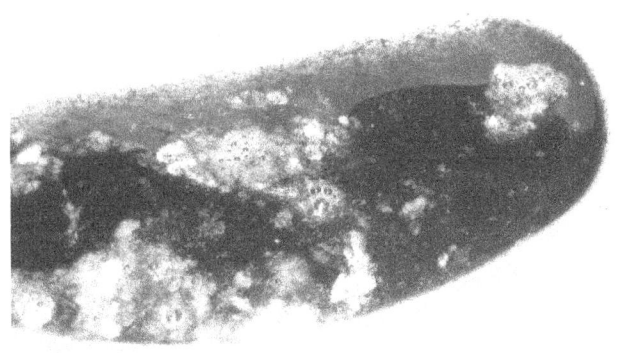

QUESTIONS

126. What is the likely diagnosis?

    a. Cholecystitis

    b. Gastroparesis

    c. Pancreatitis

    d. Peptic Ulcer Disease

    e. Variceal Bleed

127. What is the likely cause of this condition in this patient?

    a. Alcohol Binge

    b. Chronic low-dose prednisone that she is taking daily and forgot to tell you about.

    c. Helicobacter Pylori

    d. Non-Steroidal Anti-Inflammatory Drugs

    e. Tobacco Use

128. Which of the following intervention is likely to decrease mortality risk in this patient?

    a. Erythromycin IV before Endoscopy

    b. Endoscopic Therapy

    c. Nasogastric Tube Cold Water Irrigation

    d. Proton Pump Inhibitor IV Bolus

    e. Proton Pump Inhibitor IV Bolus Followed by a Continuous Drip

ANSWERS

126. d

127. d

128. b

VISUAL STIMULUS REVIEW

The image shows coffee ground gastric content.

REFERENCES

- Holster IL, Kuipers EJ. Management of acute nonvariceal upper gastrointestinal bleeding: current policies and future perspectives. World J Gastroenterol. 2012 Mar 21;18(11):1202-7.

- Laine L, Jensen DM. Management of patients with ulcer bleeding. Am J Gastroenterol. 2012 Mar;107(3):345-60.

CASE #40: WATERY DIARRHEA

CASE

A 72-year-old woman develops watery diarrhea and crampy abdominal pain on hospital day number four after she is hospitalized for management of right-sided pyelonephritis. Her vital signs are temperature 102.3F (39C), heart rate 104/min, respirations 19/min, blood pressure 110/60, and O_2Sat 96% on room air. On physical examination she has diffuse abdominal tenderness with guarding and rebound over her right lower, right middle, and right upper quadrants. A CT scan is obtained.

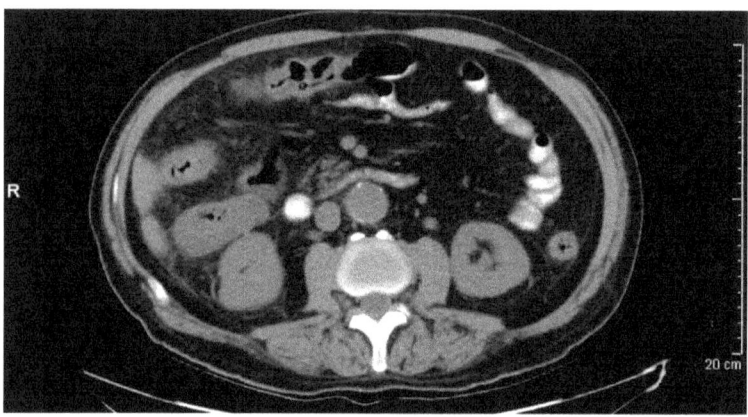

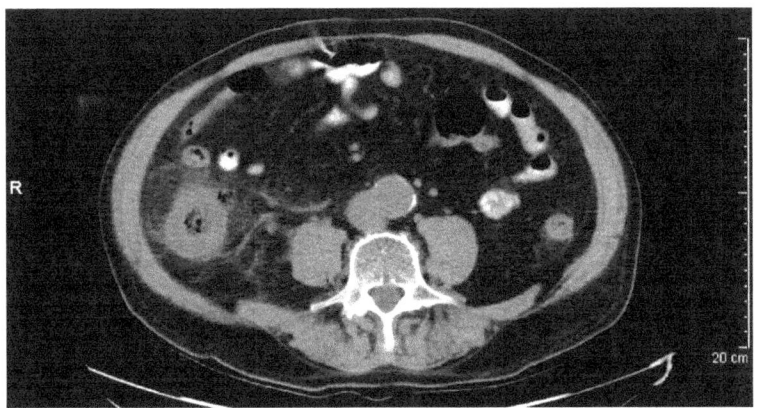

QUESTIONS

129. What is the likely diagnosis?

    a. Appendicitis

    b. Clostridium Difficile Colitis

    c. Crohn's Disease

    d. Emphysematous Pyelonephritis

    e. Toxic Megacolon

    f. Ulcerative Colitis

130. What is the most sensitive test for diagnosing this condition?

    a. Abdominal Ultrasound

    b. CT Abdomen and Pelvis with IV Contrast

    c. Direct Microscopy of Colon Biopsy

    d. Enzyme Immunoassay (EIA)

    e. Real Time PCR

    f. Stool Culture

131. What is the likely cause of this condition?
    a. Autoimmune
    b. Bacterial Invasion into Mucosa
    c. Bacterial Toxins
    d. Colonic Perforation
    e. Necrotizing Renal Infection
    f. Obstruction of Colonic Appendage
132. Which of the following may be used for the treatment of this condition?
    a. Appendectomy
    b. Ceftriaxone (Rocephin)
    c. Nephrectomy
    d. Pulse IV Steroid Therapy
    e. Stool Transplant
    f. Vancomycin IV

ANSWERS

129. b
130. f
131. c
132. e

VISUAL STIMULUS REVIEW

The CT images demonstrate markedly thickened ascending colon with surrounding stranding.

REFERENCES

- Moudgal V, Sobel JD. Clostridium difficile colitis: a review. Hosp Pract (Minneap). 2012 Feb;40(1):139-48.

- Kachrimanidou M, Malisiovas N. Clostridium difficile infection: a comprehensive review. Crit Rev Microbiol. 2011 Aug;37(3):178-87.

CASE #41: PAINFUL SORE

CASE

A 30-year-old man presents to his family doctor complaining of a painful sore to his lower lip for two days. He has no past medical history and is taking no medications. He recalls that two days prior he noticed some tingling to the center of his lower lip that progressed into burning pain before the lesion appeared earlier that morning.

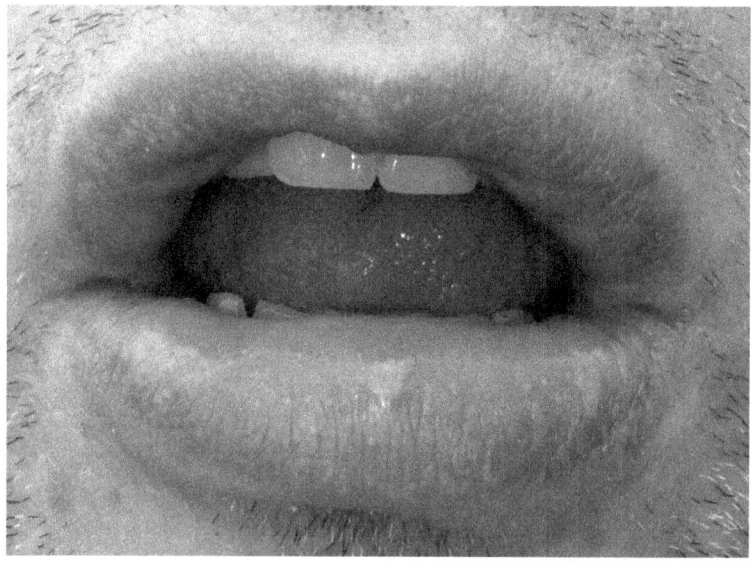

QUESTIONS

133. What is the likely diagnosis?
    a. Chancre
    b. Chancroid
    c. Hand Foot and Mouth Disease
    d. Herpes Labialis
    e. Primary Varicella Infection

134. What is the likely cause?
    a. Coxsackievirus Virus
    b. Hemophilus Ducreyi
    c. Herpes Simplex Virus Type 1
    d. Herpes Simplex Virus Type 2
    e. Treponema Pallidum

135. This presentation likely represents?
    a. Direct Inoculation
    b. Latent Infection
    c. Primary Infection
    d. Reactivation

ANSWERS

133. d

134. c

135. d

VISUAL STIMULUS REVIEW

The image shows intraepidermal vesicles to the lower lip.

REFERENCES

- Arduino PG, Porter SR. Oral and perioral herpes simplex virus type 1 (HSV-1) infection: review of its management. Oral Dis. May 2006;12(3):254-70.
- Spruance SL, Overall JC Jr, Kern ER, Krueger GG, Pliam V, Miller W. The natural history of recurrent herpes simplex labialis: implications for antiviral therapy. N Engl J Med. Jul 14 1977;297(2):69-75.

CASE #42: WRIST PAIN

CASE

A 62-year-old woman presents to the emergency department complaining of right wrist pain after falling on an outstretched hand an hour ago. On physical examination she has severe tenderness over proximal wrist. An X-ray is obtained.

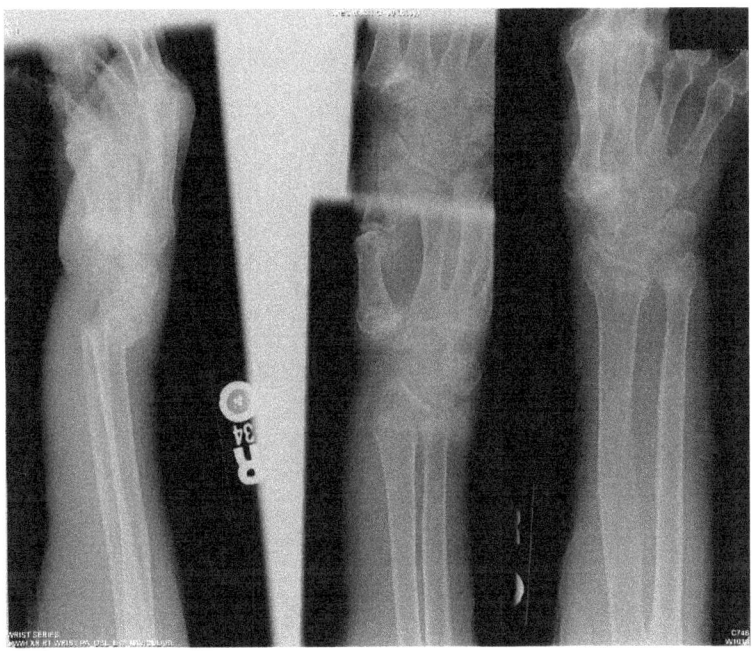

QUESTIONS

136. What is the likely diagnosis?
     a. Barton Fracture
     b. Colles Fracture
     c. Hutchinson Fracture
     d. Scaphoid Fracture
     e. Smith Fracture
     f. Wrist Dislocation

137. What is the usual mechanism that causes this condition?
     a. Direct Blow
     b. Hyperextension
     c. Hyperflexion
     d. Pathological Fracture

138. Numbness to the volar thumb, index, and middle fingers in this patient will suggest injury to which of the following nerves?
     a. Median
     b. Radial
     c. Superficial Branch of the Radial Nerve
     d. Ulnar

ANSWERS

136. b

137. b

138. a

VISUAL STIMULUS REVIEW

The radiograph shows fractures to the distal radius and ulna with dorsal displacement of the distal fragments.

REFERENCES

- Krishnan J. Distal radius fractures in adults. Orthopedics. 2002 Feb;25(2):175-9; discussion 179-80.
- Davis DI, Baratz M. Soft tissue complications of distal radius fractures. Hand Clin. 2010 May;26(2):229-35.

CASE #43: LEG PAIN

CASE

A 27-year-old man who has no past medical history presents to the emergency department complaining of severe pain to his left lower leg. He was hit by a car the night before, suffering what he recalls a minor injury to his left posterior lower leg. He did not fall and was able to ambulate and did not seek any medical attention. Overnight, his pain intensified, and he noticed swelling and discoloration. On examination, his calf is tense to the touch, his pain worsens on passive foot dorsiflexion, and he has decreased two points discrimination to his foot. The patient reports 10/10 burning-type pain.

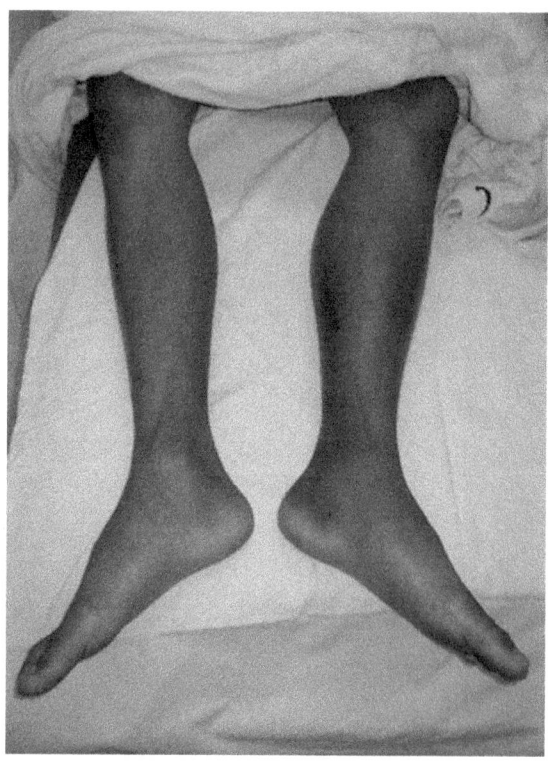

QUESTIONS

139. What is the likely diagnosis?

   a. Acute Gastrocnemius Muscle Teat
   b. Compartment Syndrome
   c. Deep Venous Thrombosis
   d. Popliteal Artery Thrombosis
   e. Pyomyositis

140. Which of the following findings is likely to be present in this patient?

   a. Absent Tibialis Posterior Pulse (left)
   b. Absent Dorsalis Pedis Pulse (left)
   c. Decreased Capillary Refill (left lower leg)
   d. Point Tenderness (left lower leg)
   e. Warm Skin (left lower leg)

141. Which of the following studies should be used to confirm the above diagnosis?

   a. CT Angiogram
   b. Doppler, Duplex Ultrasound
   c. Intracompartmental Pressure Measurement
   d. MRI

ANSWERS

139. b

140. c

141. c

VISUAL STIMULUS REVIEW

The left lower leg seems mildly swollen and ecchymotic.

REFERENCES

- Shadgan B, Menon M, Sanders D et al. Current thinking about acute compartment syndrome of the lower extremity. Can J Surg. 2010 Oct;53(5):329-34.

- Kirk KL, Hayda R. 129.Compartment syndrome and lower-limb fasciotomies in the combat environment. Foot Ankle Clin. 2010 Mar;15(1):41-61.

CASE #44: SMALL BUMPS

CASE

A 28-year-old woman presents to her family doctor complaining of painless bumps to her lower vagina that she noticed two months ago. She has no past medical history and denies history of sexually transmitted illnesses or current vaginal pain or discharge.

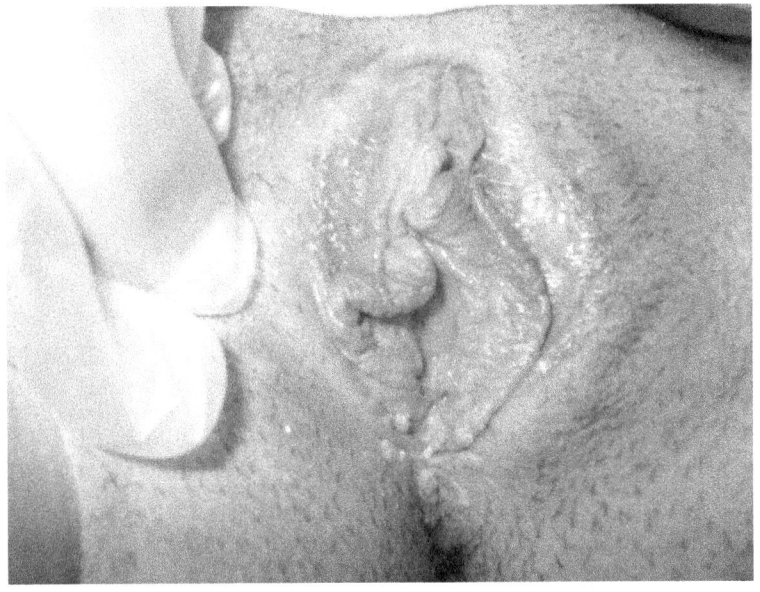

QUESTIONS

142. What is the likely diagnosis?
- a. Chancre
- b. Genital Warts
- c. Herpetic Ulcers
- d. Malignant Melanoma
- e. Molluscum Contagiosum

    f. Squamous Cell Carcinoma

143. What is the likely cause of this condition?

    a. Hemophilus Ducreyi
    b. Herpes Simplex Virus
    c. Human Papilloma Virus
    d. Treponema Pallidum
    e. Sun Exposure

144. The cause of this condition is also a leading cause for?

    a. Cervical Cancer
    b. Encephalitis
    c. Uterine Cancer
    d. Vasculitis

145. Which of the following is true regarding this condition?

    a. Male circumcision reduces the risk to acquire this condition by 35 percent.
    b. Vaccination after natural onset of this condition is highly protective against recurrences.
    c. Vaccination after natural onset is highly effective in producing regression of those lesions.
    d. Oral and perioral lesions are common presentation of this condition.

ANSWERS

142. b

143. c

144. a

145. a

VISUAL STIMULUS REVIEW

The image shows pearly papular eruption to the inferior vulva and anterior perineum.

REFERENCES

- Stanley MA. Genital human papillomavirus infections: current and prospective therapies. J Gen Virol. 2012 Apr;93(Pt 4):681-91.
- Juckett G, Hartman-Adams H. Human papillomavirus: clinical manifestations and prevention. Am Fam Physician. 2010 Nov 15;82(10):1209-13.

CASE #45: RED EYE

CASE

A 23-year-old woman presents to her family doctor complaining of red eye for two days. She has no past medical history, is not taking any medications, and is not using glasses or contact lenses. The patient complains of redness and copious watery discharge from her right eye. The patient denies eye pain, purulent discharge, photophobia, or any vision changes to her right eye. Her visual acuity is 20/20 OD and OS.

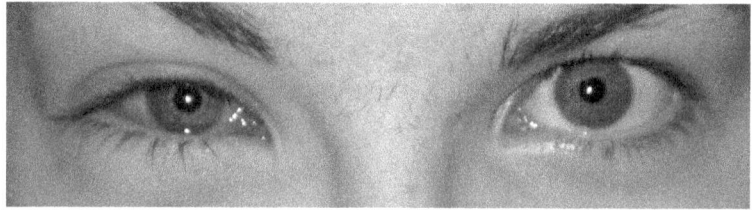

QUESTIONS

146. What is the likely diagnosis?

   a. Acute Angle Closure Glaucoma

   b. Blepharitis

   c. Conjunctivitis

   d. Corneal Abrasion

   e. Episcleritis

   f. Keratitis

147. What is the likely cause of this condition in this patient?

   a. Autoimmune

   b. Bacterial

   c. Foreign Body

   d. Pupillary Block

   e. Trauma

   f. Viral

148. Which of the following causes should be considered in a similar patient with a similar exam and additional complaint of a large amount of yellow/green purulent discharge?

   a. Adenovirus

   b. Herpes Simplex Virus

   c. Neisseria Gonorrhea

   d. Staphylococcus Aureus

   e. Rheumatoid Arthritis

   f. Ultraviolet-Light Exposure

ANSWERS

146. c

147. f

148. c

VISUAL STIMULUS REVIEW

The image demonstrates severe conjunctival injection and edema with clear and normal appearing cornea. The pupils seem to be round and symmetric.

REFERENCES

- Richards A, Guzman-Cottrill JA. Conjunctivitis. Pediatr Rev. 2010 May;31(5):196-208.
- Cronau H, Kankanala RR, Mauger T. Diagnosis and management of red eye in primary care. Am Fam Physician. 2010 Jan 15;81(2):137-44.

CASE #46: ITCHY RASH

CASE

A 30-year-old woman presents to her family doctor complaining of pruritic rash to both her arms for the last three days. She has no medical history, is taking no medications, and reports no new exposure and no history of similar rash. Her hands, feet, face, and torso show no lesions.

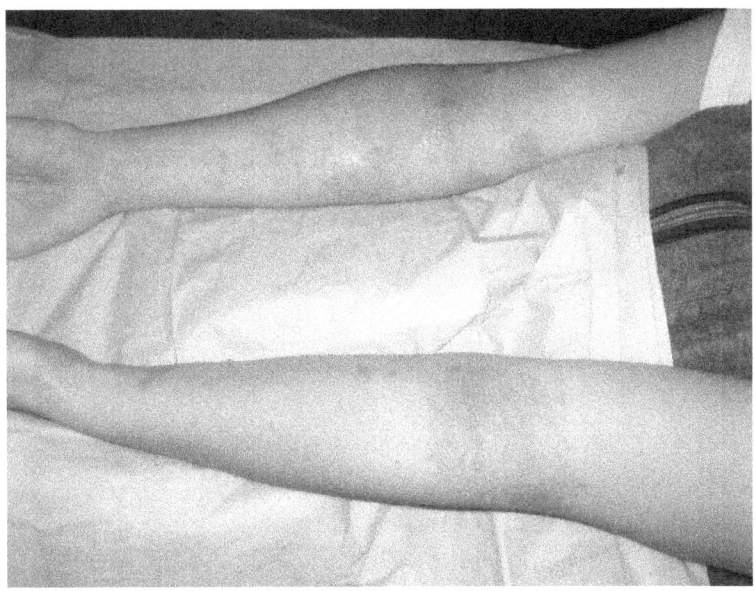

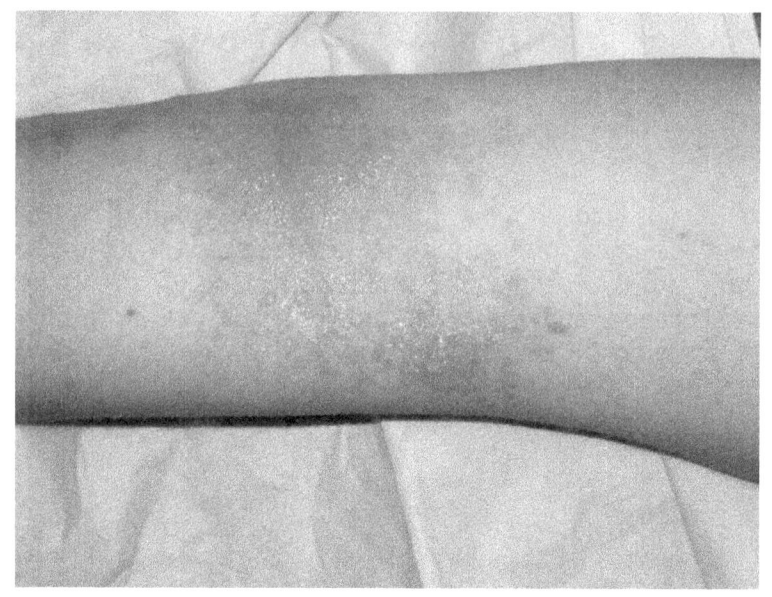

QUESTIONS

149. What is the likely diagnosis?
    a. Allergic Contact Dermatitis
    b. Cellulitis
    c. Erythema Multiforme
    d. Scabies
    e. Tinea Corporis
    f. Urticaria

150. What is the likely mechanism causing this condition?
    a. Autoimmune
    b. Bacterial Infection
    c. Fungal Infection
    d. Histamine Release
    e. Type IV Hypersensitivity

151. What is the most common cause for this condition in the United States?
    a. Candida Albicans
    b. Malassezia Furfur
    c. Nickel
    d. Poison Ivy
    e. Streptococcus Pyogenes

ANSWERS

149. a

150. e

151. d

VISUAL STIMULUS REVIEW

The images show papules and vesicles on an erythematous base.

REFERENCES

- Prakash AV, Davis MD. Contact dermatitis in older adults: a review of the literature. Am J Clin Dermatol. 2010 Dec 1;11(6):373-81.

- Usatine RP, Riojas M. Diagnosis and management of contact dermatitis. Am Fam Physician. 2010 Aug 1;82(3):249-55.

CASE #47: EYE PAIN

CASE

A 42-year-old woman presents to the emergency department complaining of right eye pain and foreign body feeling that prevents her from opening her eye. She recalls walking outdoors and feeling a wind blowing on her face with the sudden onset of pain about an hour ago. She has no past medical history, is not taking any medications, and is not using contact lenses. After an instillation of anesthetic drops into her right eye, her visual acuity is 20/20. Careful slit lamp exam, including eyelid eversion, fails to demonstrate any foreign body and shows clear cornea and normal anterior chamber. The following image is taken after fluorescin dye is used.

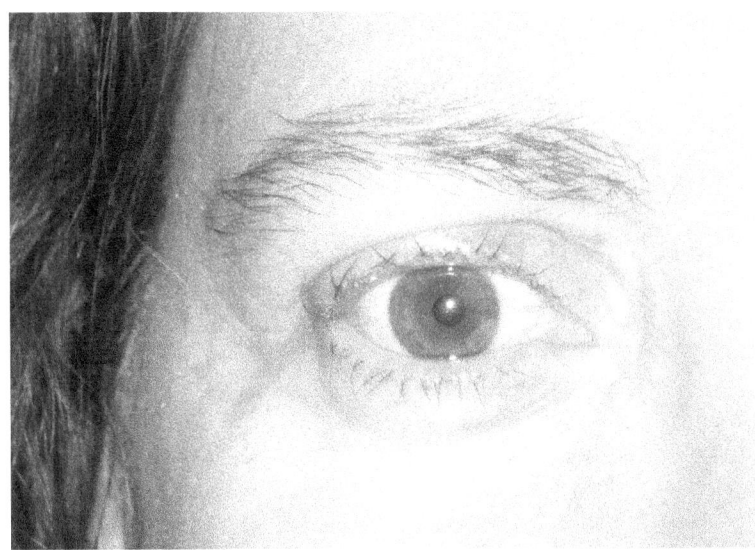

QUESTIONS

152. What is the likely diagnosis?

   a. Acute Angle Closure Glaucoma

   b. Conjunctivitis

   c. Corneal Abrasion

   d. Corneal Laceration

   e. Corneal Ulcer

153. What is the likely cause of this condition?

   a. Chlamydia Trachomatis

   b. Direct Trauma

   c. Herpes Simplex Virus

   d. Pupillary Block

   e. Pseudomonas Aeruginosa

154. Which of the following causes should be considered in patients with a similar presentation who wear contact lenses?

   a. Chlamydia Trachomatis

   b. Herpes Simplex Virus

   c. Herpes Zoster Virus

   d. Pupillary Block

   e. Pseudomonas Aeruginosa

ANSWERS

152. c

153. b

154. e

VISUAL STIMULUS REVIEW

The image shows Fluorescin stain uptake to the medial upper cornea of the right eye.

REFERENCES

- Cronau H, Kankanala RR, Mauger T. Diagnosis and management of red eye in primary care. Am Fam Physician. 2010 Jan 15;81(2):137-44.
- Dargin JM, Lowenstein RA. The painful eye. Emerg Med Clin North Am. 2008 Feb;26(1):199-216, viii.

CASE #48: PAINFUL EYE

CASE

A 63-year-old woman presents to her ophthalmologist complaining of right eye pain eight days following cataract surgery. She reports gradual worsening of her vision following initial post-surgical improvement with two days of severe pain and yellow drainage from the eye. Her vision is 20/200 OD and 20/30 OS.

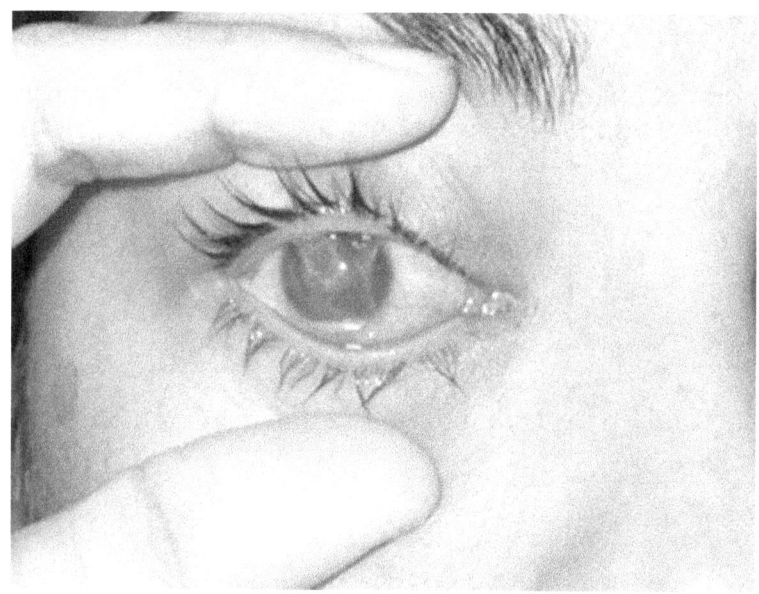

QUESTIONS

155. What is the likely diagnosis?
    a. Conjunctivitis
    b. Corneal Abrasion
    c. Endophthalmitis
    d. Herpes Zoster Ophthalmicus
    e. Purulent Retinitis

156. What clinical finding is shown in the image?
    a. Anterior Chamber Flare
    b. Hyphema
    c. Hypopyon
    d. Corneal Pseudomembranes

157. What is the likely cause of this condition?
    a. Adenovirus
    b. Candida Albicans
    c. Cytomegalovirus
    d. Escherichia Colli
    e. Staphylococcus Aureus

ANSWERS

155. c

156. c

157. e

VISUAL STIMULUS REVIEW

The image shows injected sclera and conjunctiva, purulent conjunctival discharge, hazy cornea, and layering of pus in the anterior chamber (Hypopyon).

REFERENCES

- Garg P. Fungal, Mycobacterial, and Nocardia infections and the eye: an update. Eye (Lond). 2012 Feb;26(2):245-51
- Packer M, Chang DF, Dewey SH et al. Prevention, diagnosis, and management of acute postoperative bacterial endophthalmitis. J Cataract Refract Surg. 2011 Sep;37(9):1699-714.

CASE #49: BARKING COUGH

CASE

An 18-month-old boy is brought to the emergency department for acute onset of hoarseness and barking cough. He has no past medical history but had a cold the previous couple of days with a runny nose and a sore throat. His vital signs are temp 100.9F (38.2), blood pressure 90/60 mmHg, respiration 26/min, heart rate 130/min, and O_2Sat 99% on room air. On exam he is awake and alert and is well-appearing with normal skin color. He is in mild respiratory distress, but he is not drooling. He has inspiratory stridor with clear breath sounds on both lungs without retractions, and his oropharynx appears mildly erythematous but without any exudates.

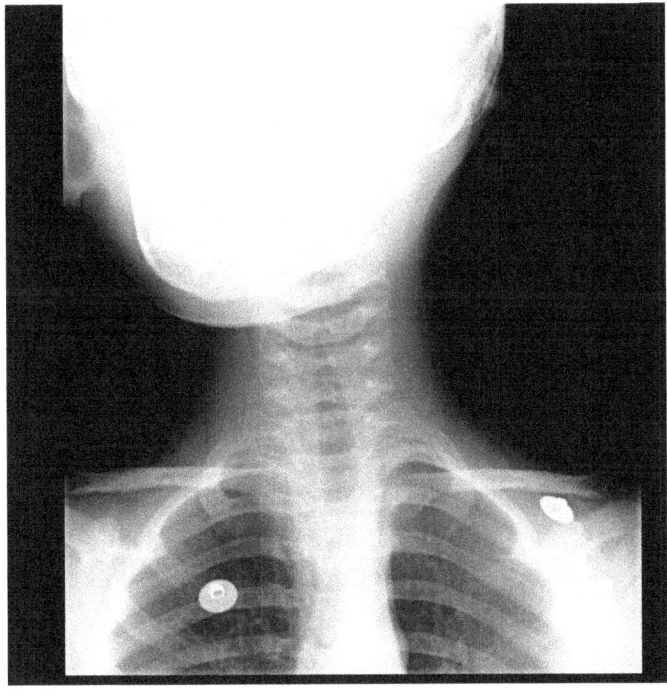

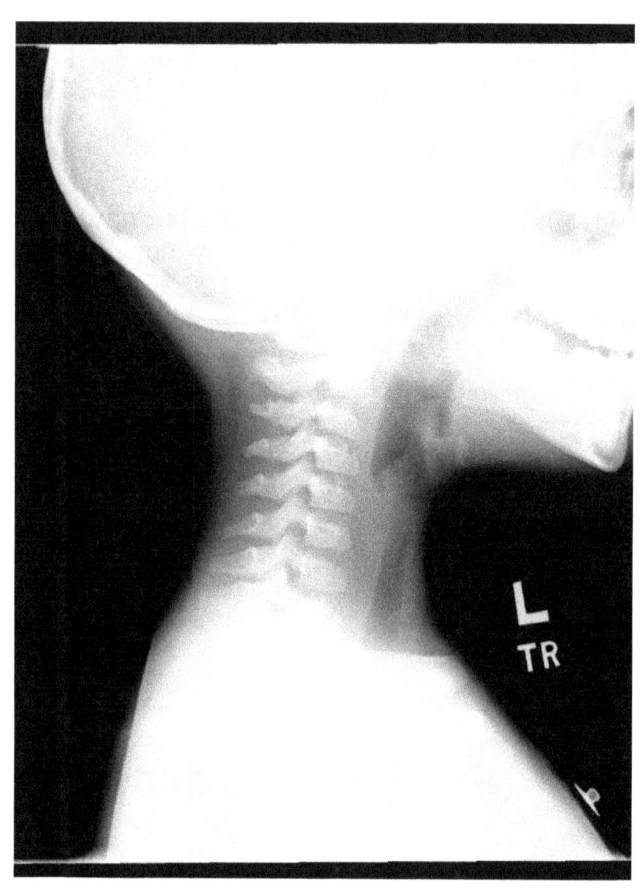

QUESTIONS

158. What is the likely diagnosis?

    a. Bronchiolitis
    b. Croup
    c. Diphtheria
    d. Epiglottitis
    e. Pneumonia

159. What sign is visible in the radiographs?

    a. Hypopharyngeal Narrowing
    b. Steeple Sign
    c. Subglottic Widening
    d. Thumbprint Print

160. What is the most common cause of this condition?

    a. Influenza Virus
    b. Metapneumovirus
    c. Parainfluenza Virus
    d. Respiratory Syncytial Virus
    e. Streptococcus Pneumonia

161. Corner stone treatment of this condition includes:

    a. Cool Mist
    b. Corticosteroids
    c. Heliox
    d. Hot Steam Humidifier
    e. Oral Antibiotics

ANSWERS

158. b

159. b

160. c

161. b

VISUAL STIMULUS REVIEW

The AP radiograph shows the steeple sign (subglottic narrowing) and the lateral radiograph shows ballooning of the hypopharynx. The epiglottis appears normal on the lateral radiograph.

REFERENCES

- Choi J, Lee GL. Common pediatric respiratory emergencies. Emerg Med Clin North Am. 2012 May;30(2):529-63, x.
- Zoorob R, Sidani M, Murray J. Croup: an overview. Am Fam Physician. 2011 May 1;83(9):1067-73.
- Russell KF, Liang Y, O'Gorman K, Johnson DW, Klassen TP. Glucocorticoids for croup. Cochrane Database Syst Rev. 2011 Jan 19;(1):CD001955.

CASE #50: DYSPNEA

CASE

A 72-year-old man is brought to the emergency department after he suffered smoke inhalation in his home. He is not sure what happened, but he was cooking dinner when his kitchen caught on fire. He immediately left the house but was still exposed to the smoke and fumes. He started to wheeze immediately and was unable to catch his breath using his Albuterol MDI. He has a past medical history of COPD and is using Albuterol, Atrovent inhalers as needed, and twice daily salmeterol/fluticasone Diskus Inhaler. He still smokes a pack of cigarettes a day. His vital signs are temp 99.3F (37.4C), blood pressure 160/80, respiratory rate 24/min and O_2Sat 83% on room air. He is wheezing bilaterally on lung exam.

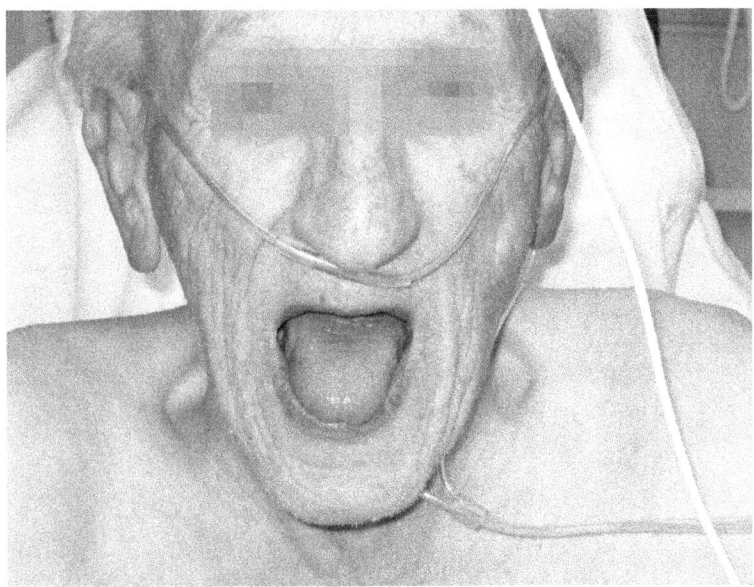

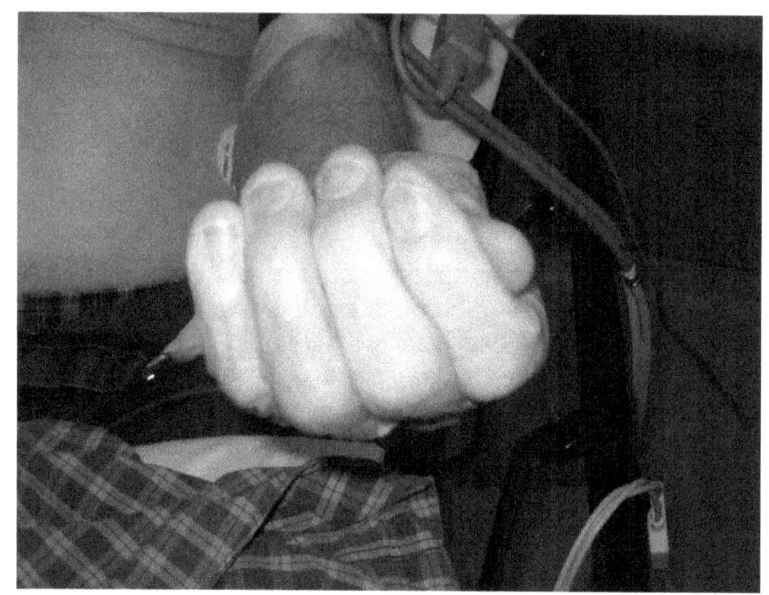

QUESTIONS

162. What is the likely diagnosis?

    a. Carbon Monoxide Poisoning

    b. Cyanide Poisoning

    c. Hypoxemia

    d. Methemoglobinemia

163. What is the likely Capillary Deoxygenated Hemoglobin concentration in this patient?

    a. < 1 g/dl

    b. 1 – 2 g/dl

    c. 2 – 3 g/dl

    d. 3 – 4 g/dl

    e. > 5 g/dl

164. Which of the following sentences is true?

   a. Anemic patients develop cyanosis at lower PaO2 levels than patients with normal hemoglobin concentrations.

   b. Cyanosis is a common feature of acute cyanide poisoning.

   c. Hyperbaric oxygen therapy is recommended in cases of idiopathic methemoglobinemia.

   d. Patients with methemoglobinemia are likely to have normal SaO2 and low PaO2.

ANSWERS

162. c

163. e

164. a

VISUAL STIMULUS REVIEW

The images demonstrate cyanosis of the lips and fingertips.

REFERENCES

- Mizutani T, Hojo M. Severe hypoxaemia due to methaemoglobinaemia and aspiration pneumonia. Emerg Med J. Jan 2012;29(1):74-6.

- Martin L, Khalil H. How much reduced hemoglobin is necessary to generate central cyanosis? Chest. Jan 1990;97(1):182-5.

- Baernstein A, Smith KM, Elmore JG. Singing the blues: is it really cyanosis? Respir Care. Aug 2008;53(8):1081-4.

CASE #51: WEAKNESS

CASE

A 67-year-old woman is brought to the emergency department by ambulance complaining of generalized weakness. Her husband reports that she was in her usual health when she complained of rapid palpitations before she lost consciousness for a couple of minutes. She is awake and alert and denies any chest pain or shortness of breath or any injuries. She does report generalized weakness but has no problem talking or swallowing. Her vital signs are temp 99.7F (37.6C), blood pressure 110/60, heart rate 100/min, respiratory rate 14/min, and O$_2$Sat 99% on room air. Her physical examination is unremarkable.

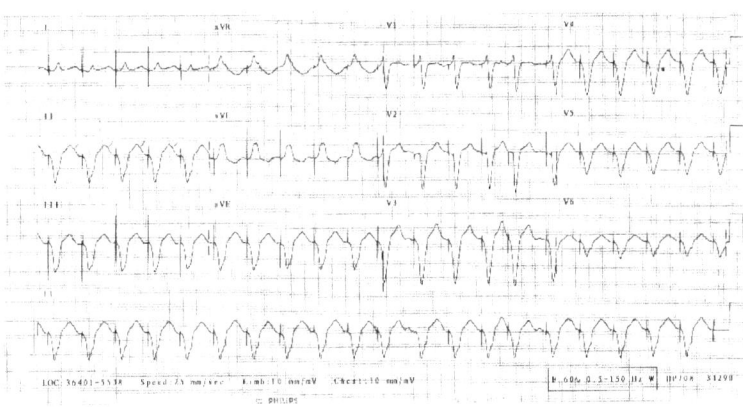

QUESTIONS

165. What is the likely diagnosis?
    a. Acute Myocardial Infarction
    b. Atrio-Ventricular Disassociation
    c. Ischemic Stroke
    d. Syncope
    e. Wolf Parkinson White Syndrome

166. What rhythm is shown on the EKG?
    a. Atrial Fibrillation
    b. Normal Sinus Rhythm
    c. Paced Rhythm
    d. Ventricular Fibrillation
    e. Ventricular Tachycardia

167. What is the likely cause of her loss of consciousness?
    a. Cardiac Arrhythmias
    b. Cardiac Ischemia
    c. Cerebral Ischemia
    d. Infection
    e. Vasovagal Response

ANSWERS

165. d

166. c

167. a

VISUAL STIMULUS REVIEW

The EKG shows paced rhythm.

REFERENCES

- Gauer RL. Evaluation of syncope. Am Fam Physician. 2011 Sep 15;84(6):640-50.
- Serrano LA, Hess EP, Bellolio MF et al. Accuracy and quality of clinical decision rules for syncope in the emergency department: a systematic review and meta-analysis. Ann Emerg Med. 2010 Oct;56(4):362-373.e1.

CASE #52: TOOTHACHE

CASE

A 37-year-old woman presents to her family doctor complaining of left upper toothache that has been progressively worsening over the past two weeks. She has no medical history and is not seeing a dentist on a regular basis. Her vital signs are all within normal limits; she has no trismus, and her pharyngeal exam is normal.

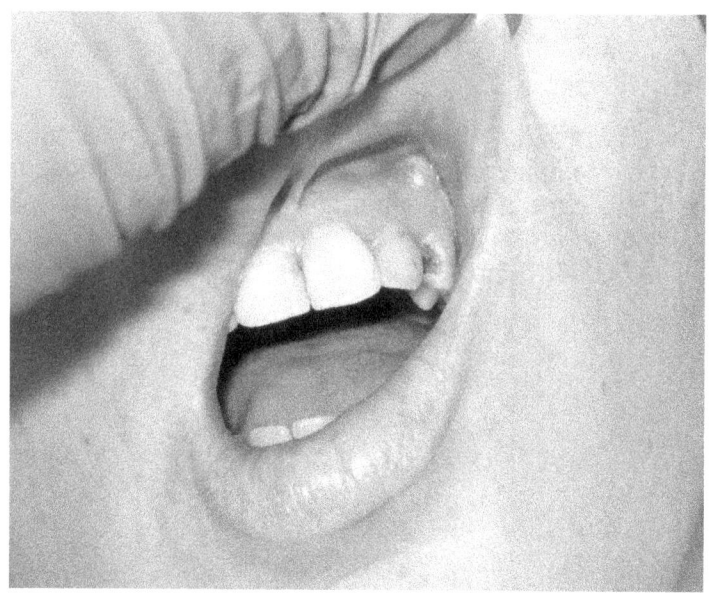

QUESTIONS

168. What is the likely diagnosis?
    a. Aphthous Ulcer
    b. Apical Abscess
    c. Buccal Cyst
    d. Necrotizing Gingivitis

169. What is the most common organism isolated from this condition?
    a. Actinomyces
    b. Fusobacterium
    c. Peptostreptococcus
    d. Prevotella Oralis

170. Which of the following is usually required for management of this condition?
    a. Antibiotic Therapy
    b. Incision and Drainage
    c. Tooth Extraction
    d. Topical Anesthetic Gel

ANSWERS

168. b

169. c

170. b

VISUAL STIMULUS REVIEW

The image shows an apical abscess to #11.

REFERENCES

- Zero DT, Zandona AF, Vail MM, Spolnik KJ. Dental caries and pulpal disease. Dent Clin North Am. 2011 Jan;55(1):29-46.

- Robertson D, Smith AJ. The microbiology of the acute dental abscess. J Med Microbiol. 2009 Feb;58(Pt 2):155-62.

CASE #53: ITCHY RASH

CASE

A four-year-old girl with history of asthma and eczema is brought to her pediatrician for a rash her parents noticed over her thighs and buttocks. She was in her normal health when she went to sleep in her underpants and a long-sleeved shirt and covered with a new blanket.

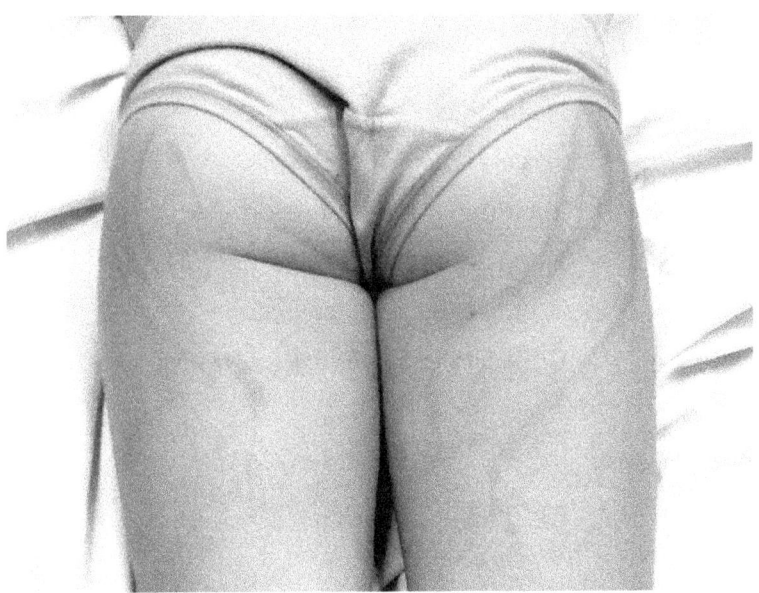

QUESTIONS

171. What is the likely diagnosis?
    a. Child Abuse
    b. Contact Dermatitis
    c. Dermographism
    d. Mastocytosis
    e. Myasis

172. What is the likely cause?
    a. External Antigen
    b. Histamine Mediated
    c. Hyperplastic Response
    d. Malignant Transformation
    e. Non-Accidental Trauma

173. Treatment of this condition includes?
    a. Child Protective Services Referral
    b. H1 Blocker
    c. Incision and Extraction
    d. Ivermectin
    e. Prednisone
    f. Psoralen plus UV-A

ANSWERS

171. c
172. b
173. b

VISUAL STIMULUS REVIEW

The image shows linear wheels.

REFERENCES

- Wallengren J, Isaksson A. Urticarial dermographism: clinical features and response to psychosocial stress. Acta Derm Venereol. 2007;87(6):493-8.
- Mahmood T. Physical urticarias. Am Fam Physician. 1994 May 1;49(6):1411-4.

CASE #54: RASH

CASE

A two-month-old baby girl is brought to her pediatrician for groin rash lasting two days. The mother reports that the patient had two episodes of watery diarrhea the day before but normally formed stool today.

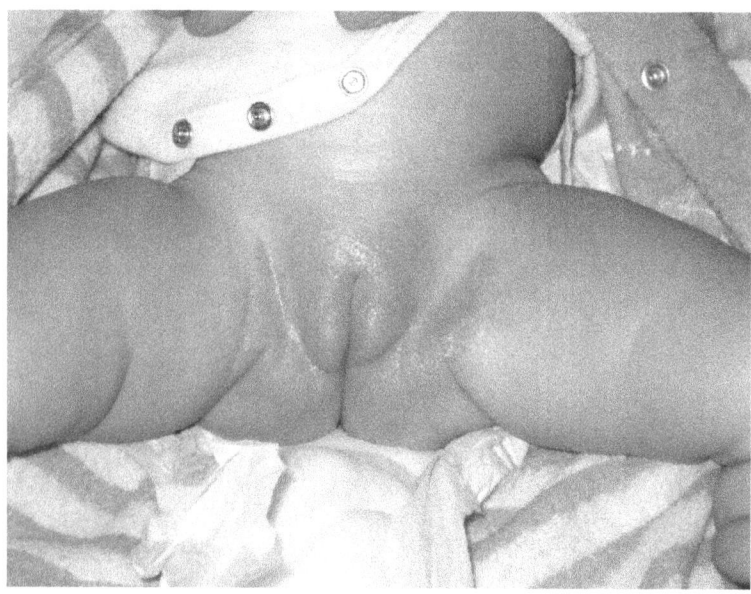

QUESTIONS

174. What is the likely diagnosis?
    a. Enterohepatic Acrodermatitis
    b. Atopic Dermatitis
    c. Diaper Rash
    d. Impetigo
    e. Scabies

175. What is the normal pH of the skin?
    a. 4.5 – 5.5
    b. 5.5 – 6.5
    c. 6.5 – 7.5
    d. 7.5 – 8.5

176. What is the most likely cause of this condition?
    a. Candida Albicans
    b. Escherichia Colli
    c. Fecal Proteases and Lipases
    d. Staphylococcus Aureus
    e. Urea

177. What is the first line treatment of this condition?
    a. Azole Cream
    b. Azole Ointment
    c. Hydrocortisone Cream
    d. White Petrolatum Ointment
    e. Zinc Oxide Ointment

ANSWERS

174. c

175. a

176. c

177. e

VISUAL STIMULUS REVIEW

The image demonstrates an erythematous scaly rash over the patient's perineum and labia as well as papules and vesicles. The eruption seems confluent.

REFERENCES

- Adam R. Skin care of the diaper area. Pediatr Dermatol. 2008 Jul-Aug;25(4):427-33.
- Scheinfeld N. Diaper dermatitis: a review and brief survey of eruptions of the diaper area. Am J Clin Dermatol. 2005;6(5):273-81.
- Wolf R, Wolf D, Tüzün B, Tüzün Y. Diaper dermatitis. Clin Dermatol. 2000 Nov-Dec;18(6):657-60.

CASE #55: LLQ PAIN

CASE

A 65-year-old woman presents to the emergency department complaining of left-lower-quadrant pain, bloating, and nausea for three days. She has a past medical history of hypertension and hyperlipidemia. Her temperature is 102.F (38.9C), heart rate of 103/min, respirations 16/min, blood pressure of 140/80 mmHg, and O_2Sat of 99% on room air. On physical examination, she has severe left-lower-quadrant tenderness with guarding. A CT scan is ordered.

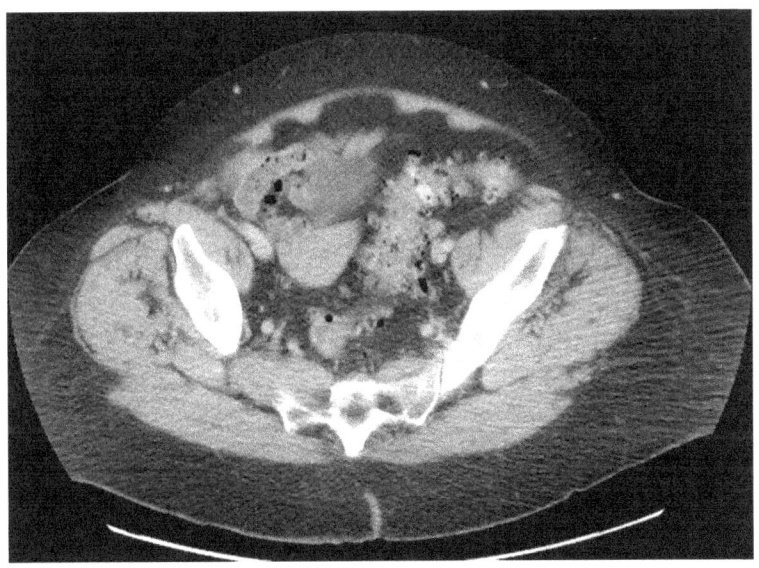

QUESTIONS

178. What is the likely diagnosis?
    a. Colon Cancer
    b. Diverticulitis
    c. Mesenteric Ischemia
    d. Pancreatitis
    e. Perforated Duodenal Ulcer
    f. Pyelonephritis

179. Which of the following diagnostic procedures should be performed at the time of presentation to the ED or shortly thereafter?
    a. Barium Enema
    b. Colonoscopy
    c. Flexible Sigmoidoscopy
    d. Laparoscopy
    e. Mesenteric Angiogram
    f. None of the Above

180. Early management of this condition includes:
    a. Azithromycin
    b. High Fiber Diet
    c. High Osmolarity Enema
    d. Ciprofloxacin and Metronidazole
    e. Left Hemicolectomy

ANSWERS

178. b
179. f
180. d

VISUAL STIMULUS REVIEW

The CT image shows diverticula and pericolonic fat stranding of the sigmoid colon as well as some extraluminal air bubbles.

REFERENCES

- Weizman AV, Nguyen GC. Diverticular disease: epidemiology and management. Can J Gastroenterol. 2011 Jul;25(7):385-9.

- Hammond NA, Nikolaidis P, Miller FH. Left lower-quadrant pain: guidelines from the American College of Radiology appropriateness criteria. Am Fam Physician. 2010 Oct 1;82(7):766-70.

- Hemming J, Floch M. Features and management of colonic diverticular disease. Curr Gastroenterol Rep. 2010 Oct;12(5):399-407.

CASE #56: SHORTNESS OF BREATH

CASE

An 18-year-old man was found underwater in a chlorinated water pool during a paternity party. His friends pulled him out of the water, performed immediate CPR, and by the time the EMS crew arrived he was already breathing on his own. His vitals are temperature 95.7F (35.3C), respiratory rate of 30/min, heart rate 110/min, BP 150/80, and O_2Sat 92% on room air. He is awake and alert and complains of shortness of breath. He reports consuming alcohol before falling into the pool. A chest X-ray is obtained.

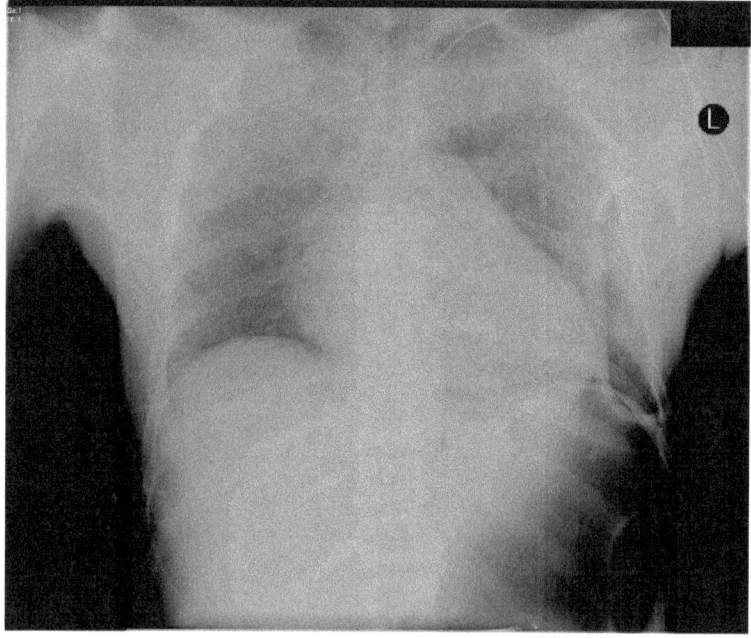

QUESTIONS

181. What is the likely diagnosis?
    a. Acute Respiratory Distress Syndrome
    b. Pneumonia
    c. Pneumonitis
    d. Pulmonary Edema
    e. Pulmonary Hypertension

182. What is the most common cause of electrolyte abnormalities following immersion injuries?
    a. Hypoxemia Related Acidosis
    b. Neurogenic SIADH
    c. Water Aspiration
    d. Water Ingestion

183. Which of the following is part of the mammalian diving reflex?
    a. Hyperventilation
    b. Laryngospasm
    c. Shivering
    d. Tachycardia
    e. Vasoconstriction

ANSWERS

181. d

182. d

183. e

VISUAL STIMULUS REVIEW

The chest radiograph shows bilateral patchy infiltrates.

REFERENCES

- Deakin CD. Drowning: more hope for patients, less hope for guidelines. Resuscitation. 2012 Sep;83(9):1051-2.

- Szpilman D, Bierens JJ, Handley AJ, Orlowski JP. Drowning. N Engl J Med. 2012 May 31;366(22):2102-10.

CASE #57: LEG PAIN

CASE

A 53-year-old man presents to the emergency department complaining of painful swelling to his left leg. He has a medical history of lymphoma for which he is being treated with chemotherapy. He is afebrile, and his vital signs are within normal limits. His left leg is warm to the touch and swollen from the mid-thigh and distally. He has good symmetric femoral, popliteal, dorsalis pedis, and tibialis posterior pulses. An ultrasound is ordered.

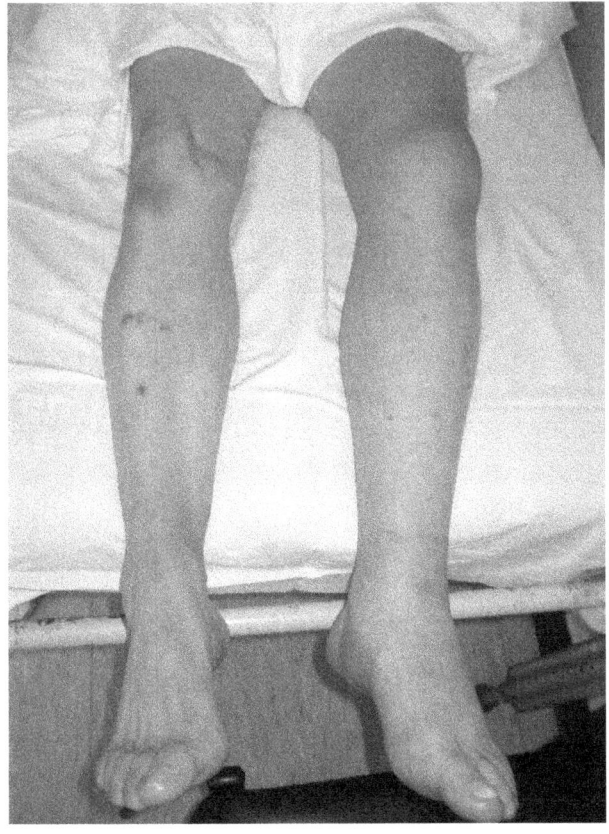

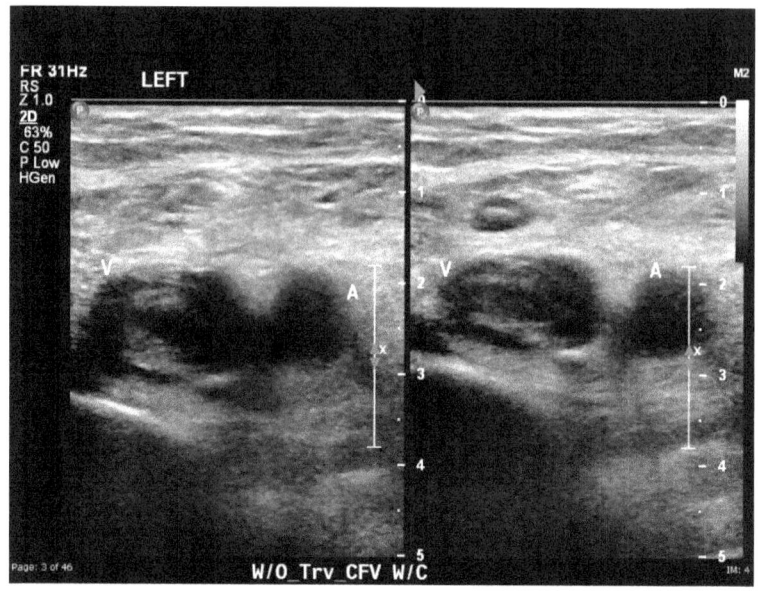

QUESTIONS

184. What is the likely diagnosis?
    a. Arterial Thrombosis
    b. Cellulitis
    c. Deep Venous Thrombosis
    d. Necrotizing Fasciitis
    e. Pyomyositis

185. Which of the following is a first line therapy for this condition?
    a. Aspirin PO
    b. Catheter Guided Aspiration
    c. Catheter Guided Thrombolysis
    d. Heparin
    e. Incision and Drainage
    f. Vancomycin IV

186. Which of the following is the most common abnormality found in patients with this condition?
    a. Factor C Deficiency
    b. Factor S Deficiency
    c. Factor V Leiden Mutation
    d. Hemophilia A
    e. Von Willebrand Disease

ANSWERS

184. c

185. d

186. c

VISUAL STIMULUS REVIEW

The gross image shows a swollen and erythematous left lower leg.

The ultrasound image demonstrates an uncompressible left common femoral vein suggesting the presence of a thrombus in that vein.

REFERENCES

- Ho WK. Deep vein thrombosis--risks and diagnosis. Aust Fam Physician. 2010 Jul;39(7):468-74.
- Somarouthu B, Abbara S, Kalva SP. Diagnosing deep vein thrombosis. Postgrad Med. 2010 Mar;122(2):66-73.

CASE #58: SEIZURES AND VISION LOSS

CASE

A nine-year-old girl who lives in a small rural village in Argentina presents to a neurologist's office for evaluation of seizures. The patient is developmentally delayed with severe mental retardation and known seizure disorder since early childhood, which is partially controlled on Phenytoin. The parents reports that over the past three months they noticed loss of vision, decrease in appetite, and increase in the frequency of her generalized seizures up to eight seizures a day. The patient is afebrile with normal vital signs. On exam she is found to have a dilated and nonreactive left pupil. A CT of her head is obtained.

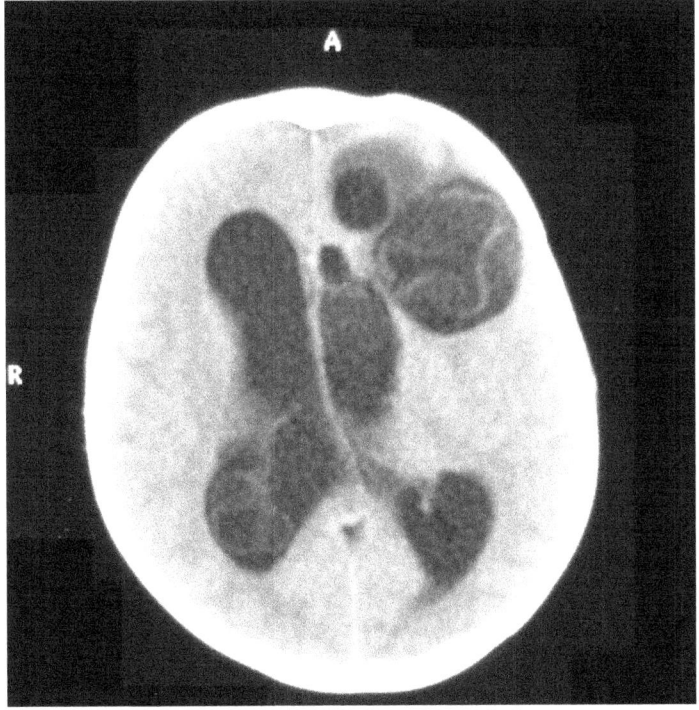

QUESTIONS

187. What is the likely diagnosis?
    a. Brain Abscess
    b. Cysticercosis
    c. Echinococcal Cysts
    d. Lymphoma
    e. Metastatic Cancer to Brain

188. Which of the following signs is pathognomonic for this condition?
    a. Crescent Sign
    b. Outer Rim Enhancement Sign
    c. Water Lily Sign
    d. Zipper Amygdala Sign

189. What is the treatment of choice of this condition?
    a. Albendazole
    b. Amphotericin
    c. Dexamethasone
    d. Surgical Drainage
    e. Vancomycin

ANSWERS

187. c

188. c

189. a

VISUAL STIMULUS REVIEW

The CT scan shows three cysts with the largest one demonstrating the pathognomonic internal split wall (floating membrane or water lily sign).

REFERENCES

- Brunetti E, Kern P, Vuitton DA,. Expert consensus for the diagnosis and treatment of cystic and alveolar echinococcosis in humans. Acta Trop. Apr 2010;114(1):1-16.

- Brunetti E, Junghanss T. Update on cystic hydatid disease. Curr Opin Infect Dis. Oct 2009;22(5):497-502.

CASE #59: UNRESPONSIVENESS

CASE

A 23-year-old man suffered a baseball bat injury to his head. His temperature is 97.8F (36.5C), heart rate 42/min, blood pressure 190/80 mmHg, respirations of 6/min, and O₂Sat 99% on room air. He opens his eyes to painful stimulation, mumbles incomprehensible words, and is able to localize to pain with his right arm.

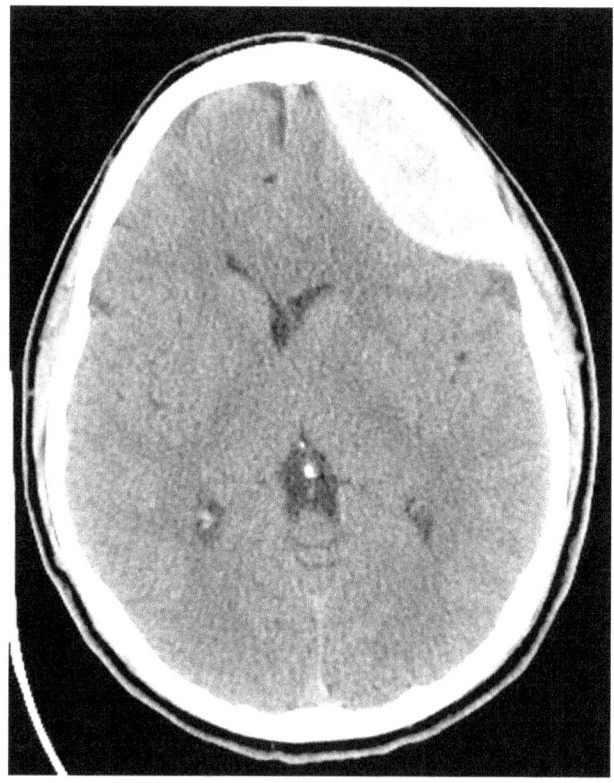

QUESTIONS

190. What is the likely diagnosis?
    a. Epidural Hemorrhage
    b. Subarachnoid Hemorrhage
    c. Subdural Hemorrhage
    d. Traumatic Hygroma

191. What other condition is present?
    a. Beck's Triad
    b. Behçet's Triad
    c. Charcot's Triad
    d. Cushing's Triad
    e. Virchow's Triad

192. What is the most common cause of this condition?
    a. Arachnoid Capillaries Bleed
    b. Arterial Bleed
    c. Venous Bleed
    d. Venous Sinus Bleed

ANSWERS

190. a

191. d

192. b

VISUAL STIMULUS REVIEW

The CT image shows an extra-axial, smoothly marginated, lenticular, or biconvex homogenous hyperdensity.

REFERENCES

- Kubal WS. Updated imaging of traumatic brain injury. Radiol Clin North Am. 2012 Jan;50(1):15-41.
- Rosenfeld JV, Maas AI, Bragge P et al. Early management of severe traumatic brain injury. Lancet. 2012 Sep 22;380(9847):1088-98.

CASE #60: ELBOW PAIN

CASE

A 43-year-old man presents to his family doctor's office complaining of left elbow pain following a fall during a basketball game. He has no medical history and is taking no medications. On exam the patient's skin is intact; he has normal left wrist and hand neuro, muscular, and vascular exam. He has tenderness to his left elbow, mostly laterally with limited supination and pronation.

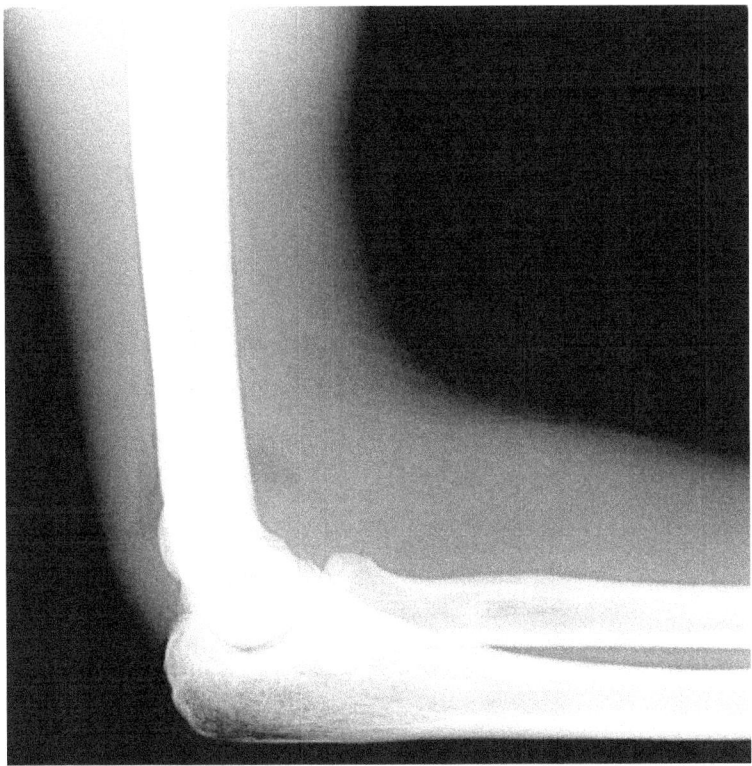

QUESTIONS

193. What is the likely diagnosis?

    a. Elbow Dislocation

    b. Medial Condyle Fracture

    c. Olecranon Avulsion Fracture

    d. Radial Head Fracture

    e. Radial Neck Fracture

194. What is the most common etiology for this condition?

    a. Direct Blow to the Lateral Condyle

    b. Direct Blow to the Olecranon

    c. Fall on an Outstretched Arm

    d. Osteoporosis Leading to a Pathological Fracture

195. Management recommendations for this patient should include:

    a. Analgesia and Early Mobilization

    b. Analgesia and Casting for Four Weeks

    c. Closed Reduction

    d. Open Reduction and Internal Fixation

    e. Internal Fixation

ANSWERS

193. c

194. c

195. a

VISUAL STIMULUS REVIEW

This lateral elbow X-ray image shows a posterior fat pad (should be absent in normal films) and an anteriorly displaced anterior fat pat.

REFERENCES

- Edwards SG, Weber JP, Baecher NB. Proximal forearm fractures. Orthop Clin North Am. 2013 Jan;44(1):67-80.
- Black WS, Becker JA. Common forearm fractures in adults. Am Fam Physician. 2009 Nov 15;80(10):1096-102.

CASE #61: ABDOMINAL PAIN

CASE

An 89-year-old woman presents to the emergency department complaining of abdominal pain, nausea, and vomiting for 48 hours. She has a history of hypertension, diabetes mellitus type 2, coronary artery disease, and atrial fibrillation. Her vital signs are temperature of 96.8F (36.0C), blood pressure of 100/67 mmHg, pulse of 100/min, respirations of 18/min, and an O_2Sat of 96%. The abdominal exam reveals a distended abdomen that is tender to palpation mostly on the right upper and lower quadrants with guarding but without rebound tenderness. The rest of the physical exam is unremarkable. Please examine the following CT image.

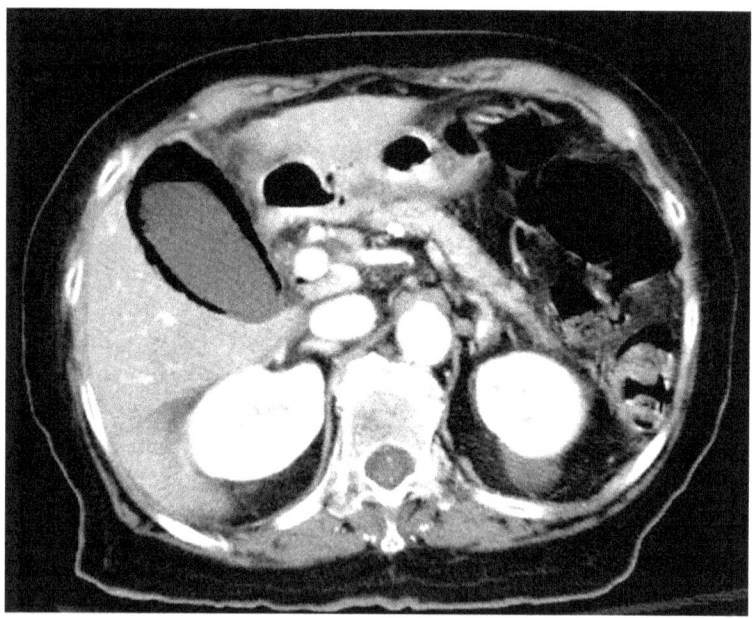

QUESTIONS

196. What is the likely diagnosis?
    a. Diverticulitis
    b. Emphysematous Cholecystitis
    c. Mesenteric Ischemia
    d. Perforated Duodenal Ulcer
    e. Sigmoid Volvulus

197. Which of the following is a common risk factor for this condition?
    a. Alcoholism
    b. Atrial Fibrillation
    c. Constipation
    d. Diabetes Mellitus
    e. Fiber Rich Diet

198. What is the first line treatment for this condition?
    a. Air Enema
    b. Angiography
    c. Cholecystectomy
    d. Colonoscopy
    e. Intravenous Antibiotics
    f. Omental Patching

ANSWERS

196. b

197. d

198. c

VISUAL STIMULUS REVIEW

Abdominal CT image shows an air-fluid level in a distended gallbladder with no visible gallstones but with gallbladder wall emphysema.

REFERENCES

- Wu JM, Lee CY, Wu YM. Emphysematous cholecystitis. Am J Surg 2010;200:e53–4.
- Chiu HH, Chen CM, Mo LR. Emphysematous cholecystitis. Am J Surg 2004;188:325–6.
- Jolly BT, Love JN. Emphysematous cholecystitis in an elderly woman: case report and review of the literature. J Emerg Med. 1993 Sep-Oct;11(5):593-7.

CASE #62: SORE THROAT

CASE

A 63-year-old man presents to the emergency department complaining of sore throat, odynophagia, and hoarseness for three days. His vital signs are temperature of 102.5F (39.2C), blood pressure of 150/90, heart rate of 108/min, respiratory rate of 20/min, and O_2Sat of 98%. Physical examination reveals minimal pharyngeal erythema and no stridor or drooling. His lung exam is normal. A lateral neck X-ray is obtained.

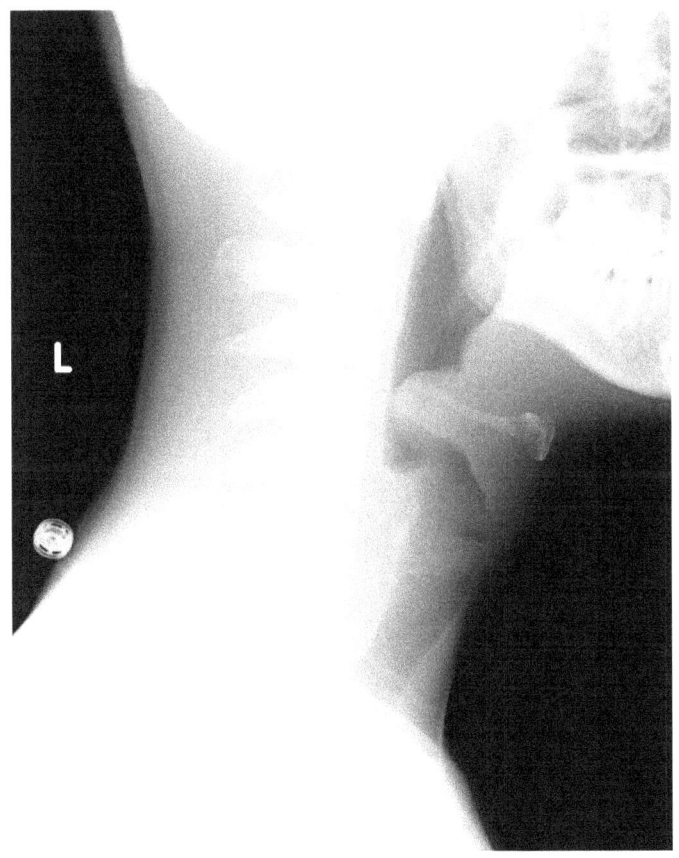

QUESTIONS

199. What is the likely diagnosis?

   a. Bronchiolitis

   b. Croup

   c. Epiglottitis

   d. Laryngitis

   e. Retropharyngeal Abscess

200. What is the most common organism causing this condition?

   a. Hemophilus Influenza B

   b. Influenza A

   c. Parainfluenza

   d. Staphylococcus Aureus

   e. Streptococus Spc

201. Which of the following is contraindicated in this patient?

   a. Clindamycin IV

   b. Dexamethasone IV

   c. Emergent Tracheostomy

   d. Oropharyngeal Examination Using a Tongue Depressor

   e. Orotracheal Intubation

   f. Racemic Epinephrine Neb.

ANSWERS

199. c

200. e

201. d

VISUAL STIMULUS REVIEW

The X-ray image demonstrates an enlarged and swollen epiglottis (thumb sign).

REFERENCES

- Derber CJ, Troy SB. Head and neck emergencies: bacterial meningitis, encephalitis, brain abscess, upper airway obstruction, and jugular septic thrombophlebitis. Med Clin North Am. 2012 Nov;96(6):1107-26.

- Isakson M, Hugosson S. Acute epiglottitis: epidemiology and Streptococcus pneumoniae serotype distribution in adults. J Laryngol Otol. 2011 Apr;125(4):390-3.

CASE #63: RASH

CASE

A three-year-old boy is brought to his pediatrician's office for a progressive rash that started on his arms and legs two days ago. The patient had a recent cough and fever about a week go that resolved. He is well-appearing and active and has no problem tolerating food. He doesn't itch, and his vital signs are normal. His hands and feet appear somewhat swollen and are mildly tender. He has no mucosal lesions.

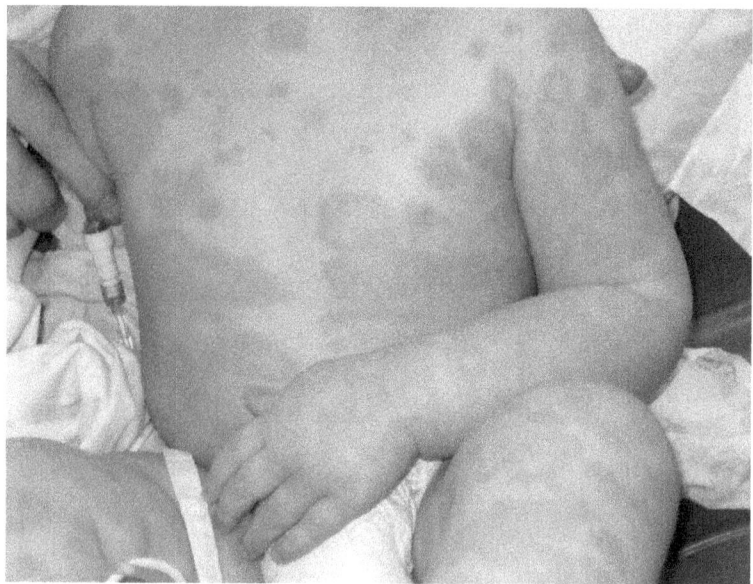

QUESTIONS

202. What is the likely diagnosis?
    a. Atopic Dermatitis
    b. Erythema Multiforme
    c. Steven Johnson's Syndrome
    d. Urticaria

203. Which of the following is a known cause of this condition?
    a. Dust Mite Droppings
    b. Herpes Zoster Virus
    c. Mycoplasma Pneumonia infection
    d. Peanuts
    e. Poison Ivy Exposure

204. The recommended first line treatment for this child includes?
    a. Acyclovir
    b. Azithromycin
    c. Dexamethasone
    d. Prednisone
    e. Symptomatic Care

ANSWERS

202. b

203. c

204. e

VISUAL STIMULUS REVIEW

The image shows macules, patches, and target lesions, which are the characteristic cutaneous finding seen in this disorder.

REFERENCES

- Sokumbi O, Wetter DA. Clinical features, diagnosis, and treatment of erythema multiforme: a review for the practicing dermatologist. Int J Dermatol. 2012 Aug;51(8):889-902.

- Hosaka H, Ohtoshi S, Nakada T, Iijima M. Erythema multiforme, Stevens-Johnson syndrome and toxic epidermal necrolysis: frozen-section diagnosis. J Dermatol. 2010 May;37(5):407-12.

CASE #64: ALTERED MENTAL STATUS

CASE

A 53-year-old man who is a known alcoholic is brought to the emergency department by EMS after he was found to be unresponsive. He is lethargic but opens his eyes to painful stimuli; he is not making any sounds and will localize to pain. His vitals are temp of 99.8F (37.7C), BP 85/50 mmHg, hear rate 120/min, respiratory rate 32/min, and O_2Sat 94% on room air. His pupils are 4 mm and reactive to light bilaterally. The paramedic reports that the patient had an empty (unlabeled) bottle next to him. After initial stabilization, a Foley catheter is inserted, and a urine sample (with saline control) is exposed to ultraviolet light.

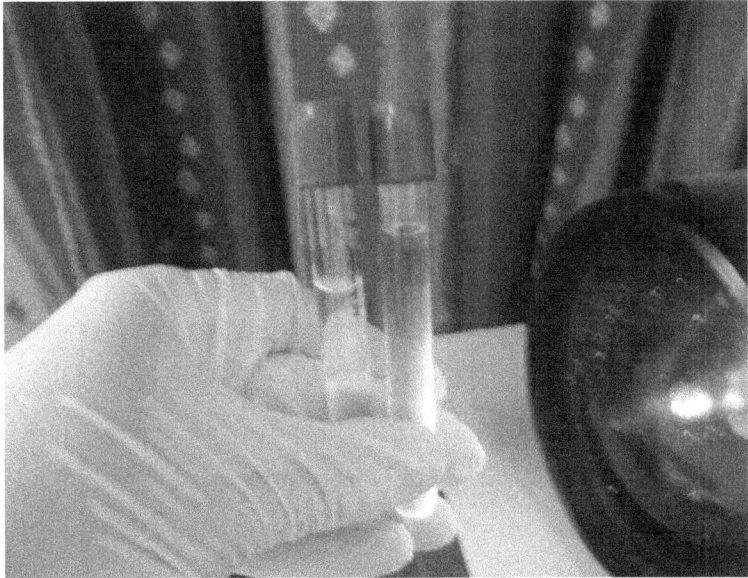

QUESTIONS

205. What is the likely diagnosis?

   a. Ethyl Alcohol Poisoning

   b. Ethylene Glycol Poisoning

   c. Isopropyl Alcohol Poisoning

   d. Methanol Poisoning

206. What is the metabolite responsible for the toxidrome described in the above clinical vignette?

   a. Acetaldehyde

   b. Acetone

   c. Formaldehyde

   d. Glyoxylic Acid

207. Which of the following laboratory finding will support the diagnosis?

   a. Hyperglycemia

   b. Hypernatremia

   c. Hypocalcemia

   d. Hypokalemia

   e. Hyponatremia

208. Definitive treatment of this condition includes:

   a. Alcohol Dehydrogenase Inhibition

   b. Alcohol Dehydrogenase Stimulation

   c. Aldehyde Dehydrogenase Inhibition

   d. Aldehyde Dehydrogenase Stimulation

ANSWERS

205. b

206. d

207. c

208. a

VISUAL STIMULUS REVIEW

The visual stimulus demonstrates positive fluorescence of the patient's urine as compared with normal saline placed in the same glass tube.

REFERENCES

- Jammalamadaka D, Raissi S. Ethylene glycol, methanol and isopropyl alcohol intoxication. Am J Med Sci. Mar 2010;339(3):276-81.
- Brent J. Fomepizole for ethylene glycol and methanol poisoning. N Engl J Med. 2009 May 21;360(21):2216-23.

CASE #65: RESPIRATORY DISTRESS

CASE

A 60-year-old woman presents to the emergency department for severe respiratory distress. She is immediately intubated for airway protection and ventilatory support. A post-intubation chest X-ray is obtained.

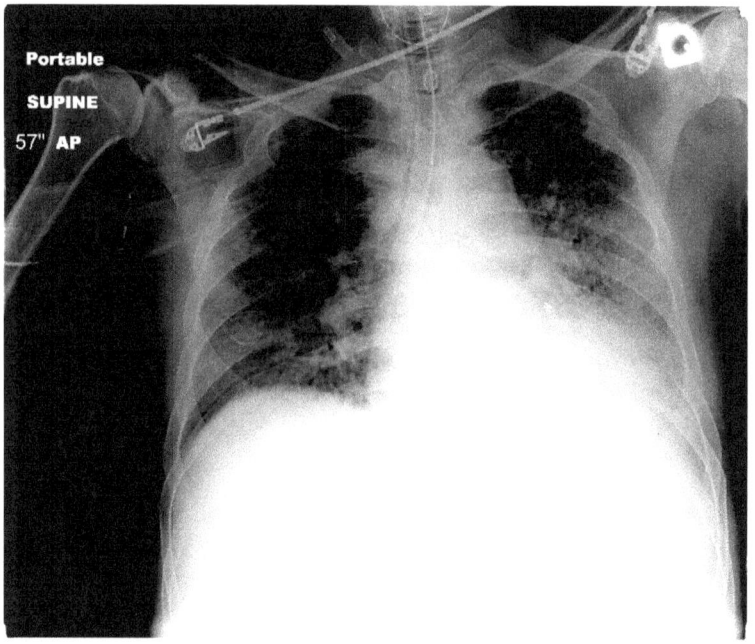

QUESTIONS

209. What is the likely diagnosis?
- a. Adequate ETT Positioning
- b. Esophageal Intubation
- c. Post Intubation Pulmonary Edema
- d. Right Mainstem Intubation

210. The treatment of this condition includes:
- a. Emergent Bronchoscopy
- b. Increasing the PEEP Setting
- c. Re-intubation
- d. Withdrawal of the ETT by 4 cm.

ANSWERS

209. d

210. d

VISUAL STIMULUS REVIEW

The chest radiogram shows an endotracheal tube that passes through the trachea but ends in the right mainstem bronchus.

REFERENCES

- Pesola GR, Filangeri J. Mechanisms for preferential right or left mainstem bronchus intubation. Am J Emerg Med. 1995 May;13(3):380.

CASE #66: NECK SWELLING

CASE

A 28-year-old male presents to his family physician complaining of painless swelling to his neck that developed over the last three months. He also reports occasionally spitting out small granules. The patient is afebrile and has normal vital signs. His physical exam shows poor dentition and woody hard nodular swelling to his left angle of his mandible. The patient has no trismus; his voice is unchanged, and he has no trouble swallowing. A CT scan is ordered.

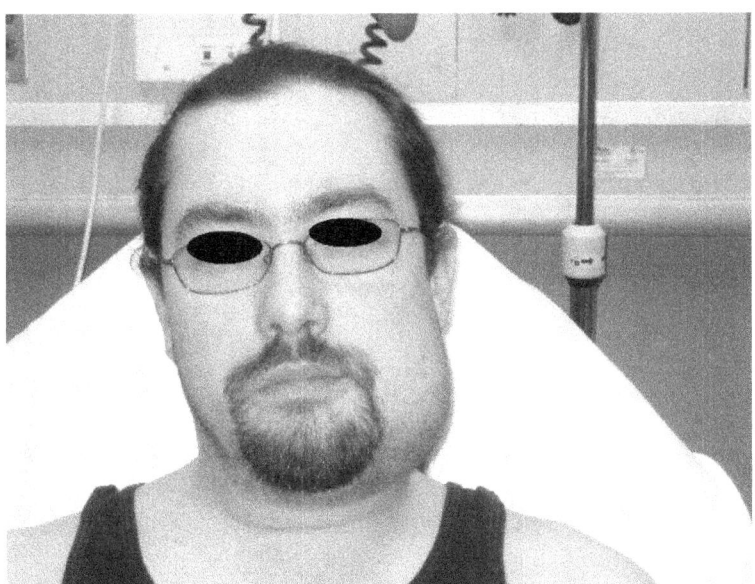

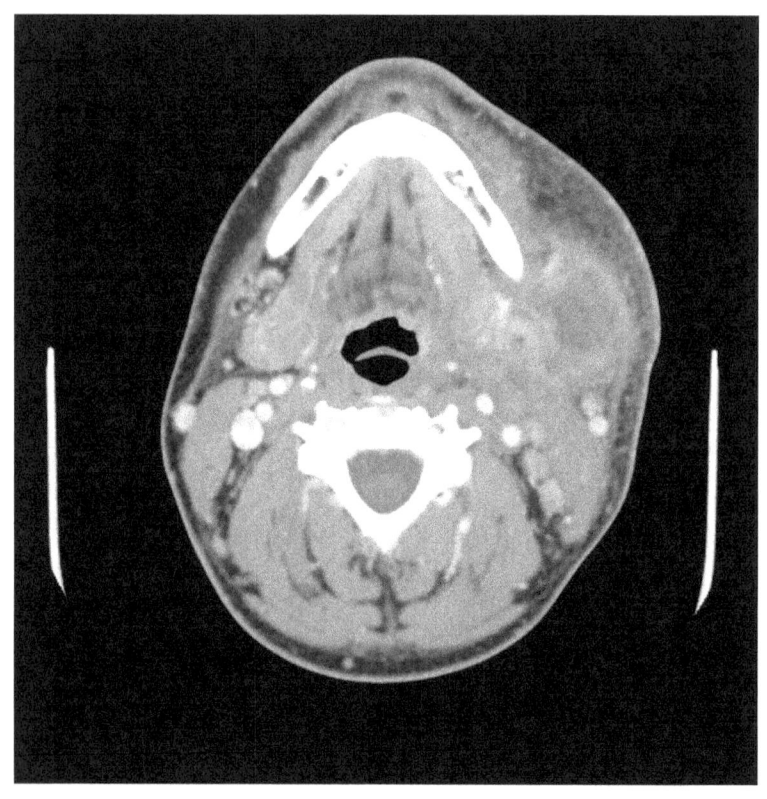

QUESTIONS

211. What is the likely diagnosis?

    a. Actinomycosis

    b. Blastomycosis

    c. Nocardiosis

    d. Staphylococcosis

    e. Tuberculosis

212. What is the usual color of the granules mentioned by the patients?

    a. Blue

    b. Green

    c. Red

    d. White

    e. Yellow

213. What is the treatment of choice of this condition?

    a. Incision and Drainage

    b. Isoniazid

    c. Metronidazole

    d. Penicillin G

    e. Trimethoprim/Sulfamethoxazole

ANSWERS

211. a

212. e

213. d

VISUAL STIMULUS REVIEW

The clinical image demonstrates a "lumpy" jaw and the CT image shows left submandibular areas of low attenuation (abscesses).

REFERENCES

- Wong VK, Turmezei TD, Weston VC. Actinomycosis. BMJ. 2011 Oct 11;343:d6099.
- Sharkawy AA. Cervicofacial actinomycosis and mandibular osteomyelitis. Infect Dis Clin North Am. 2007 Jun;21(2):543-56, viii

CASE #67: FACIAL WEAKNESS

CASE

A 70-year-old female with known history of hypertension and noninsulin dependent diabetes presents to the emergency department complaining of difficulty closing her left eye since she woke up this morning. Her vital signs are remarkable for blood pressure of 190/85 mmHg. She denies headaches, vision changes, unsteady gait, or any difficulty speaking.

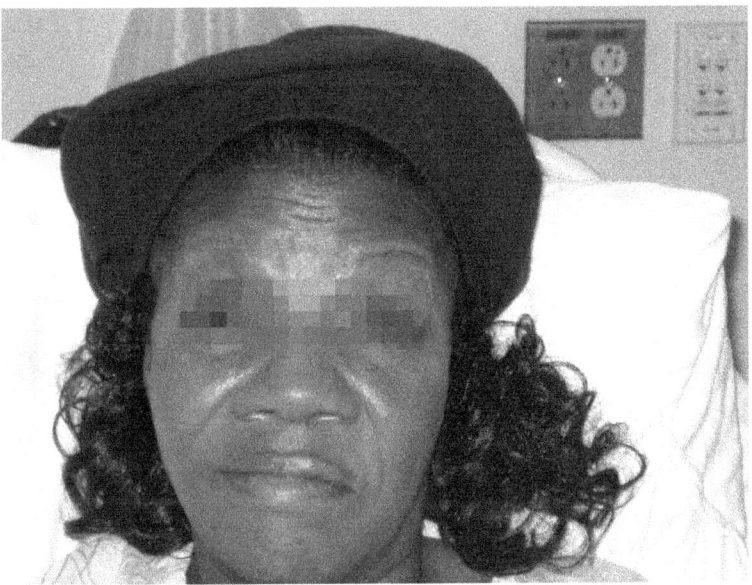

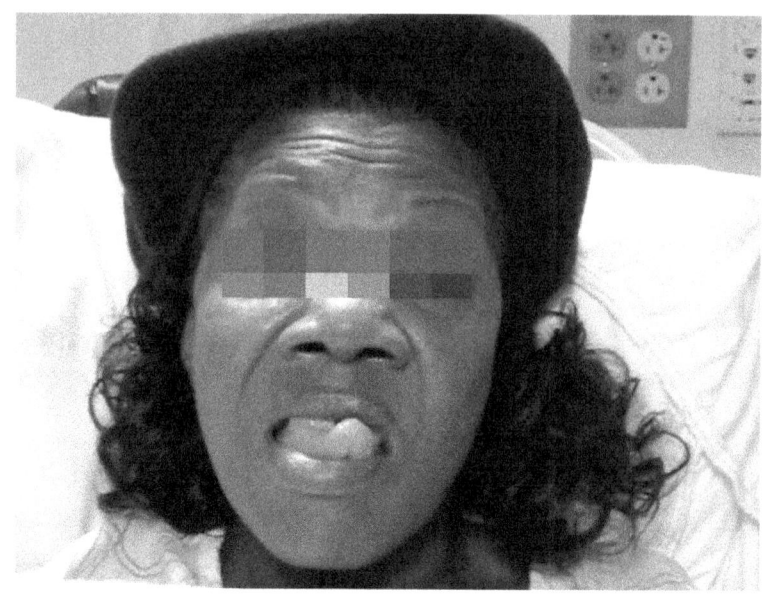

QUESTIONS

214. What is the likely diagnosis?
    a. Bell's Palsy
    b. Central CN VII Palsy
    c. Peripheral CN VII Palsy
    d. Trigeminal Neuralgia

215. What other finding is shown in the above pictures?
    a. CN II Palsy
    b. CN III Palsy
    c. CN IV Palsy
    d. CN VIII Palsy
    e. CN XII Palsy

216. What is the likely cause of this condition?
    a. Acute Varicella Virus Infection
    b. Hypoglycemia
    c. Ischemic Stroke
    d. Reactivation of Herpes 1 Virus
    e. Reactivation of Varicella Virus

ANSWERS

214. b

215. e

216. c

VISUAL STIMULUS REVIEW

The first image shows central CN VII Palsy (left facial droop with preservation of forehead motor innervation). The second image demonstrates CN XII Palsy (tongue deviated to the left).

REFERENCES

- Jauch EC, Saver JL, Adams HP Jr, Bruno A, Connors JJ, Demaerschalk BM, et al. Guidelines for the Early Management of Patients With Acute Ischemic Stroke: A Guideline for Healthcare Professionals From the American Heart Association/American Stroke Association. Stroke. 2013 Mar;44(3):870-947.

- Kasner SE, Grotta JC. Emergency identification and treatment of acute ischemic stroke. Ann Emerg Med. Nov 1997;30(5):642-53.

CASE #68: COUGH

CASE

An 18-month-old girl is brought by her parents to the emergency department for evaluation of cough. They report that the patient went to sleep in her crib in normal health and that two hours later they woke up as she had a severe coughing and wheezing spell. The patient has normal vital signs, her lungs and oropharyngeal exams are normal; she is not drooling and appears to be in no distress. A chest X-ray is obtained.

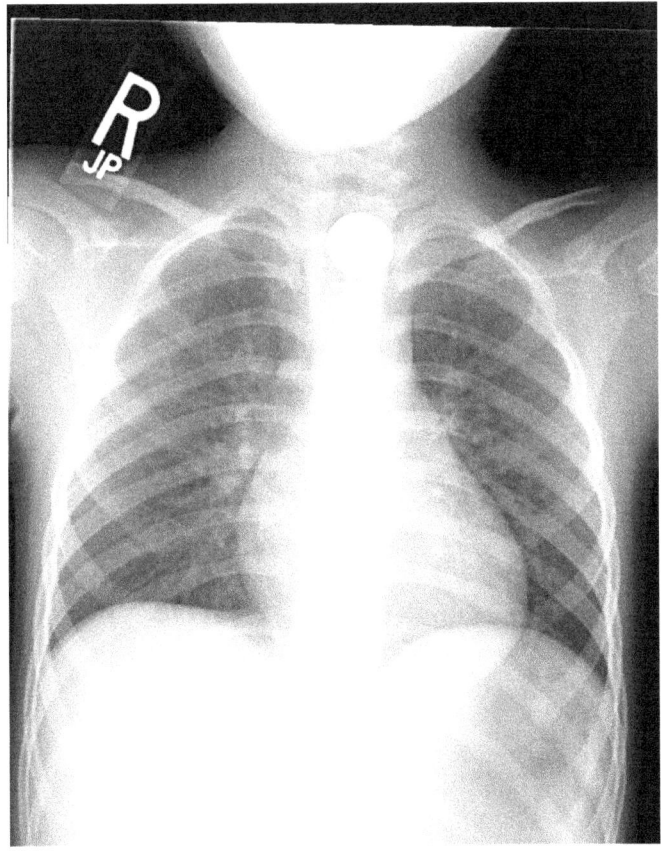

QUESTIONS

217. What is the likely diagnosis?
    a. Esophageal Foreign Body
    b. Laryngeal Foreign Body
    c. Nasopharyngeal Foreign Body
    d. Oropharyngeal Foreign Body

218. Which of the following foreign bodies is likely to cause rapid esophageal necrosis if not removed promptly?
    a. Aluminum Coins
    b. Button Batteries
    c. Copper Coins
    d. Nickel Coins

219. Which of the following modalities is most sensitive in detecting nonradiopaque ingested foreign bodies?
    a. Barium Swallow
    b. CT Scanning
    c. Gastrografin Swallow
    d. Handheld Metal Detector
    e. Ultrasound

ANSWERS

217. a
218. b
219. b

VISUAL STIMULUS REVIEW

The radiogram shows a rounded radiopaque object in a coronal plane at the level of the proximal esophagus.

REFERENCES

- Triadafilopoulos G, Roorda A, Akiyama J. Update on foreign bodies in the esophagus: diagnosis and management. Curr Gastroenterol Rep. 2013 Apr;15(4):317.
- Waltzman ML. Management of esophageal coins. Curr Opin Pediatr. 2006 Oct;18(5):571-4.

CASE #69: FINGER PAIN

CASE

A 32-year-old male patient with no past medical history presents to his doctor's office complaining of throbbing pain to his left index finger. He reports progressive swelling to his fingertip. He denies any history of trauma or splinters.

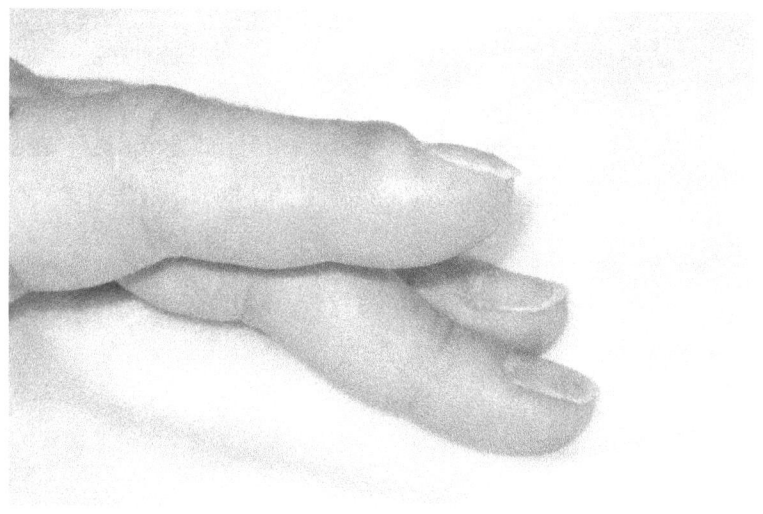

QUESTIONS

220. What is the likely diagnosis?
    a. Felon
    b. Fingertip Hematoma
    c. Paronychia
    d. Herpetic Whitlow
    e. Raynaud's Syndrome

221. What is the anatomical structure of the fingertip pulp?
    a. The pulp is divided into numerous small compartments by horizontal septa.
    b. The pulp is divided into numerous small compartments by vertical septa.
    c. The pulp is divided into three compartments by horizontal septa.
    d. The pulp is divided into three compartments by vertical septa.

222. What is the most common cause of this condition?
    a. Blunt Trauma
    b. Gram Negative Cocci
    c. Ingrown Fingernail
    d. Staphylococcus Aureus
    e. Vasospasm

ANSWERS

220. a

221. b

222. d

VISUAL STIMULUS REVIEW

The image shows significant edema and tension to the fingertip pulp of the left index finger.

REFERENCES

- McDonald LS, Bavaro MF, Hofmeister EP, Kroonen LT. Hand infections. J Hand Surg Am. 2011 Aug;36(8):1403-12.
- Clark DC. Common acute hand infections. Am Fam Physician. 2003 Dec 1;68(11):2167-76.
- Imahara SD, Friedrich JB. Community-acquired methicillin-resistant Staphylococcus aureus in surgically treated hand infections. J Hand Surg Am. 2010 Jan;35(1):97-103.
- Ong YS, Levin LS. Hand infections. Plast Reconstr Surg. 2009 Oct;124(4):225e-233e.

CASE #70: RASH

CASE

A five-year-old boy is brought to his pediatrician for evaluation of a mildly pruritic rash over his face arms and torso that developed over the last two days. The patient has no past medical history and is taking no medications. He is afebrile with normal vital signs. His mother reports runny nose, mild cough, and sore throat as well as low-grade fever that he had about a week ago but resolved by now.

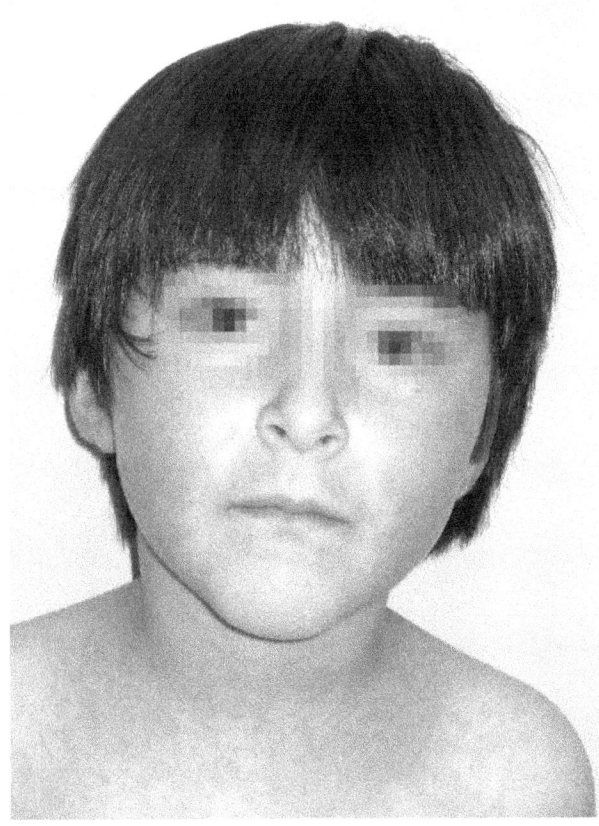

QUESTIONS

223. What is the likely diagnosis?
    a. Fifth Disease
    b. Measles
    c. Mumps
    d. Roseola Infantum
    e. Scarlet Fever

224. What is the cause of this condition?
    a. Group A Beta-Hemolytic Streptococci
    b. Human Herpesvirus Type 6
    c. Human Parvovirus B19
    d. Measles Virus
    e. Rubella Virus

225. Which of the following is a common additional finding in this condition?
    a. Arthralgias
    b. Diarrhea
    c. Enanthems
    d. Vomiting

ANSWERS

223. a

224. c

225. a

VISUAL STIMULUS REVIEW

The image shows a bright red facial rash that spares the nasolabial folds and perioral skin. The image also shows a lacy rash over the torso.

REFERENCES

- Servey JT, Reamy BV, Hodge J. Clinical presentations of parvovirus B19 infection. Am Fam Physician. 2007 Feb 1;75(3):373-6.

CASE #71: SWOLLEN HAND

CASE

A 32-year-old right-handed man presents to the emergency department complaining of right-hand pain and progressive swelling that have been progressing over the last three days s/p fall. The patient will not elaborate on the circumstances of the injury. He is febrile to 102.F (38.9C) with heart rate of 110/min.

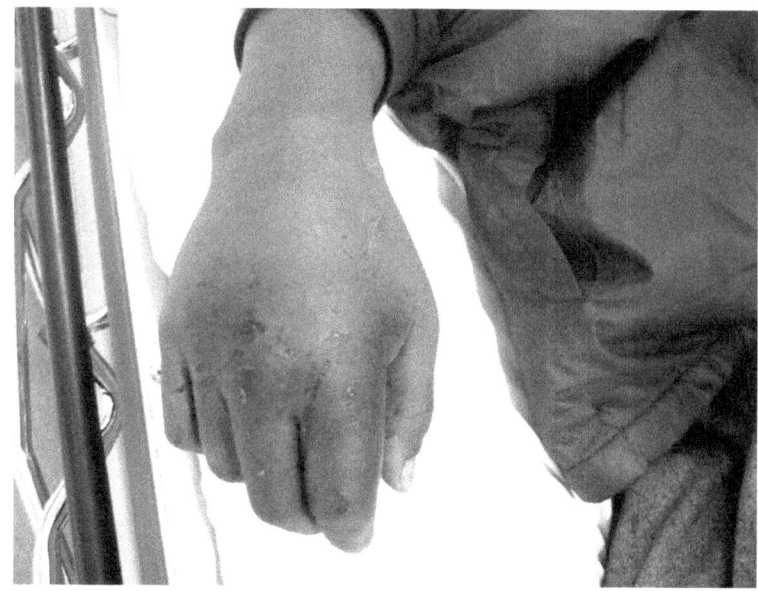

QUESTIONS

226. What is the likely diagnosis?
    a. Extensor Tenosynovitis
    b. Flexor Tenosynovitis
    c. Human Bite
    d. Metacarpal Fracture

227. What is the most common gram positive organism isolated in this type of injury?
    a. Eikenella Corrodens
    b. Peptostreptococcus
    c. Staphylococcus Aureus
    d. Streptococcus Pyogenes

228. What is the most common gram negative organism isolated in this type of injury?
    a. Bacteroides Fragilis
    b. Eikenella Corrodens
    c. Escherichia Colli
    d. Peptostreptococcus

ANSWERS

226. c

227. c

228. b

VISUAL STIMULUS REVIEW

The clinical image demonstrates swollen right hand and fingers (Septic Hand) with small horizontal lacerations over the dorsal 2nd and 3rd metacarpophalangeal joints.

REFERENCES

- McDonald LS, Bavaro MF, Hofmeister EP, Kroonen LT. Hand infections. J Hand Surg Am. 2011 Aug;36(8):1403-12.

- Harrison M. A 4-year review of human bite injuries presenting to emergency medicine and proposed evidence-based guidelines. Injury. Aug 2009;40(8):826-30.

CASE #72: FINGER PAIN

CASE

A 23-year-old (left-handed) man presents to the emergency department complaining of severe pain to his right middle finger. He worked at a body shop and was using a high-pressure paint injector when he accidentally injected paint directly into his right middle finger. He reports that he had no pain initially, so he continued to work for a couple of hours until he developed severe pain and swelling. On examination, his right middle finger is swollen and remarkably tender and tense. A plain film of his hand is obtained.

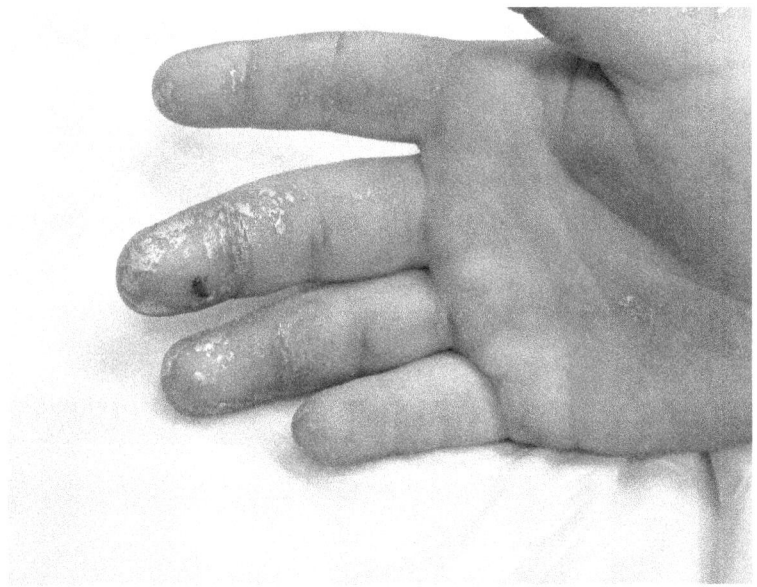

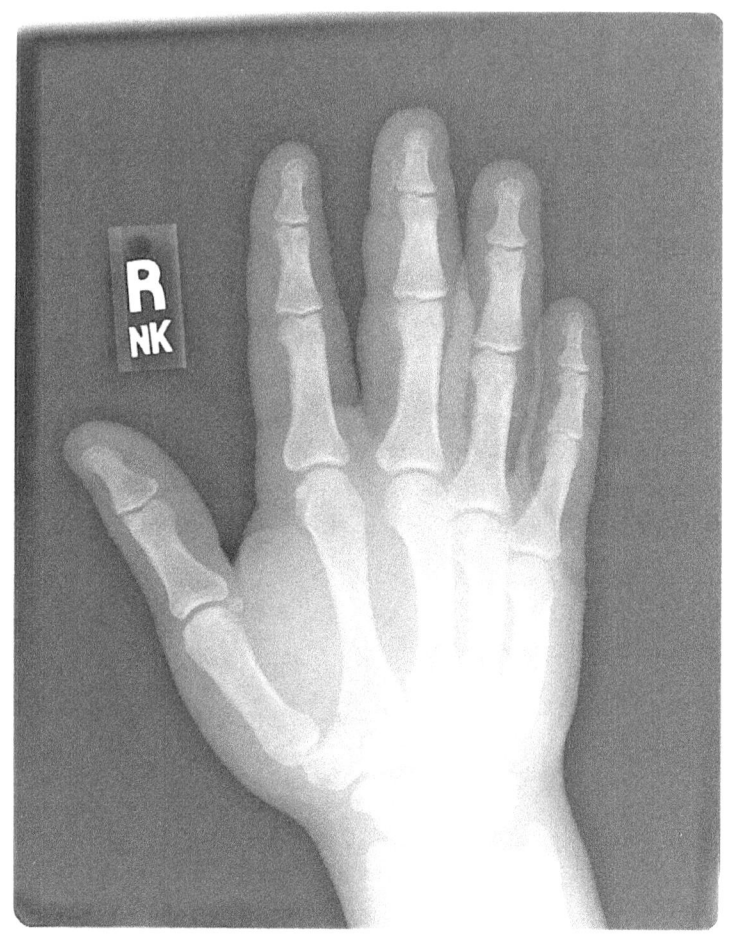

QUESTIONS

229. What is the likely diagnosis?
 a. Extensor Tenosynovitis
 b. Felon
 c. Finger Abscess
 d. Flexor Tenosynovitis
 e. High Pressure Injection Injury

230. Which of the following options describes the correct management approach for this condition?
    a. Bier Block.
    b. CT angiogram of the hand to evaluate blood supply and tissue viability.
    c. Emergent incision, drainage, and irrigation in the operating room.
    d. Intravenous antibiotics with incision and drainage if no improvement in 24 hrs.
    e. Oral antibiotics and hand elevation with 24 hrs hand surgeon follow up.
231. Which of the following statements regarding this condition is correct?
    a. Air and water injection may be treated conservatively.
    b. Grease and paint injections rarely lead to soft tissue necrosis and need for amputation.
    c. This condition is more common in the dominant hand.
    d. This condition rarely manifests as an innocuous lesion.

ANSWERS

229. e

230. c

231. a

VISUAL STIMULUS REVIEW

The gross image shows a swollen right middle finger with a puncture wound to the volar aspect of the middle finger. The plain film shows a radiopaque material in the soft tissue anterior to the distal and middle phalanxes of the right middle finger.

REFERENCES

- Soyuncu S, Bektas F, Dinc S. High-pressure Air Injection Injury to the Upper Extremity. J Emerg Med. 2013 Mar 5.

- Pappou IP, Deal DN. High-pressure injection injuries. J Hand Surg Am. 2012 Nov;37(11):2404-7.

- Verhoeven N, Hierner R. High-pressure injection injury of the hand: an often underestimated trauma: case report with study of the literature. Strategies Trauma Limb Reconstr. 2008 Apr;3(1):27-33.

CASE #73: EPIGASTRIC PAIN

CASE

A 54-year-old man with a history of alcoholism presents to the emergency department complaining of epigastric pain and vomiting for two days. On exam he has epigastric pain with some guarding and appears to be jaundiced.

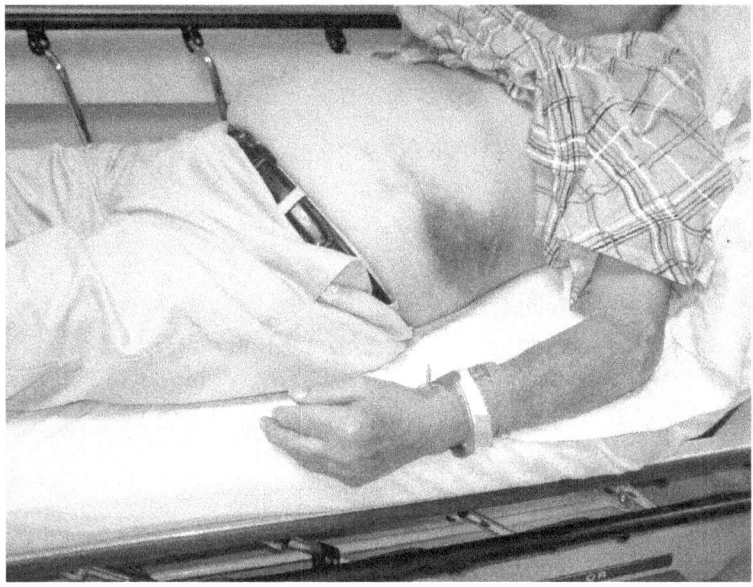

QUESTIONS

232. What is the likely diagnosis?

    a. Acute Alcoholic Cholecystitis (AAC)

    b. Acute Pancreatitis

    c. Aortic Dissection

    d. Ascending Cholangitis

    e. Necrotizing Pancreatitis

233. What sign is seen in the image above?

    a. Cullen Sign

    b. Grey Turner Sign

    c. McBurney's Sign

    d. Murphy's Sign

    e. Rovsing's Sign

234. What sign might accompany this sign?

    a. Cullen Sign

    b. Grey Turner Sign

    c. McBurney's Sign

    d. Murphy's Sign

    e. Rovsing's Sign

235. Which of the following vital signs is likely to represent this patient's condition?

    a. T: 101F (38.3C); HR: 80/min; BP: 130/70

    b. T: 97.5F (36.4C); HR: 80/min; BP: 130/70

    c. T: 101F (38.3C); HR: 110/min; BP: 90/60

    d. T: 97.5F (36.4C); HR: 80/min; BP: 90/60

    e. T: 97.5F (36.4C); HR: 80/min; BP: 110/60

ANSWERS

232. e

233. b

234. a

235. c

VISUAL STIMULUS REVIEW

The image shows a left flank hematoma.

REFERENCES

- Chung KM, Chuang SS. Cullen and Grey Turner signs in idiopathic perirenal hemorrhage. CMAJ. 2011 Nov 8;183(16):E1221.

- Wu BU, Banks PA. Clinical management of patients with acute pancreatitis. Gastroenterology. 2013 Jun;144(6):1272-81.

CASE #74: FINGER PAIN

CASE

A 47-year-old carpenter presents to his family doctor three days after he suffered a puncture wound to his right middle finger. On exam his right middle finger tender to palpation over the plantar aspect. Passive extension of the finger causes severe pain.

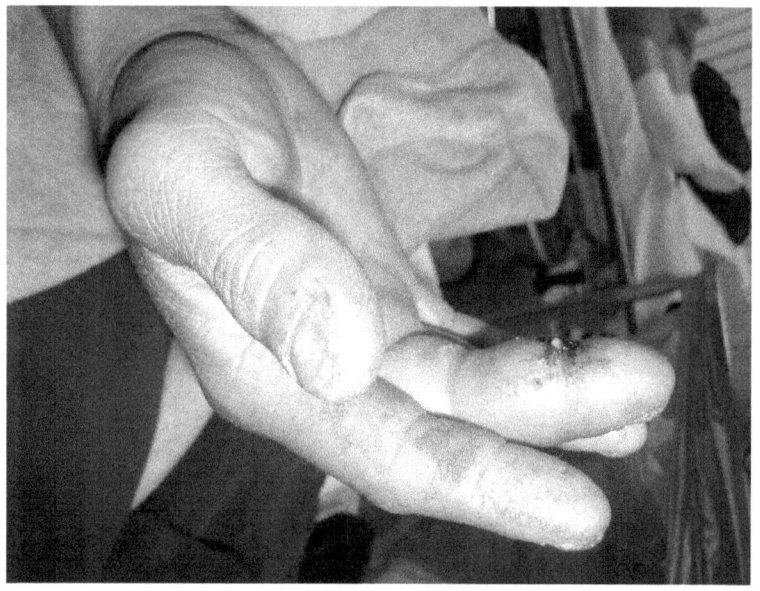

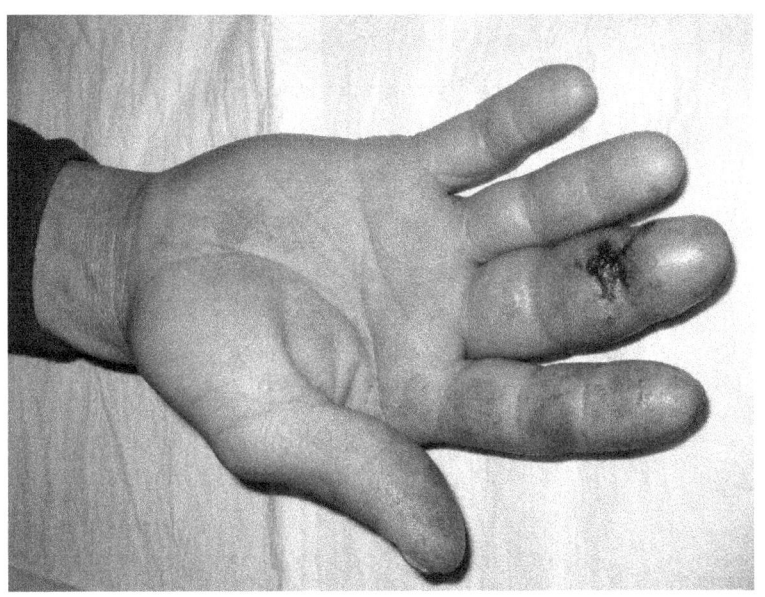

QUESTIONS

236. What is the likely diagnosis?

    a. de Quervain's Disease

    b. Finger Abscess

    c. Flexor Tenosynovitis

    d. Felon

    e. Paronychia

237. Which of the following findings is expected in this condition?

a. Fever

b. Severe Pain on Palpation of the Fingertip

c. Severe Pain with Passive Extension

d. Severe Pain with Passive Flexion

238. Which of the following options describes the correct management approach for this condition?

a. Bier Block.

b. CT angiogram of the hand to evaluate blood supply and tissue viability.

c. Emergent incision, drainage, and irrigation in the operating room.

d. Intravenous antibiotics with incision and drainage if no improvement in 24 hrs.

e. Oral antibiotics and hand elevation with 24 hrs hand surgeon follow up.

ANSWERS

236. c

237. c

238. c

VISUAL STIMULUS REVIEW

The gross images show fusiform swelling and erythema of the right middle finger that is held in the flexed position.

REFERENCES

- Nikkhah D, Rodrigues J, Osman K, Dejager L. Pyogenic flexor tenosynovitis: one year's experience at a UK hand unit and a review of the current literature. Hand Surg. 2012;17(2):199-203.

- Henry M. Septic flexor tenosynovitis. J Hand Surg Am. 2011 Feb;36(2):322-3.

CASE #75: FACIAL RASH

CASE

A 19-year-old man presents to his family doctor complaining of mildly pruritic rash to his face that developed over the last week. He lives on a farm, has a dog that shares a room with him, and reports no past medical history.

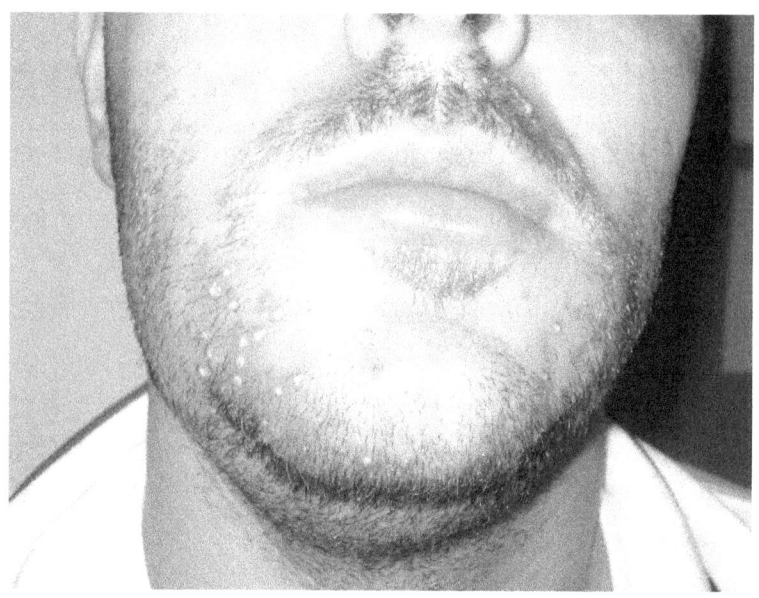

QUESTIONS

239. What is the likely diagnosis?

   a. Acne Vulgaris

   b. Bacterial Folliculitis

   c. Perioral Dermatitis

   d. Seabather's Eruption

   e. Tinea Barbae

240. What is the most likely cause of this patient's condition?

   a. Propionibacterium Acnes

   b. Sebum Impaction

   c. Staphylococcus Aureus

   d. Streptococus Group A

   e. Trichophyton Rubrum

241. Definitive treatment of this condition includes which of the following?

   a. Hair Depilation

   b. Oral Anti-Fungal Antibiotics

   c. Oral Anti-Staphylococcal Antibiotics

   d. Oral Anti-Streptococcal Antibiotics

   e. Topical Anti-Staphylococcal Antibiotic Cream

ANSWERS

239. e
240. e
241. b

VISUAL STIMULUS REVIEW

The image shows papules and pustules involving the bearded facial skin with surrounding erythema.

REFERENCES

- Hainer BL. Dermatophyte infections. Am Fam Physician. 2003 Jan 1;67(1):101-8.
- Luelmo-Aguilar J, Santandreu MS. Folliculitis: recognition and management. Am J Clin Dermatol. 2004;5(5):301-10.

CASE #76: POOR FEEDING

CASE

A 14-days-old, full-term (40 weeks), planned, uneventful cesarean section delivery, baby boy is brought to the pediatrician's office for poor feeding and irritability. The baby had an unremarkable neonate exam, received all recommended vaccinations, and was discharged home on his third day of life. The parents report two days of decreased PO intake and mild cough. The patient is lethargic with temp of 101.F (38.7C), respirations of 40/min, HR of 160/min, BP of 70/40 mmHg, and O_2Sat of 100% on room air. His lungs are clear; he has normal retinas on funduscopy, and his skin exam shows no rash. Both his tympanic membranes appear mildly erythematous.

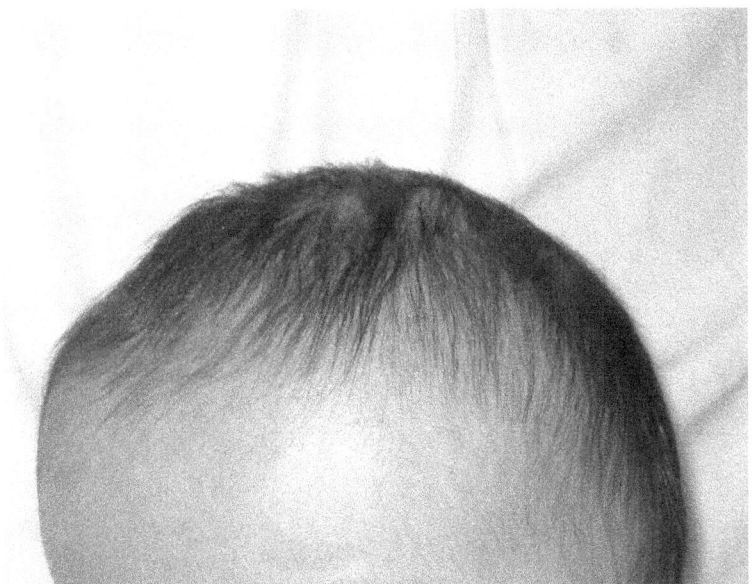

QUESTIONS

242. What is the likely diagnosis?

    a. Epidural Hematoma

    b. Hydrocephalus

    c. Pneumonia

    d. Scalp Abscess

    e. Scalp Hematoma

243. What is the likely cause of this condition?

    a. Accidental Trauma

    b. Bacterial Meningitis

    c. Non-Accidental Trauma

    d. Spontaneous

    e. Staphylococcus Aureus

244. What is the first line of treatment for this condition?

    a. Emergent CT of the Head with IV Contrast

    b. Emergent CT of the Head without IV Contrast

    c. Incision and Drainage of Hematoma

    d. Intravenous Antibiotics

    e. Ventriculoperitoneal Shunt

ANSWERS

242. b

243. b

244. d

VISUAL STIMULUS REVIEW

The image shows a bulging frontal fontanel.

REFERENCES

- Galiza EP, Heath PT. Improving the outcome of neonatal meningitis. Curr Opin Infect Dis. 2009 Jun;22(3):229-34.
- Heath PT, Nik Yusoff NK, Baker CJ. Neonatal meningitis. Arch Dis Child Fetal Neonatal Ed. May 2003;88(3):F173-8
- Shacham S, Kozer E, Bahat H, Mordish Y, Goldman M. Bulging fontanelle in febrile infants: is lumbar puncture mandatory? Arch Dis Child. 2009 Sep;94(9):690-2.
- Kimberlin DW. Meningitis in the Neonate. Curr Treat Options Neurol. 2002 May;4(3):239-248.

CASE #77: FOOT PAIN

CASE

A 30-year-old construction worker presents to his family doctor after stepping on a 3-inch rusted nail through a pair of rubber sole construction shoes about two hours ago. He is able to ambulate with minimal pain.

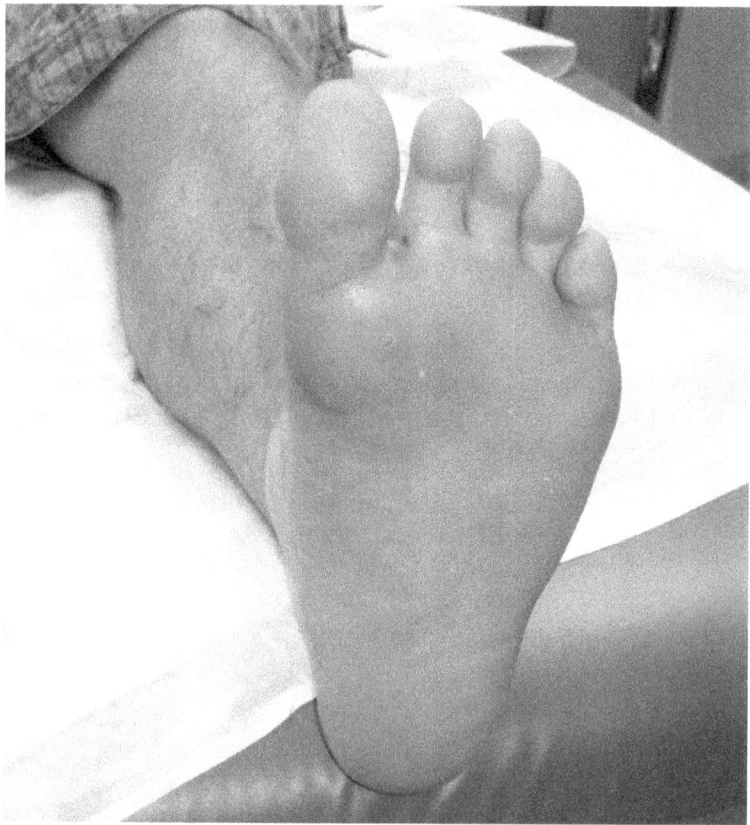

QUESTIONS

245. What is the likely diagnosis?

   a. Cellulitis

   b. Necrotizing Fasciitis

   c. Osteomyelitis

   d. Plantar Puncture Wound

246. What is the most common cause of infection in this context?

   a. Methicillin Resistant Staphylococcus Aureus

   b. Pasteurella Multocida

   c. Pseudomonas Aeruginosa

   d. Streptococcus Viridans

247. Which of the following statement is correct?

   a. Inoculation of the deep spaces of the foot is uncommon in this scenario.

   b. Only patients who complain about foreign body sensation should be x-rayed.

   c. Pain out of proportion to the injury strongly indicates that an infection has developed.

   d. Pseudomonas aeruginosa is the usually responsible organism cultured after nail puncture through bare foot.

ANSWERS

245. d

246. c

247. c

VISUAL STIMULUS REVIEW

The image demonstrates a plantar puncture wound without swelling or erythema.

REFERENCES

- Belin R, Carrington S. Management of pedal puncture wounds. Clin Podiatr Med Surg. 2012 Jul;29(3):451-8.

- Haverstock BD. Puncture wounds of the foot. Clin Podiatr Med Surg. 2012 Apr;29(2):311-22.

CASE #78: PAINFUL SCROTUM

CASE

A 43-year-old man with a past medical history of diabetes mellitus presents to the emergency department complaining of painful scrotal swelling. He is well-appearing, and his vitals are temp of 99.7F (37.6C), blood pressure of 120/70 mmHg, heart rate of 92 beats/min, respiratory rate of 19 per minute, and pulse oximetry of 99% on room air. His scrotum is swollen and erythematous with no skin breakdown or crepitus. The erythema extends toward his lower abdominal wall.

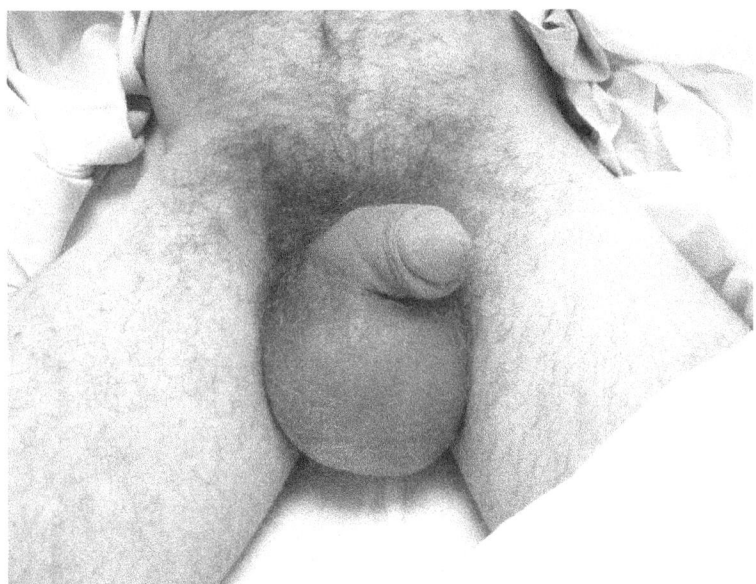

QUESTIONS

248. What is the likely diagnosis?
   a. Balanitis
   b. Fournier's Gangrene

c. Scrotal Abscess
   d. Scrotal Cellulitis

249. Which of the following is the most common predisposing factor for this condition?
   a. Alcoholism
   b. Chronic Corticosteroid Therapy
   c. Cirrhosis of Liver
   d. Diabetes Mellitus
   e. HIV Infection

250. Which of the following is the most common microbiological result when cultures are obtained from patients with this condition?
   a. Bacteroides
   b. Clostridium Difficile
   c. Escherichia Coli
   d. Polymicrobial Infection
   e. Staphylococcus Aureus

251. Which of the following statements is correct?
   a. Broad spectrum intravenous antibiotics and admission for monitoring of disease progression are the first line therapies for this condition.
   b. Most cases have an identifiable cause.
   c. CT scan with IV contrast provides the gold standard for the diagnosis of this condition.
   d. Hyperbaric oxygen therapy should be provided as soon as possible after initiation of IV antibiotics therapy for the treatment of this condition.

ANSWERS

248. b

249. d

250. d

251. b

VISUAL STIMULUS REVIEW

The image shows scrotal erythema and edema with progression of the erythema to the penile shaft, supra pubic area, and anterior abdominal wall.

REFERENCES

- Benjelloun el B, Souiki T, Yakla N, et al. Fournier's gangrene: our experience with 50 patients and analysis of factors affecting mortality. World J Emerg Surg. 2013 Apr 1;8(1):13.

- Koukouras D. et al. Fournier's gangrene, a urologic and surgical emergency: presentation of a multi-institutional experience with 45 cases. Urol Int. 2011;86(2).

- Erol B. et al. Fournier's gangrene: overview of prognostic factors and definition of new prognostic parameter. Urology. 2010 May;75(5):1193-8.

- Levenson RB, Singh AK, Novelline RA. Fournier gangrene: role of imaging. Radiographics. 2008 Mar-Apr;28(2):519-28.

CASE #79: EPIGASTRIC PAIN

CASE

A 47-year-old man presents to the emergency department complaining of severe epigastric pain that started a couple hours ago. The pain radiates to his back and is associated with nausea and vomiting of nonbilious and nonbloody content. On exam the patient appears ill-appearing with heart rate of 107/min, BP of 100/60, and O_2Sat of 97% on room air. His abdominal exam shows diffuse abdominal tenderness with guarding over the epigastrium. A chest X-ray is obtained.

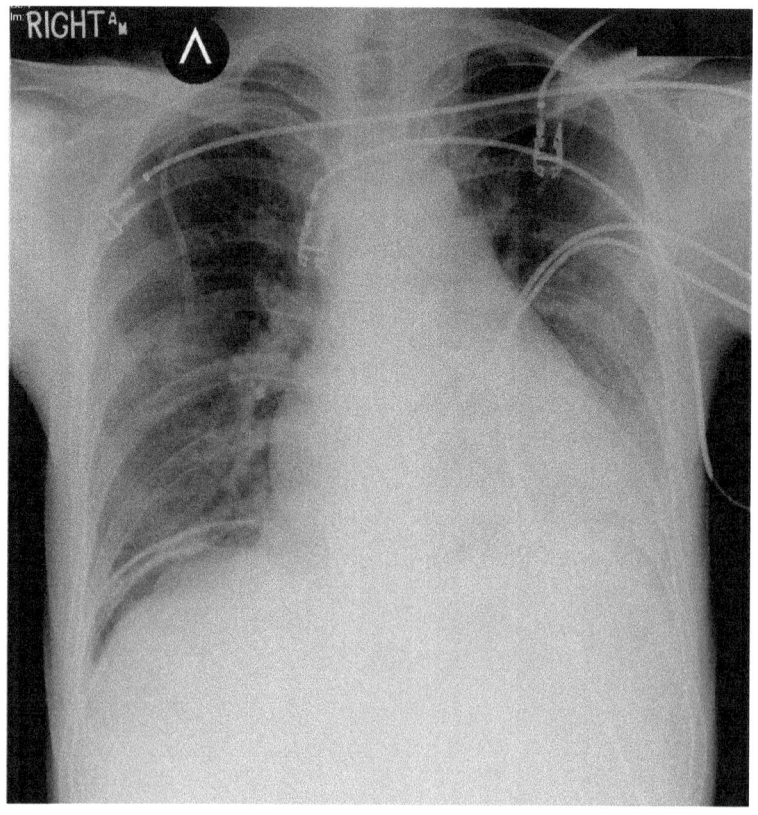

QUESTIONS

252. What is the likely diagnosis?

    a. Abdominal Aortic Dissection

    b. Cholecystitis

    c. Gastritis

    d. Pancreatitis

    e. Perforated Viscous

253. What is the most common cause of this condition?

    a. Alcoholism

    b. Aneurismal Dilation of the Abdominal Aorta

    c. Chronic NSAID Use

    d. Helicobacter Pylori

    e. Obstruction of the Cystic Duct

    f. Staphylococcal Exotoxins

254. Which of the following is included in the first line therapy for this condition?

    a. Endovascular Aortic Stent Graft

    b. Intravenous Proton Pump Inhibitors

    c. Intravenous Thiamin

    d. Laparotomy or Laparoscopy

    e. Oral Proton Pump Inhibitors

255. Which of the following is indicated after initial management of this condition?

    a. Annual CT Angiogram or Abdominal Ultrasound

    b. Helicobacter Pylori Eradication

    c. Oral Anticoagulation

d. Oral Antihypertensive Therapy
e. Oral Statin Therapy

ANSWERS

252. e

253. c

254. d

255. b

VISUAL STIMULUS REVIEW

The radiogram shows free air under the right hemidiaphragm.

REFERENCES

- Tomtitchong P, Siribumrungwong B, Vilaichone RK. Et al. Systematic review and meta-analysis: Helicobacter pylori eradication therapy after simple closure of perforated duodenal ulcer. Helicobacter. 2012 Apr;17(2):148-52.
- Bertleff MJ, Lange JF. Perforated peptic ulcer disease: a review of history and treatment. Dig Surg. 2010 Aug;27(3):161-9.

CASE #80: FOOT PAIN

CASE

A 56-year-old man patient presents to the emergency department complaining of one day of severe, sudden onset pain and swelling to his left foot. He has a history of diabetes and peripheral vascular disease. He also reports a puncture wound to his left big toe that he suffered two days prior. The patient is afebrile, ill-appearing, and tachycardic. He complains of 10/10 pain to his left foot that extends to his mid-lower leg. A plain film of his foot is shown below.

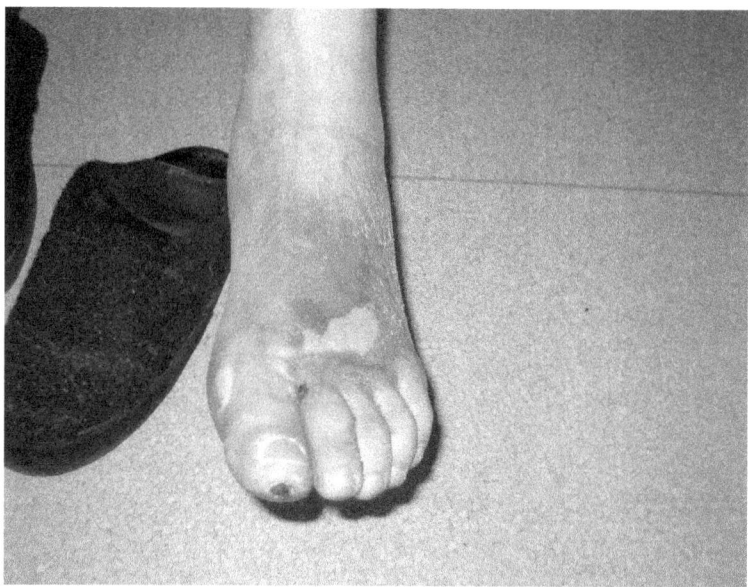

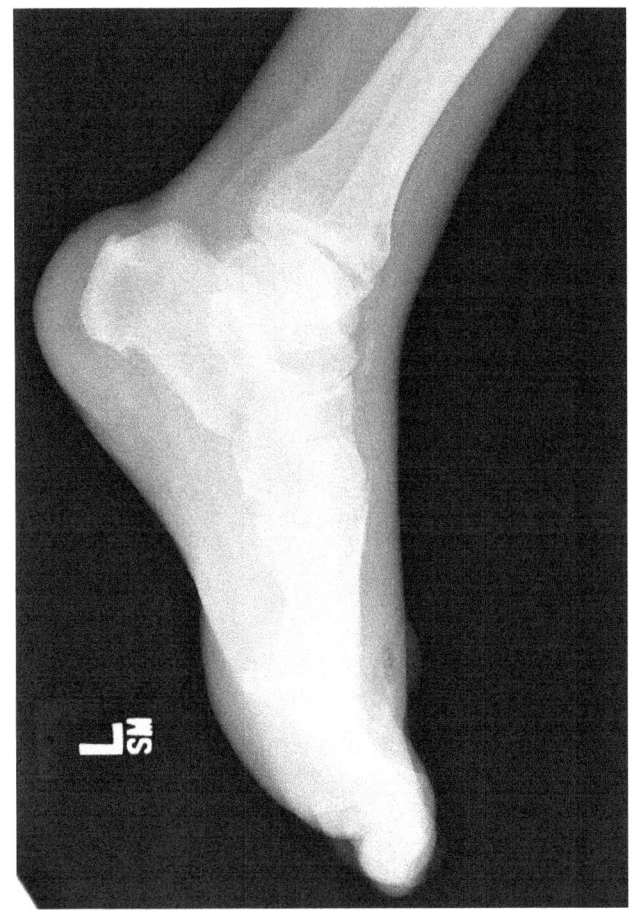

QUESTIONS

256. What is the likely diagnosis?
    a. Arterial Embolism
    b. Deep Vein Thrombosis
    c. Diabetic Foot Infection
    d. Gas Gangrene
    e. Toxic Shock Syndrome

257. What is the likely cause of this condition?
    a. Atrial Fibrillation
    b. Clostridium Perfringens
    c. Hypercoagulable State
    d. Staphylococcus Aureus
    e. Streptococcus Group A

258. Which of the following should be included in the first line therapy of condition?
    a. Clindamycin IV
    b. Heparin IV
    c. Penicillin G IV
    d. Vancomycin IV
    e. A and C

259. Which of the following should also be included in the first line therapy of this condition?
    a. Angiogram and Embolectomy
    b. Femoral Popliteal Arterial Bypass
    c. Beta Blockers IV
    d. Surgical Debridement
    e. Tissue Plasminogen Activator (TPA) IV

ANSWERS

256. d

257. b

258. e

259. d

VISUAL STIMULUS REVIEW

The image shows a black scab to the left big toe with erythema to the dorsal foot with a large hemorrhagic bullae to the dorsal foot with a blue/black border. The radiogram shows gas in the soft tissue of the dorsal left foot.

REFERENCES

- Stevens DL, Aldape MJ, Bryant AE. Life-threatening clostridial infections. Anaerobe. 2012 Apr;18(2):254-9.

- Dedemadi G, Sakellariou I, Kolinioti A, Lazaridis P, Anagnostou E. Clostridium septicum myonecrosis: a destructive and lethal condition. Am Surg. 2011 Jun;77(6):e101-2.

- Bryant AE, Stevens DL. Clostridial myonecrosis: new insights in pathogenesis and management. Curr Infect Dis Rep. 2010 Sep;12(5):383-91.

- Headley AJ. Necrotizing soft tissue infections: a primary care review. Am Fam Physician. Jul 15 2003;68(2):323-8.

CASE #81: FINGER PAIN

CASE

A six-year-old girl is brought to her pediatrician for right index finger and mouth pain for two days. She is well-appearing with normal vital signs.

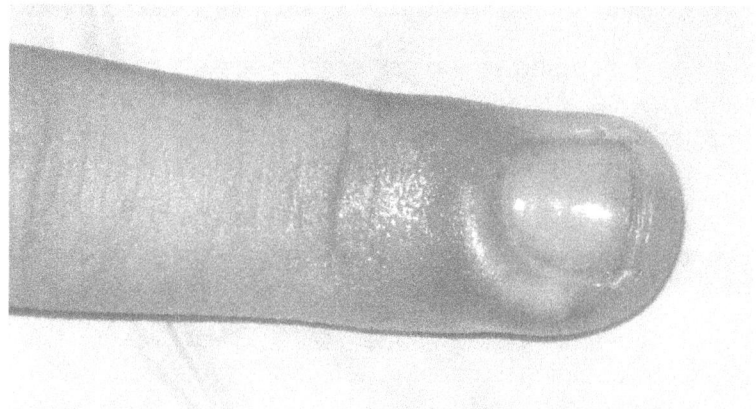

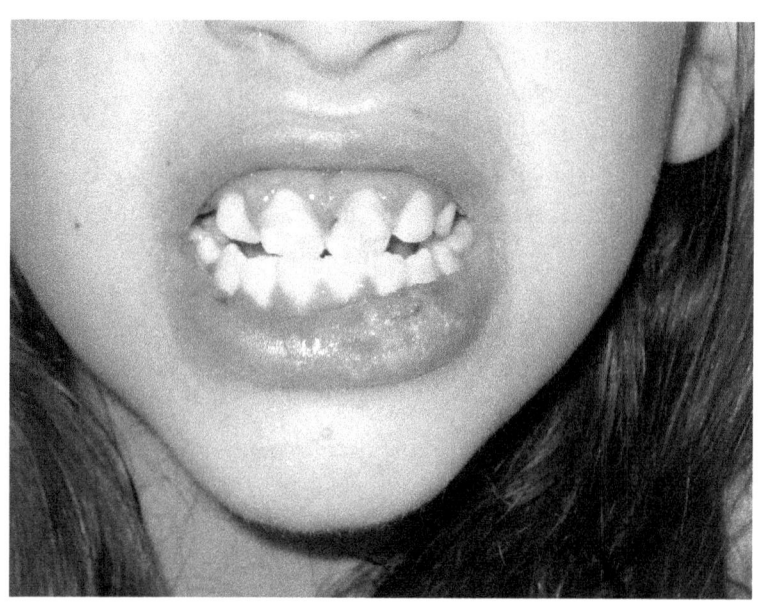

QUESTIONS

260. What is the likely diagnosis?
    a. Felon
    b. Hand Foot and Mouth Disease
    c. Herpetic Whitlow
    d. Ingrown Fingernail

261. What is the most likely cause of this condition?
    a. Coxsackie Virus
    b. Herpes Simplex Virus Type 1
    c. Streptococcus Group A
    d. Staphylococcus Aureus
    e. Too Short Nail Clipping

262. What is the recommended treatment for this condition?
    a. Acyclovir
    b. Finger Immersion in Betadine Solution
    c. Ibuprofen
    d. Incision and Drainage
    e. Sulfamethoxazole-Trimethoprim (Bactrim)

263. Which of the following treatment is contraindicated for this condition?
    a. Acyclovir
    b. Finger Immersion in Betadine Solution
    c. Ibuprofen
    d. Incision and Drainage
    e. Sulfamethoxazole-Trimethoprim (Bactrim)

ANSWERS

260. c

261. b

262. a

263. d

VISUAL STIMULUS REVIEW

The finger images shows erythematous distal phalanx of the right index finger with multiple vesicles on an erythematous base just proximal to the nail fold with purulent material accumulation underneath the ulnar nail fold. The face image shows erythematous swollen gums with crust covering the lower lip.

REFERENCES

- Rubright JH, Shafritz AB. The herpetic whitlow. J Hand Surg Am. 2011 Feb;36(2):340-2.
- Clark DC. Common acute hand infections. Am Fam Physician. 2003 Dec 1;68(11):2167-76.

CASE #82: EYE PAIN

CASE

A 60-year-old woman presents to the emergency department complaining of sudden onset severe left eye pain and blurry vision for the last two hours. She walked into her dark bedroom when she felt a sudden onset left eye pain and left retro orbital headache, nausea, and vomited once. She also reports seeing halos around objects intermittently over the past couple of weeks. On physical examination the patient had normal vital signs, unreactive left pupil, and her visual acuity was OD: 20/20; OS: hand motion.

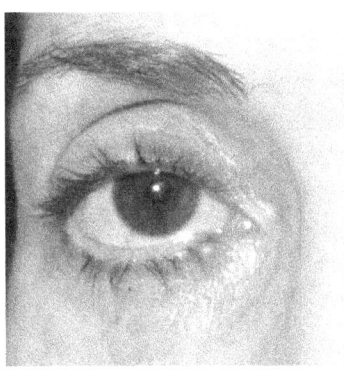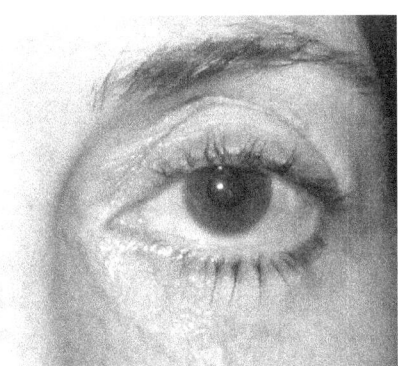

QUESTIONS

264. What is the likely diagnosis?
    a. Acute Angel Closure Glaucoma
    b. Acute Stroke
    c. Iritis
    d. Retinal Detachment
    e. Vitreous Hemorrhage

265. What is the likely cause of this condition?
    a. Increase in Intracranial Pressure
    b. Increase in Intraocular Pressure
    c. Iris Inflammation
    d. Retinal Hemorrhage
    e. Posterior Vitreous Detachment

266. What is the gold standard test for confirming the diagnosis in this condition?
    a. MRI Brain
    b. Ocular Ultrasound
    c. Slit Lamp Examination
    d. Tonometry

267. Which of the following is the definitive treatment of this condition?
    a. Cerebral Angiogram with Clot Retrieval
    b. Laser Peripheral Iridotomy
    c. Pars Plana Vitrectomy
    d. Pneumatic Retinopexy
    e. Steroid Ocular Solution

ANSWERS

264. a

265. b

266. d

267. b

VISUAL STIMULUS REVIEW

The image shows a mid-dilated left pupil with scleral injection.

REFERENCES

- Chang RT, Singh K. Myopia and glaucoma: diagnostic and therapeutic challenges. Curr Opin Ophthalmol. 2013 Mar;24(2):96-101.

- Rahim SA, Sahlas DJ, Shadowitz S. Blinded by pressure and pain. Lancet. Jun 25-Jul 1 2005;365(9478):2244.

CASE #83: FOOT PAIN

CASE

A 58-year-old man presents to an urgent care center complaining of severe pain to his right foot and big toe for two days that is not relieved with acetaminophen. His vital signs are all within normal limit. His right foot is extremely tender to the touch over his first metatarsophalangeal joint. Both his hands had soft nodules, with the nodule over his right fifth metacarpophalangeal joint being mildly erythematous and tender.

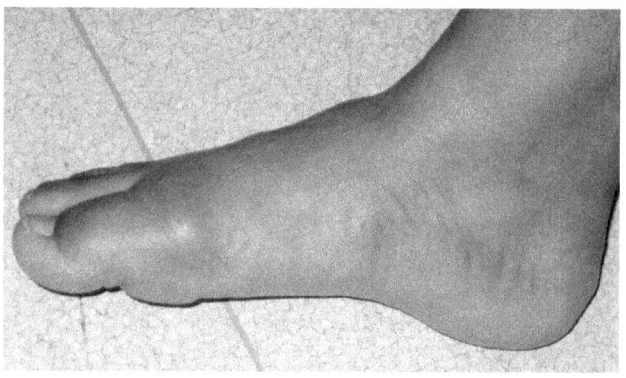

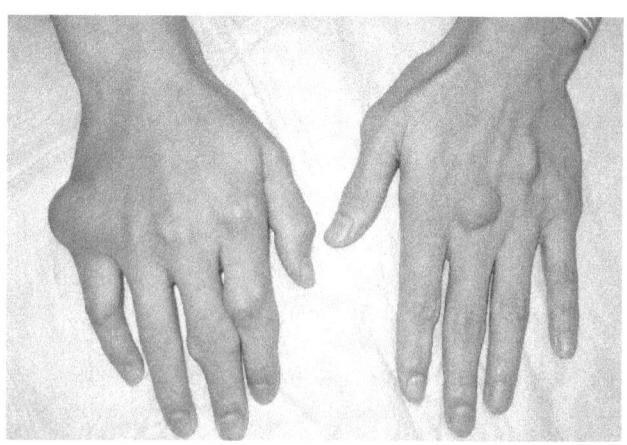

QUESTIONS

268. What is the likely diagnosis?

   a. Gout

   b. Pseudogout

   c. Rheumatoid Arthritis

   d. Septic Arthritis

   e. Systemic Lupus Erythematosus

269. What is the likely cause of this condition?

   a. Auto Antibodies

   b. Neisseria Gonorrhea

   c. Calcium Pyrophosphate Crystals Deposition

   d. Monosodium Urate Monohydrate Crystals Deposition

270. Which of the following is expected to be elevated in patients who suffer from this condition?

   a. Double Stranded Antibodies

   b. Ionized Calcium

   c. Rheumatoid Factor

   d. Uric Acid

ANSWERS

268. a

269. d

270. d

VISUAL STIMULUS REVIEW

The foot image shows swelling and erythema to the right first metatarsophalangeal joint and big toe. The hands image shows erythema of a tophaceous nodule to the right fifth metacarpophalangeal joint.

REFERENCES

- Doghramji PP, Wortmann RL. Hyperuricemia and gout: new concepts in diagnosis and management. Postgrad Med. 2012 Nov;124(6):98-109.

- Ruoff G. The treatment of gout. J Fam Pract. 2012 Jun;61(6 Suppl):S11-5.

CASE #84: RASH AND FEVER

CASE

A five-year-old girl presents to her pediatrician complaining of sore throat and painful rash to her hands and feet over the last three days. On exam she has a temp of 101.2F (38.4C), heart rate of 100/min, respirations 18/min, blood pressure 90/55 mmHg, and O₂Sat 99% on room air.

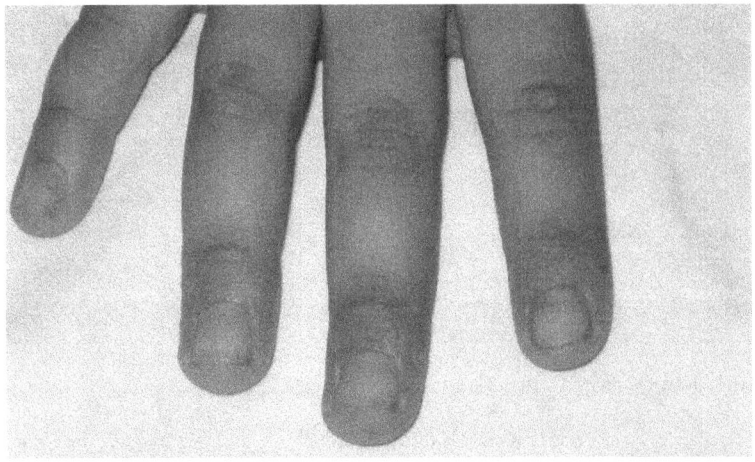

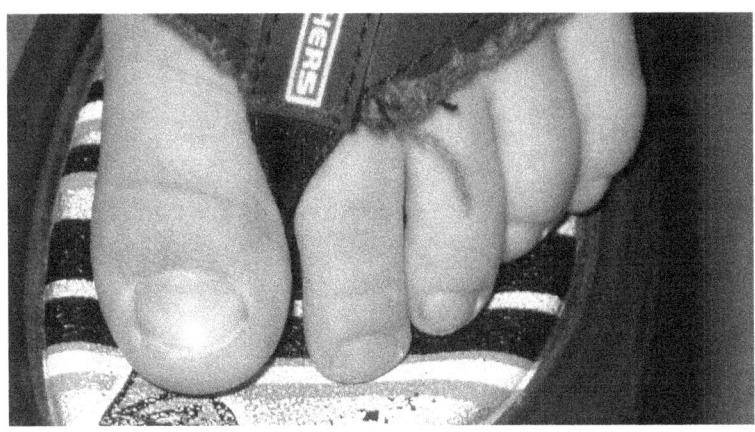

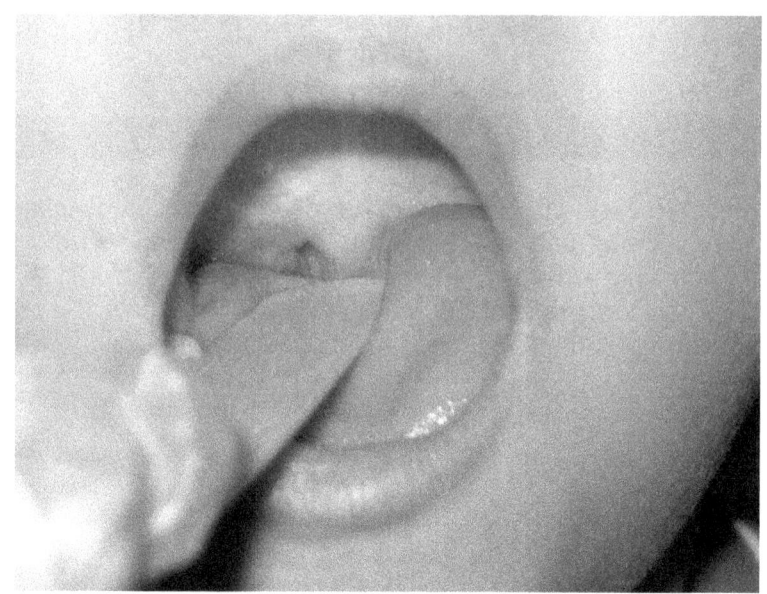

QUESTIONS

271. What is the likely diagnosis?
    a. Erythema Multiforme
    b. Hand Foot and Mouth Disease
    c. Herpangina
    d. Kawasaki Disease
    e. Pharyngitis

272. What is the most likely cause of this condition?
    a. Autoantibodies
    b. Coxsackie Virus
    c. Herpes Simplex Virus Type 1
    d. Streptococcus
    e. Staphylococcus Aureus

273. Which of the following provides the highest diagnostic yield?
    a. Rectal Swabs
    b. Serum Antibody Titers
    c. Sputum Culture
    d. Skin Lesions Swab
    e. Urine Antigen

274. Which of the following is part of the first line therapy of this condition?
    a. Acyclovir IV
    b. Acyclovir PO
    c. Amoxicillin PO
    d. Prednisone PO
    e. Symptomatic Care

ANSWERS

271. b

272. b

273. a

274. e

VISUAL STIMULUS REVIEW

The images show pharyngeal erythema with vesicular rash over the soft palate as well as around the nail folds of the hands and feet.

REFERENCES

- Lee TC, Guo HR, Su HJ.et al. Diseases caused by enterovirus 71 infection. Pediatr Infect Dis J. 2009 Oct;28(10):904-10.

- Frydenberg A, Starr M. Hand, foot and mouth disease. Aust Fam Physician. 2003 Aug;32(8):594-5.

CASE #85: HEMATURIA

CASE

An eight-year-old boy is brought to his pediatrician's office by his parents because of decreased appetite and gross hematuria. He reports an episode of sore throat two weeks prior that resolved without any residual symptoms. Over the past week the parents noticed facial and lower extremity swelling. On exam the patient is afebrile with heart rate on 96/min and blood pressure of 160/90 mmHg. His has clear breath sounds on auscultation with significant periorbital and anterior tibial edema.

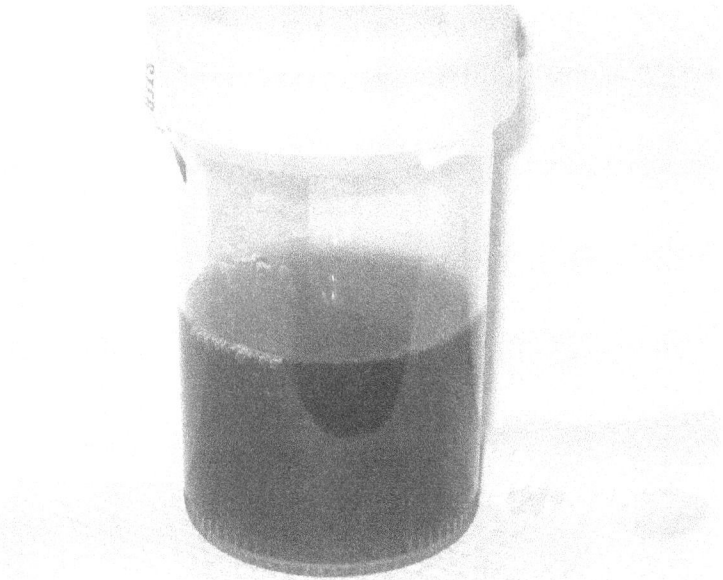

QUESTIONS

275. What is the likely diagnosis?
    a. Cryoglobulinemia
    b. Glomerulonephritis
    a. Hemorrhagic Cystitis
    b. Renal Cell Carcinoma

276. What is the likely cause of this condition?
    a. Escherichia Coli
    b. Malignant Transformation
    c. Renal Crystals Deposition
    d. Streptococus Group A

277. Which of the following is part of the first line of treatment?
    a. Hemodialysis
    b. IVIG
    c. Nephrectomy
    d. Prednisone PO
    e. Symptomatic Care

ANSWERS

275. b

276. d

277. e

VISUAL STIMULUS REVIEW

The image shows gross dark red-colored urine.

REFERENCES

- Marshall CS, Cheng AC, Markey PG et al. Acute post-streptococcal glomerulonephritis in the Northern Territory of Australia: a review of 16 years data and comparison with the literature. Am J Trop Med Hyg. 2011 Oct;85(4):703-10.

- Eison TM, Ault BH, Jones DP et al. Post-streptococcal acute glomerulonephritis in children: clinical features and pathogenesis. Pediatr Nephrol. 2011 Feb;26(2):165-80.

CASE #86: PAINFUL LUMP

CASE

A 47-year-old man presents to his family doctor complaining of sudden onset severe pain to his anus. The pain started while the patient was straining to have a bowel movement. He reports history of similar pain but never that severe.

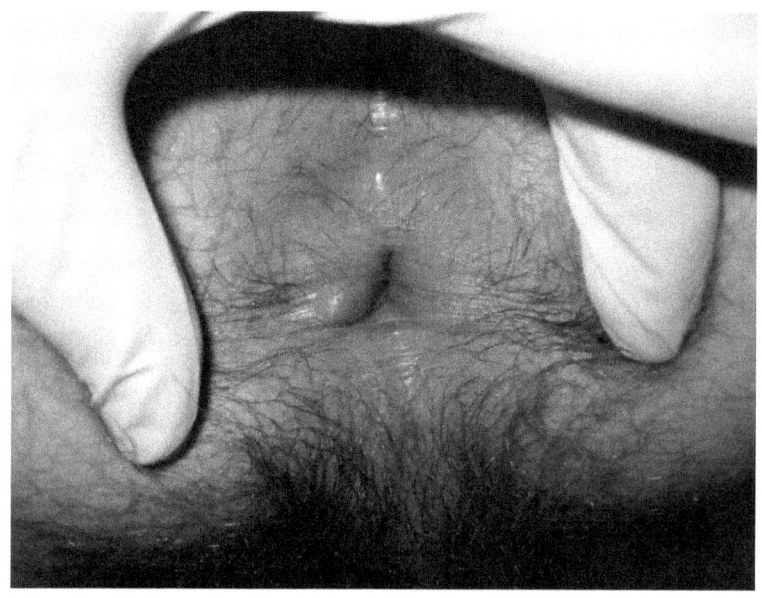

QUESTIONS

278. What is the likely diagnosis?

    a. Anal Carcinoma

    b. Anal Fissure

    c. Anal Wart

    d. Prolapsed Internal Hemorrhoid

    e. Thrombosed External Hemorrhoid

279. Which of the following statements is correct?
    a. Anal carcinoma is more common in patients with chronic diarrhea.
    b. Anal fissures are more common in patients with chronic diarrhea.
    c. External hemorrhoids are located distal to the dentate line and are covered by modified squamous epithelium.
    d. Internal hemorrhoids are located proximal to the dentate line and are not covered by epithelium.

280. Which of the following statements is correct?
    a. Anal fissures commonly cause painless bright red blood per rectum.
    b. Anal skin tags are the result of old thrombosed external hemorrhoids.
    c. Anal warts commonly cause painless bright-red blood per rectum.
    d. Prolapsed internal hemorrhoid rarely cause painless bright-red blood per rectum.

ANSWERS

278. e

279. c

280. b

VISUAL STIMULUS REVIEW

The image shows a thrombosed external hemorrhoid.

REFERENCES

- Ross NP, Hildebrand DR, Tiernan JP et al. Haemorrhoids: 21st-century management. Colorectal Dis. 2012 Aug;14(8):917-9.

- Sneider EB, Maykel JA. Diagnosis and management of symptomatic hemorrhoids. Surg Clin North Am. 2010 Feb;90(1):17-32.

CASE #87: GROIN SWELLING

CASE

A 57-year-old man presents to his family physician complaining of painless masses to his groin increasing in size over the last year. He has no past medical history and is taking no medications. On examination he has normal vital signs and has bilateral nontender, hard, nonmobile groin masses.

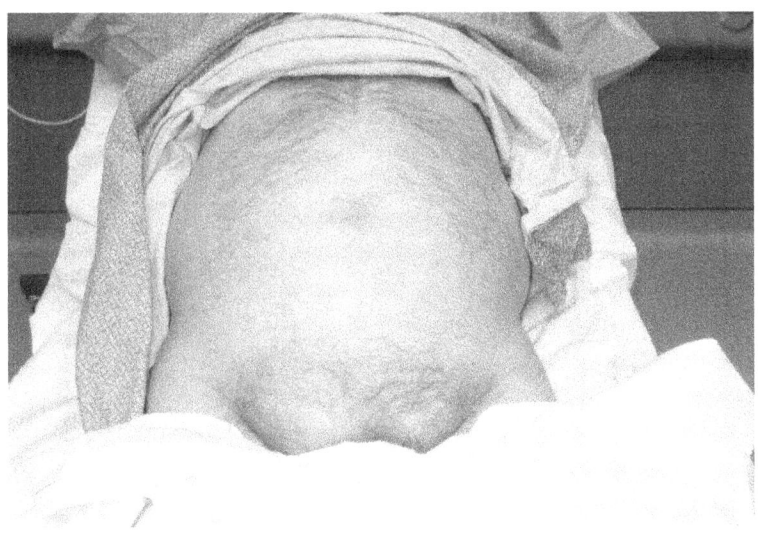

QUESTIONS

281. What is the likely diagnosis?
    a. Acute HIV Infection
    b. Incarcerated Inguinal Hernia
    c. Hodgkin's Lymphoma
    d. Infectious Mononucleosis
    e. Non-Hodgkin's Lymphoma

282. Which of the following is indicated as part of the initial workup of this patient?
    a. Complete Blood Count
    b. Comprehensive Metabolic Panel
    c. HIV Serology
    d. Excisional Lymph Node Biopsy
    e. All of the Above

ANSWERS

281. e

282. e

VISUAL STIMULUS REVIEW

The image shows bilateral groin masses with normal-appearing overlaying skin.

REFERENCES

- Shankland KR, Armitage JO, Hancock BW. Non-Hodgkin lymphoma. Lancet. 2012 Sep 1;380(9844):848-57.

CASE #88: RASH

CASE

A 14-day-old baby boy with a history of full-term spontaneous vaginal delivery and uneventful hospital stay is brought to his pediatrician's office for evaluation of a rash. The parents report that the baby has good PO intake of breast milk every two to three hours and that he wets his diapers every three hours. They describe an erythematous rash to his torso and chin with lesions changing from clear to yellow content and increasing in size over the last two days. On exam the patient has normal vital signs and is not irritable. He also has a normal eye, genital, and oral exam.

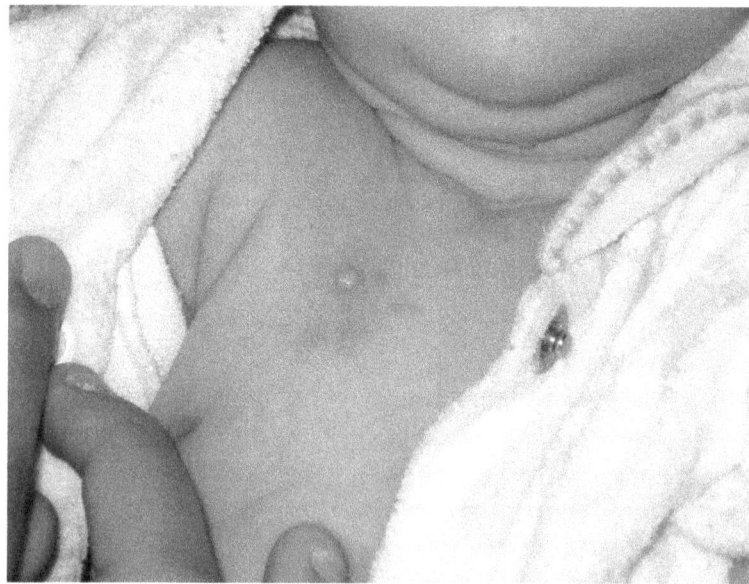

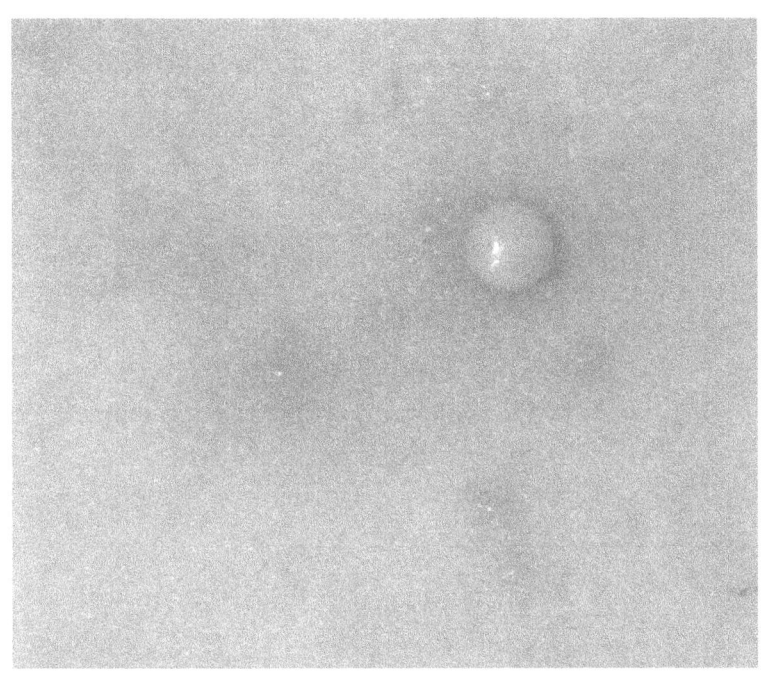

QUESTIONS

283. What is the likely diagnosis?
    a. Candidiasis
    b. Contact Dermatitis
    c. Erythema Toxicum Neonatorum
    d. Hand Foot and Mouth Disease
    e. Neonatal Herpes

284. What is the likely cause?
    a. Candida
    b. Contact Irritants
    c. Coxsackievirus
    d. Herpes Simplex Virus

285. Which of the following provides the highest sensitivity for the diagnosis of this condition?
    a. KOH Preparation
    b. PCR
    c. Punch Biopsy
    d. Serology
    e. Tzanck Smear
    f. Viral Culture

286. Which of the following is the first line therapy for this condition?
    a. Acyclovir IV
    b. Acyclovir PO
    c. Amphotericin IV
    d. Nystatin PO
    e. Prednisolone PO
    f. Symptomatic Care

ANSWERS

283. e

284. d

285. b

286. a

VISUAL STIMULUS REVIEW

The images show clustered vesicle and pustules over an erythematous base over the chin and torso of the newborn.

REFERENCES

- Berardi A, Lugli L, Rossi C et al. Neonatal herpes simplex virus. J Matern Fetal Neonatal Med. 2011 Oct;24 Suppl 1:88-90.

- Corey L, Wald A. Maternal and neonatal herpes simplex virus infections. N Engl J Med. 2009 Oct 1;361(14):1376-85.

CASE #89: SHORTNESS OF BREATH

CASE

A 57-year-old woman with a past medical history of asthma is brought to the emergency department by EMS for sudden onset dyspnea and sharp right-sided chest pain with deep inspiration. She reports no past medical history and a history of a recent road trip in which she was driving her car for 30 hours in three days. Her vital signs are temp 97.8F (36.6C), heart rate 130/min, respiratory rate 36/min, blood pressure 80/60 mmHg, and O$_2$Sat 91% on room air. On physical exam, she has rales over her left lung and mild tender swelling to her right calf.

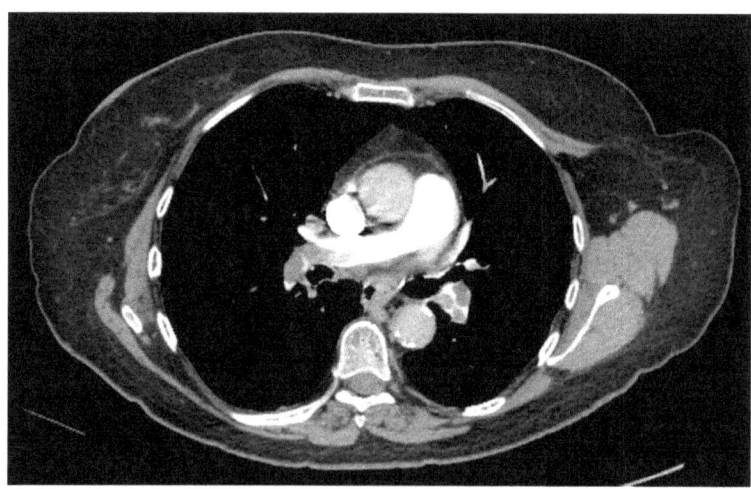

QUESTIONS

287. What is the likely diagnosis?
    a. Aortic Dissection
    b. Asthma Exacerbation
    c. Myocardial Ischemia
    d. Pulmonary Edema
    e. Pulmonary Embolism
    f. Pulmonary Hypertension

288. What is the likely cause of this patient's condition?
    a. Allergan Exposure
    b. Coagulopathy
    c. Coronary Ischemia
    d. Prolonged immobilization
    e. Vasospasm

289. What is the likely cause of this patient's hypoxia?
    a. Alveolar Fluid
    b. Atelectasis
    c. Bronchospasm
    d. Decrease in Surfactant Volume
    e. Ventilation Perfusion Mismatch

290. Which of the following is an acceptable first line therapy for management of this patient?
    a. Albuterol
    b. Aspirin
    c. Heparin IV
    d. Tissue Plasminogen Inhibitor IV
    e. Warfarin

f. Any of the above

291. Which of the following is the treatment of choice for this condition in pregnant patients?

    a. Albuterol

    b. Aspirin

    c. Heparin

    d. Low Molecular Weight Heparin

    e. Tissue Plasminogen Inhibitor

    f. Warfarin

ANSWERS

287. e

288. d

289. e

290. c

291. d

VISUAL STIMULUS REVIEW

The CT image shows a large thrombus in the right pulmonary artery. The left pulmonary artery shows multiple clots.

REFERENCES

- Takach Lapner S, Kearon C. Diagnosis and management of pulmonary embolism. BMJ. 2013 Feb 20;346:f757

- Wilbur J, Shian B. Diagnosis of deep venous thrombosis and pulmonary embolism. Am Fam Physician. 2012 Nov 15;86(10):913-9.

- Schulman S. Advances in the management of venous thromboembolism. Best Pract Res Clin Haematol. 2012 Sep;25(3):361-77.

CASE #90: HIP PAIN

CASE

A 76-year-old woman suffers a ground-level fall after slipping on a wet floor. She has a sudden onset left hip pain, and she isn't able to get up and bear weight on that leg. The patient lives independently in her home and is able to care for her activities of daily living.

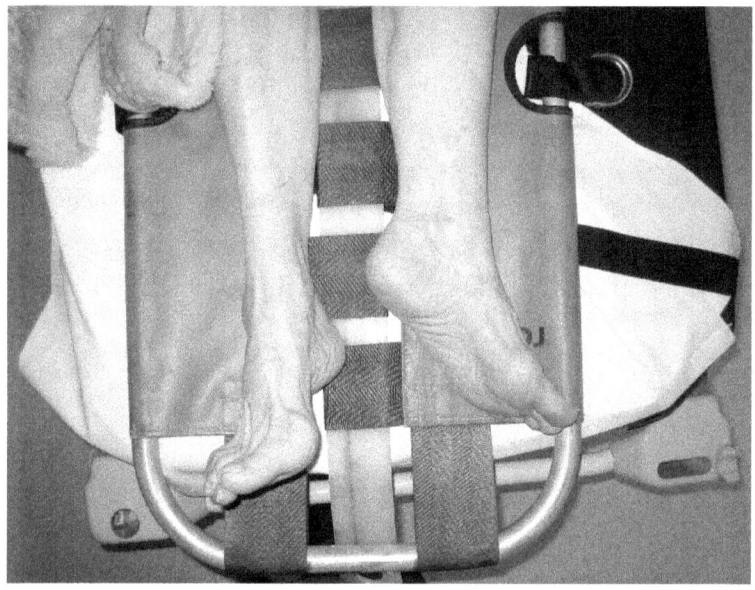

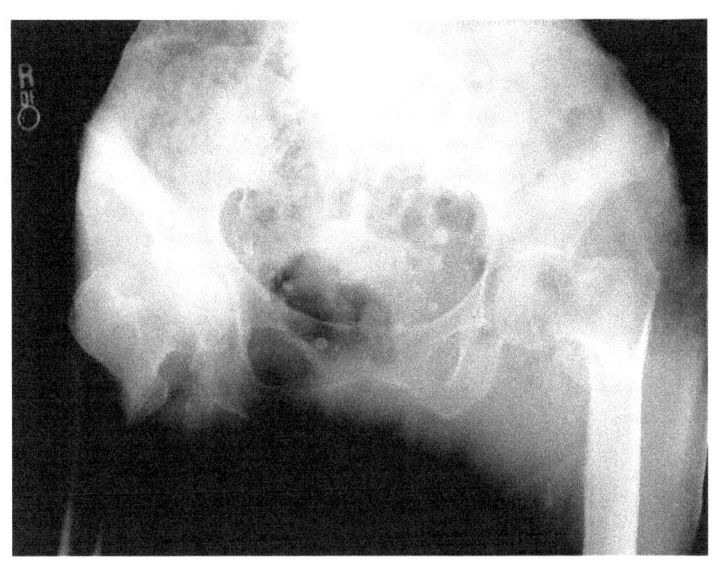
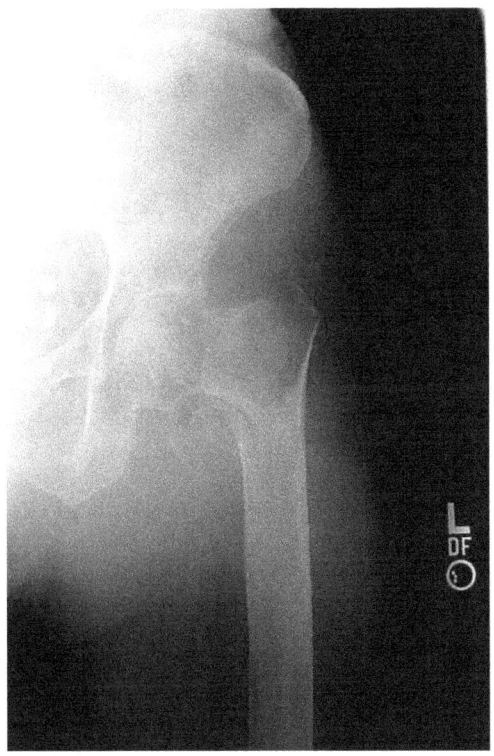

QUESTIONS

292. What is the likely diagnosis?

    a. Femoral Neck Fracture

    b. Intertrochanteric Fracture

    c. Posterior Hip Dislocation

    d. Subtrochanteric Fracture

    e. Trochanteric Fracture

293. What is the recommended treatment for this condition?

    a. Delayed Open Reduction and Internal Reduction within 7 to 14 days.

    b. Early Hemiarthroplasty within 48 hours.

    c. Early Open Reduction and Internal Fixation within 48 hours.

    d. Emergent Closed Reduction in the Emergency Department.

    e. Knee Immobilizer and Early Remobilization

294. Which of the following is a sensitive test for identifying patients with higher risk to suffer from this condition?

    a. Digital X-ray Radiogrammetry (Bone Densitometry) of the Wrist

    b. Serum Calcium (Ionized)

    c. Serum Calcium (Total)

    d. Serum Parathyroid Hormone (PTH)

    e. Serum Vitamin D

295. Which of the following conditions carries the highest risk of blood loss?

    a. Femoral Neck Fracture

b. Intertrochanteric Fracture
c. Posterior Hip Dislocation
d. Subtrochanteric Fracture
e. Trochanteric Fracture

ANSWERS

292. e

293. c

294. a

295. d

VISUAL STIMULUS REVIEW

The gross image shows a shortened left leg, which is externally rotated. The radiographs show an intertrochanteric left femoral fracture.

REFERENCES

- Della Rocca GJ, Crist BD. Hip fracture protocols: what have we changed? Orthop Clin North Am. 2013 Apr;44(2):163-82.
- Warriner AH, Saag KG. Osteoporosis diagnosis and medical treatment. Orthop Clin North Am. 2013 Apr;44(2):125-35.
- Carriero FP, Christmas C. In the clinic. Hip fracture. Ann Intern Med. 2011 Dec 6;155(11):ITC6-1-ITC6-15.

CASE #91: VISION LOSS

CASE

A 65-year-old woman with a past medical history of diabetes mellitus, atrial fibrillation, and hypertension presents to her ophthalmologist complaining that she woke up with moderate headache and loss of vision eight hour ago. The patient is awake with a normal cranial nerve exam, normal speech, and normal gait with no gross motor or sensory exam to bilateral upper and lower extremities. Visual field testing is performed.

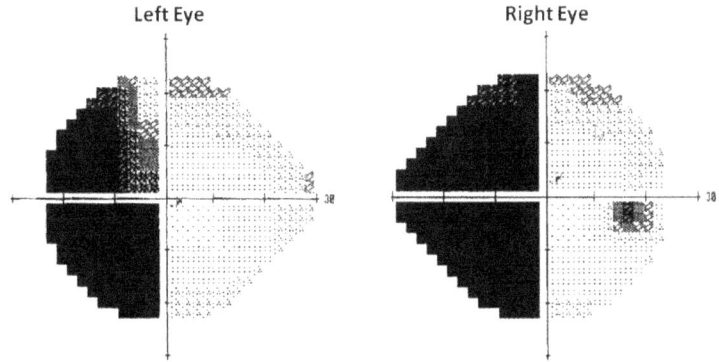

QUESTIONS

296. What is the likely diagnosis?
    a. Binasal Hemianopsia
    b. Bitemporal Hemianopsia
    c. Left Homonymous Hemianopsia
    d. Right Homonymous Hemianopsia
    e. Right Inferior Quadrantanopia

297. What is the likely cause of this condition?
    a. Brain Tumor
    b. Cysticercosis
    c. Neurosyphilis
    d. Stroke
    e. Tertiary Lyme Disease

298. What is the likely location of the pathology?
    a. Optic Chiasm
    b. Optic Tract (Left)
    c. Optic Tract (Right)
    d. Retinal Lesion (OD)
    e. Retinal Lesion (OS)

299. What should be the next diagnostic test in this patient?
    a. Carotid Ultrasound
    b. Echocardiogram
    c. Head CT
    d. Orbital CT
    e. Visual Acuity

ANSWERS

296. c

297. d

298. c

299. c

VISUAL STIMULUS REVIEW

The visual field test report shows near complete left visual field defect (left hemianopia) without macular sparing.

REFERENCES

- Fraser JA, Newman NJ, Biousse V. Disorders of the optic tract, radiation, and occipital lobe. Handb Clin Neurol. 2011;102:205-21.

- Luu S, Lee AW, Daly A, Chen CS. Visual field defects after stroke--a practical guide for GPs. Aust Fam Physician. 2010 Jul;39(7):499-503.

CASE #92: ABDOMINAL PAIN

CASE

A five-year-old boy is brought by his parents to the pediatrician's office complaining of severe abdominal cramps, recurrent vomiting, joint pain, and diffuse rash for 24 hours. The parents recall that the patient had a febrile illness with dry cough and runny nose a week prior that resolved. The patient has a temp of 101.7F (38.7C), heart rate of 128/min, respiratory rate of 24/min, blood pressure of 150/80 mmHg, and O_2Sat of 97 on room air. Physical examination shows that the skin lesions are nonblanching and are palpable and that the distribution is mostly to his bilateral lower extremities and gluteal regions. Bilateral ankle swelling is also noted. The abdomen is diffusely tender with mild guarding over the bilateral lower quadrants.

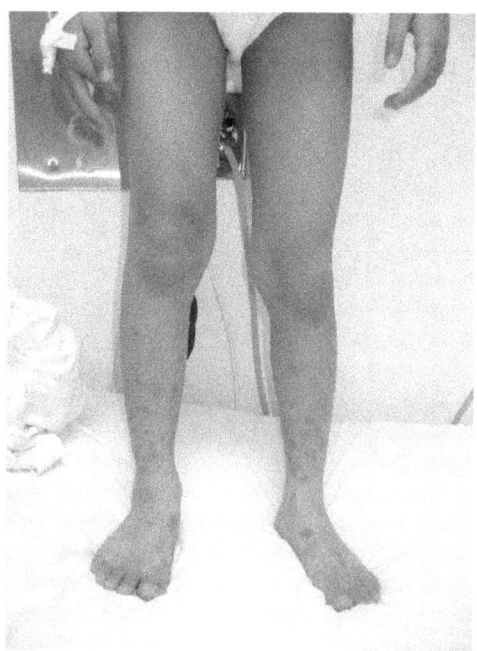

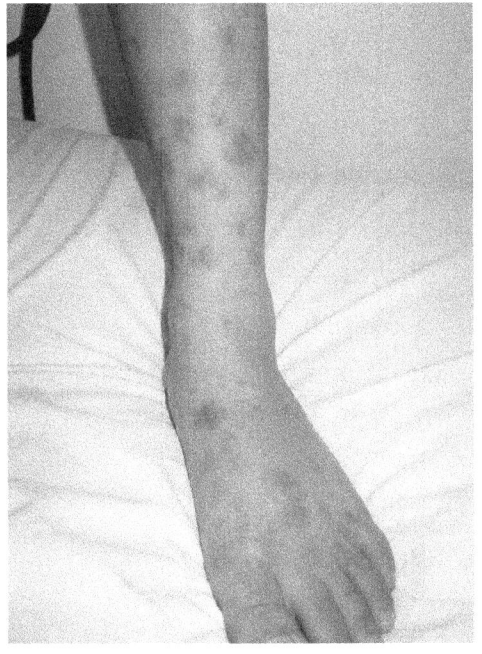

QUESTIONS

300. What is the likely diagnosis?
   a. Bacterial Meningitis
   b. Hemolytic Uremic Syndrome
   c. Henoch-Schönlein purpura
   d. Kawasaki Disease
   e. Viral Meningitis

301. What is the likely primary cause of this condition?
   a. Autoimmune Vasculitis
   b. Bacterial Toxins
   c. Primary Platelet Dysfunction
   d. Secondary Platelet Dysfunction

e. Systemic Inflammatory Response Syndrome

302. Which of the following organisms has been associated with this this condition?

a. Epstein Bar Virus

b. Escherichia coli O157:H7

c. Herpes Simplex Virus Type 1

d. Salmonella

e. Shigella Enterocolitis

303. Which of the following laboratory findings is expected to be present?

a. Hemoglobin 8.5 g/dl

b. PLT 12,000/mm^3

c. Serum Creatinine 0.7 mg/dl

d. WBC 500/μl

e. Urine RBCs >10

ANSWERS

300. c
301. a
302. a
303. e

VISUAL STIMULUS REVIEW

The images show bilateral lower extremity petechiae and purpuric lesion as well as bilateral ankle swelling.

REFERENCES

- Weiss PF. Pediatric vasculitis. Pediatr Clin North Am. 2012 Apr;59(2):407-23.
- Davin JC. Henoch-Schonlein purpura nephritis: pathophysiology, treatment, and future strategy.
- Saulsbury FT. Henoch-Schönlein purpura. Curr Opin Rheumatol. 2010 Sep;22(5):598-602.

CASE #93: PAINFUL LESIONS

CASE

A 27-year-old man presents to his family doctor complaining of severe pain to his penis lasting four days. He reports having a casual sexual encounter with a female about 10 days prior. He reports fevers up to 102.4F (39.1C), myalgias, and severe malaise and denies joint aches or other skin lesions. He reports that the lesions start as clear fluid-filled blisters that rapidly rupture and turn into painful sores. He denies having a history of sexually transmitted disease. He has a normal oropharyngeal exam and bilateral inguinal lymphadenopathy.

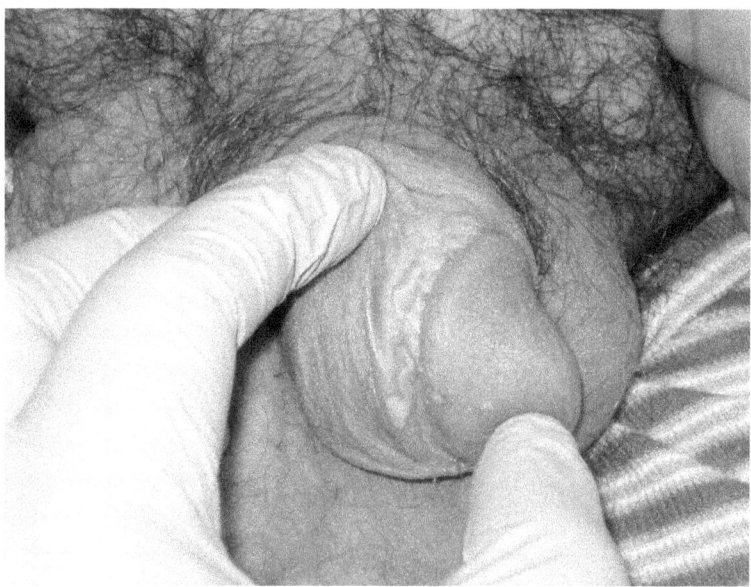

QUESTIONS

304. What is the likely diagnosis?
    a. Behçet's disease
    b. Candidiasis
    c. Chancre
    d. Chancroid
    e. Herpes Simplex

305. What is the likely cause of this condition?
    a. Autoimmunity
    b. Candida Albicans
    c. Hemophilus Ducreyi
    d. Herpes Simplex Virus
    e. Treponema Pallidum

306. Definitive diagnosis of this condition may be achieved using which of the following?
    a. Antibody Titers
    b. Dark Field Microscopy
    c. KOH Preparation
    d. Gram Stain
    e. Pathergy Test
    f. PCR of Ulcer Scraping

ANSWERS

304. e

305. d

306. f

VISUAL STIMULUS REVIEW

The image shows multiple shallow ulcers to the foreskin and glans penis.

REFERENCES

- Roett MA, Mayor MT, Uduhiri KA. Diagnosis and management of genital ulcers. Am Fam Physician. 2012 Feb 1;85(3):254-62.
- Workowski KA, Berman S; Centers for Disease Control and Prevention. Sexually transmitted diseases treatment guidelines, 2010 [published correction appears in MMWR Recomm Rep. 2011;60(1):18]. MMWR Recomm Rep. 2010;59(RR-12):1-110.

CASE #94: NECK PAIN

CASE

A 30-year-old unrestrained female driver is brought to the emergency department following a high-speed motor vehicle accident in which she was ejected from her car. She is alert and oriented and complains of some neck pain and tingling to both her hands. On physical examination she has normal vital signs and no gross motor deficit to her upper or lower extremities. She complains of subjective numbness to her bilateral upper extremities. Both her triceps reflexes are decreased.

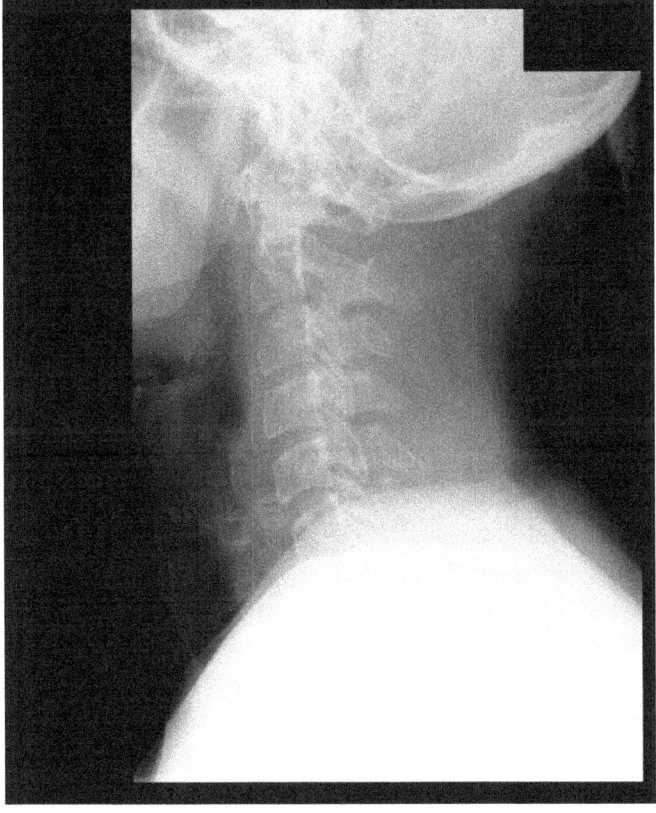

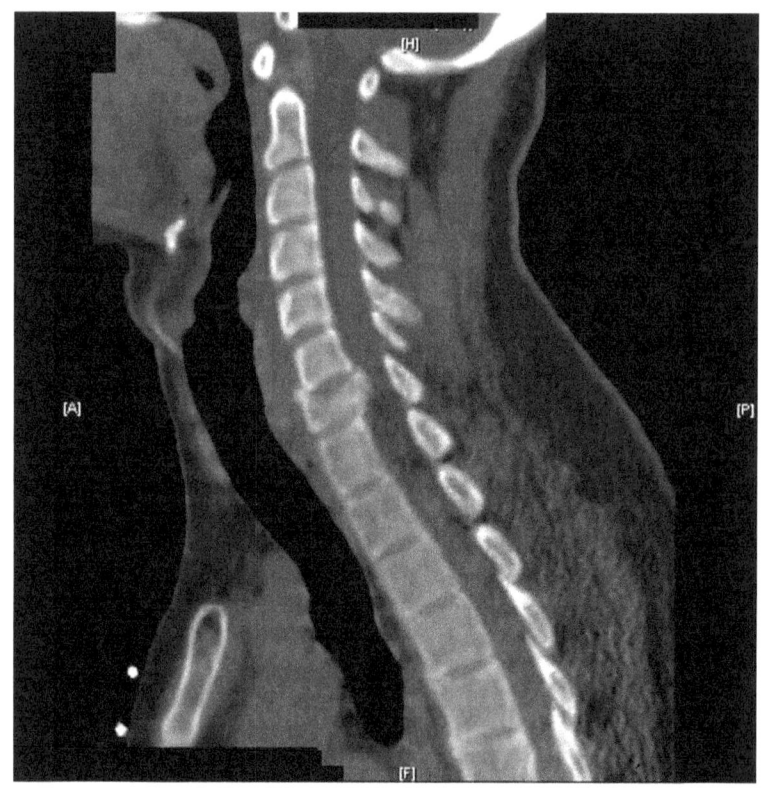

QUESTIONS

307. What is the likely diagnosis?
- a. Tear Drop Fracture
- b. C6 Fracture
- c. C7 Fracture
- d. Hangman's Fracture
- e. Jefferson's Fracture

308. What vertebral element is fractured?
    a. Articulating Surface
    b. Body
    c. Lamina
    d. Pedicle

309. What is the likely cause of her neurological symptoms?
    a. Bleeding into the Spinal Canal
    b. Direct Compression by Bony Fragments
    c. Spinal Cord Contusion
    d. Hyperflexion Mechanism and Spinal Shock Syndrome

310. Upon return from the CT suite, the patient's vital signs are blood pressure 72/40 mmHg, heart rate 36/min, respirations 12/min, O$_2$Sat 99%, and her skin is now flushed, dry, and warm to the touch. She is able to move both her feet and arms. What is the likely cause of this change?
    a. Allergic Reaction to the IV Contrast
    b. Brown-Séquard Syndrome
    c. Neurogenic Shock
    d. Spinal Shock

ANSWERS

307. c

308. b

309. b

310. c

VISUAL STIMULUS REVIEW

The plain film does not show any pathology as it is inadequate. The CT image shows a compression fracture of C7 with posterior protrusion into the spinal canal.

REFERENCES

- Pimentel L, Diegelmann L. Evaluation and management of acute cervical spine trauma. Emerg Med Clin North Am. 2010 Nov;28(4):719-38.
- Looby S, Flanders A. Spine trauma. Radiol Clin North Am. 2011 Jan;49(1):129-63.

CASE #95: WEAKNESS

CASE

A 70-year-old woman is brought to the emergency department for general fatigue and weakness as well as watery diarrhea for four days. The patient has a history of hypertension and diabetes type 2. Upon walking into the exam room, you notice that the patient just fainted on her stretcher. She is breathing comfortably, and she has a palpable weak radial pulse at about 80/min. Looking at the cardiac monitor, you notice the following rhythm.

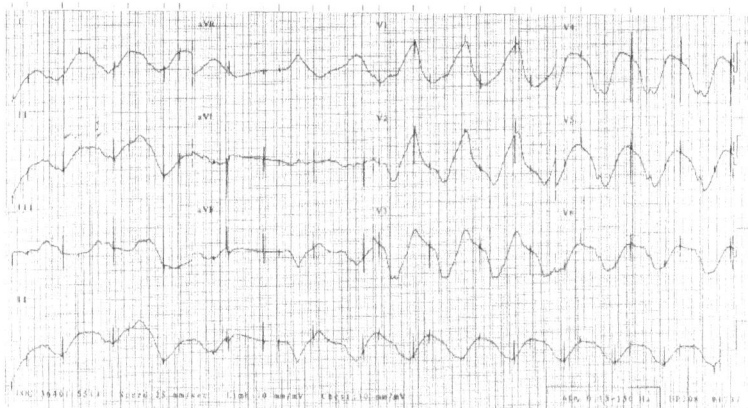

QUESTIONS

311. What is the likely diagnosis?

    a. Hypercalcemia

    b. Hyperkalemia

    c. Hypocalcemia

    d. Hypokalemia

    e. Torsade Du Point

312. Which of the following medications should be given to the patient first in an attempt to normalize her EKG?

    a. Atropine IV

    b. Calcium Chloride IV

    c. Epinephrine IV

    d. Magnesium Sulphate IV

    e. Potassium Chloride IV

313. Definitive management of this patient will likely require an emergent…

    a. Hemodialysis

    b. Infusion of Potassium Chloride 80 meq

    c. Infusion of Normal Saline 3000 ml

    d. Pacemaker Electrode Repositioning Under Fluoroscopy

    e. Plasmapheresis

ANSWERS

311. b

312. b

313. a

VISUAL STIMULUS REVIEW

The electrocardiogram shows sinusoidal tracing and pacer spikes.

REFERENCES

- Elliott MJ, Ronksley PE, Clase CM, Ahmed SB, Hemmelgarn BR. Management of patients with acute hyperkalemia. CMAJ. 2010 Oct 19;182(15):1631-5.
- Nyirenda MJ, Tang JI, Padfield PL, Seckl JR. Hyperkalaemia. BMJ. 2009 Oct 23;339:b4114.

CASE #96: EYE PAIN

CASE

A 15-year-old boy is brought to his pediatrician after suffering a baseball injury to his left eye. His vision is OS 20/20 OS 20/20, and he has no tenderness over his facial bones. He has normal and painless extra ocular movements. He denies any diplopia.

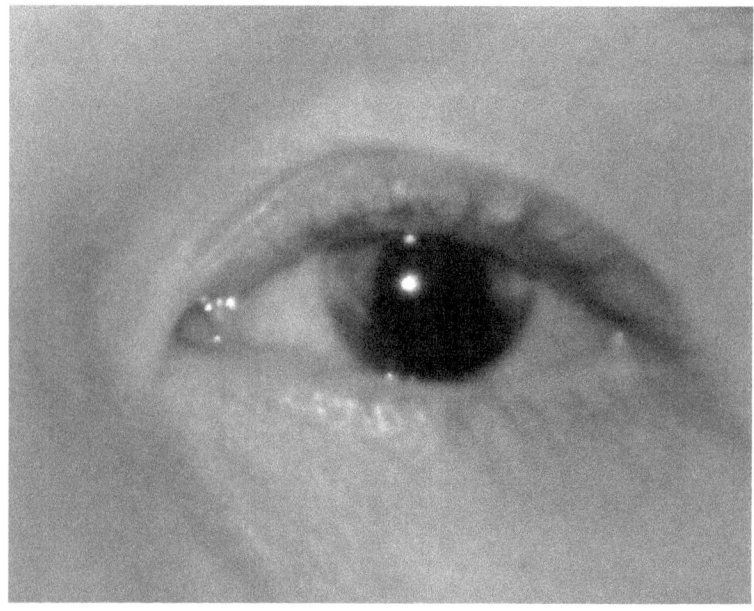

QUESTIONS

314. What is the likely diagnosis?

   a. Acute Glaucoma

   b. Hemorrhagic Conjunctivitis

   c. Hyphema

   d. Subconjunctival Hemorrhage

   e. Hypopyon

315. Which of the following conditions is a known risk factor for short- and long-term complications of this condition?

   a. Cataract

   b. Diabetes Mellitus

   c. Myopia

   d. Hypertension

   e. Sickle Cell Disease

316. Which of the following treatments is recommended for patients with this condition?

   a. Aspirin

   b. Bed Rest with Head on Bed Elevation

   c. Bed Rest in the Supine Position

   d. Eye Patching

ANSWERS

314. c

315. e

316. b

VISUAL STIMULUS REVIEW

The image shows scleral injection (erythema) and blood in the anterior chamber (hyphema).

REFERENCES

- Kirschner J, Seupaul RA. Do medical interventions for traumatic hyphema reduce the risk of vision loss? Ann Emerg Med. 2012 Aug;60(2):197-8.
- Gharaibeh A, Savage HI, Scherer RW et al. Medical interventions for traumatic hyphema. Cochrane Database Syst Rev. 2011 Jan 19;(1):CD005431.
- Cass SP. Ocular injuries in sports. Curr Sports Med Rep. 2012 Jan-Feb;11(1):11-5.

CASE #97: WEAKNESS

CASE

A 68-year-old man with a past medical history of hypertension and diabetes mellitus type 2 presents to his family doctor complaining of fatigue and severe muscle weakness that developed over the last five days. He also reports a few episodes of palpitations and near syncope earlier that morning. His vital signs are within normal limits, and his neurological exam shows symmetric generalized large and small muscles weakness with no focal motor deficit or sensory abnormalities.

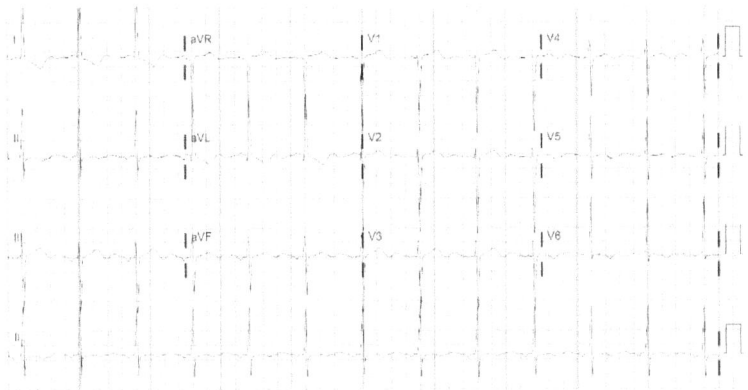

QUESTIONS

317. What is the likely diagnosis?

    a. Hypercalcemia

    b. Hypocalcemia

    c. Hyperkalemia

    d. Hypokalemia

    e. Myasthenia Gravis

318. What is the likely cause of this condition in this patient?

    a. Autoimmunity

    b. Eating Disorders

    c. Echinacea Intake

    d. Furosemide

    e. Spironolactone

319. Which of the following is part of the initial management of this condition?

    a. Normal Saline IV

    b. Calcium Gluconate IV

    c. Insulin + Glucose IV

    d. Potassium Chloride PO

    e. Neostigmine

320. Which of the following IV solutions should be avoided in this patient?

    a. D5W

    b. Normal Saline

    c. Normal Saline + KCL 20 meq/l

    d. Lactated Ringer's

    e. Saline 0.45% + KCL 20 meq/l

ANSWERS

317. d

318. d

319. d

320. a

VISUAL STIMULUS REVIEW

The electrocardiogram shows decreased amplitude of P waves and a classic u wave.

REFERENCES

- Kaplan LJ, Kellum JA. Fluids, pH, ions and electrolytes. Curr Opin Crit Care. 2010 Aug;16(4):323-31.

- Cohen JD, Neaton JD, Prineas RJ, Daniels KA. Diuretics, serum potassium and ventricular arrhythmias in the Multiple Risk Factor Intervention Trial. Am J Cardiol. 60(7):548-54.

- Materson BJ. Diuretics, potassium, and ventricular ectopy. Am J Hypertens. May 1997;10(5 Pt 2):68S-72S.

CASE #98: LLQ PAIN

CASE

A 63-year-old man presents to the emergency department for worsening left-sided abdominal pain over the last four days as well as nausea, vomiting, and bloody diarrhea. He reports an eight-month history of weight loss and constipation. On physical examination he has a temp of 98.9F (37.2C), heart rate of 106/min, blood pressure of 140/70, and O_2Sat of 99% on room air. His abdomen is distended with decreased bowel sounds and tenderness to the left lower quadrant with guarding. His rectal exam shows currant jelly stool.

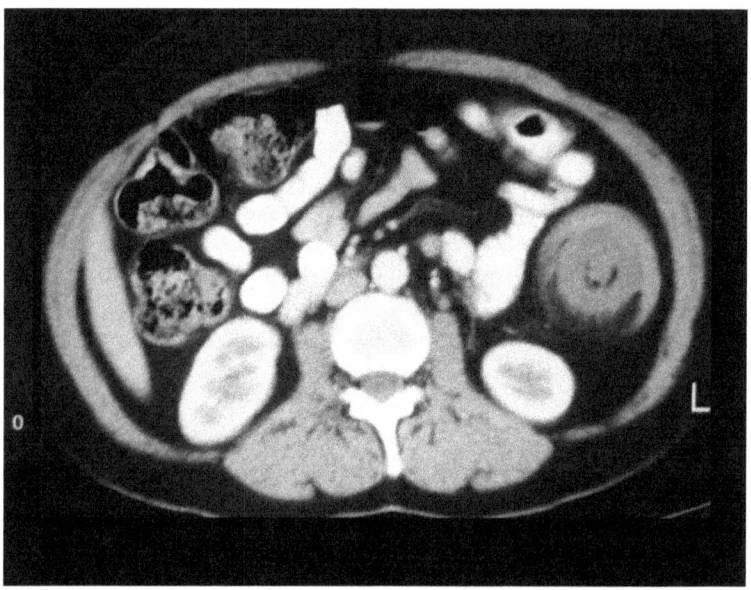

QUESTIONS

321. What is the likely diagnosis?
    a. Gastroenteritis
    b. Intussusception
    c. Mesenteric Ischemia
    d. Retroperitoneal Hematoma
    e. Volvulus

322. What is the likely cause of this condition?
    a. Atherosclerosis
    b. Chronic Constipation
    c. Colonic Tumor
    d. Low Fiber Diet
    e. Obesity

323. What is the recommended first line treatment for this condition?
    a. Air Enema
    b. Barium Enema
    c. Conservative Management
    d. Decompressing Colonoscopy
    e. Operative Reduction

ANSWERS

321. b

322. c

323. e

VISUAL STIMULUS REVIEW

The CT image shows a target appearing soft tissue mass in the left-lower quadrant.

REFERENCES

- Marinis A, Yiallourou A, Samanides L et al. Intussusception of the bowel in adults: a review. World J Gastroenterol. 2009 Jan 28;15(4):407-11.

- Kim YH, Blake MA, Harisinghani MG et al. Adult intestinal intussusception: CT appearances and identification of a causative lead point. Radiographics. 2006 May-Jun;26(3):733-44.

CASE #99: BLEEDING GUMS

CASE

A 12-year-old boy is brought to his pediatrician's office by his parents for bleeding gums and bruising for two days. He has no past medical history and is taking no medications. His parents report an influenza-like illness that he had two weeks prior with fever, sore throat, and dry cough that resolved about a week ago. He denies any nosebleed or bloody diarrhea. His vital signs are within normal limits, and he is well-appearing. Skin exam shows multiple areas of petechiae and purpura. His lungs and abdomen exam is unremarkable. A blood smear is ordered.

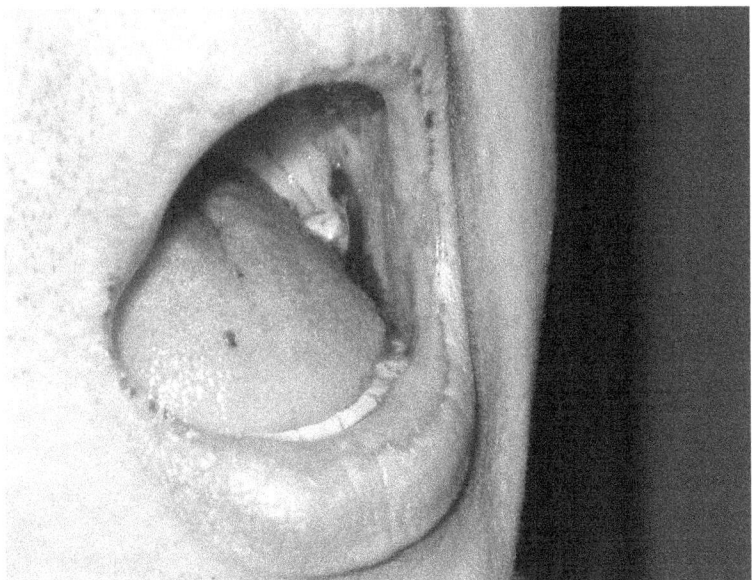

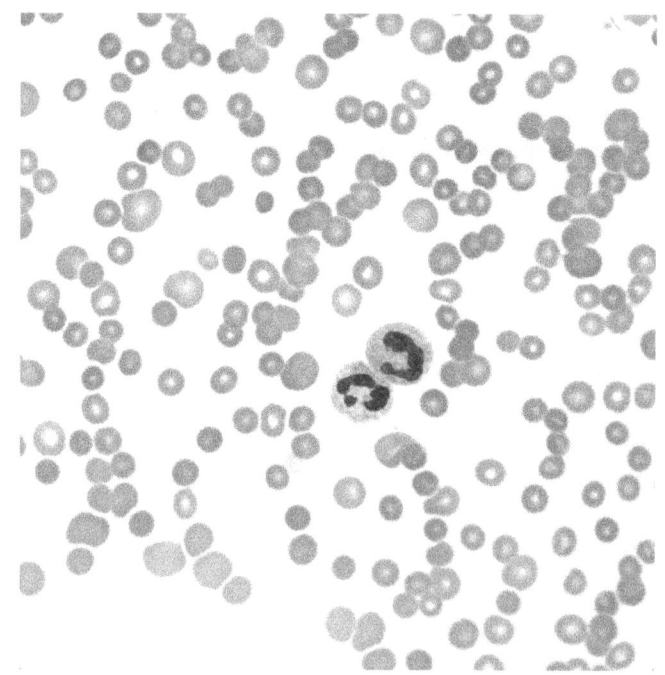

QUESTIONS

324. What is the likely diagnosis?

    a. Acute Leukemia

    b. Aplastic Anemia

    c. Disseminated Intravascular Coagulation (DIC)

    d. Immune Thrombocytopenia Purpura (ITP)

    e. Thrombotic Thrombocytopenia Purpura (TTP)

325. What is the likely cause of this condition?

   a. Bacterial Toxins
   b. Bone Marrow Malignant Transformation
   c. Epstein Bar Virus
   d. IgA Autoantibody
   e. IgG Autoantibody

326. Which of the following laboratory findings is expected to be present?

   a. Hemoglobin 6.5 g/dl
   b. PLT 12,000/mm3
   c. Serum Creatinine 3.7 mg/dl
   d. WBC 90,000/µl
   e. INR 3.8

327. Which of the following represents the first line of therapy for this condition?

   a. Antibiotics
   b. IVIG
   c. Plasma Pheresis
   d. Rituximab
   e. Splenectomy

ANSWERS

324. d

325. e

326. b

327. b

VISUAL STIMULUS REVIEW

The gross image shows bleeding from the oral mucosa. The blood smear slide shows normal morphology of red blood cells, and leukocytes is normal near absence of thrombocytes.

REFERENCES

- D'Orazio JA, Neely J, Farhoudi N. ITP in children: pathophysiology and current treatment approaches. J Pediatr Hematol Oncol. 2013 Jan;35(1):1-13.

- Neunert C, Lim W, Crowther M et al. The American Society of Hematology 2011 evidence-based practice guideline for immune thrombocytopenia. Blood. 2011 Apr 21;117(16):4190-207.

CASE #100: SHORTNESS OF BREATH

CASE

A 68-year-old man is brought to the emergency department by EMS for sudden onset shortness of breath and diaphoresis. He has a known history of hypertension and is compliant with his medications. He denies having chest pain and reports that he woke up from sleep feeling short of breath. His vital signs are temp 99.7F (37.6C), heart rate 106/min, blood pressure 210/120 mmHg, respiratory rate of 38/min, and O$_2$Sat 91% on room air. On physical examination he is awake and alert and in severe respiratory distress with bilateral rales on lungs auscultation.

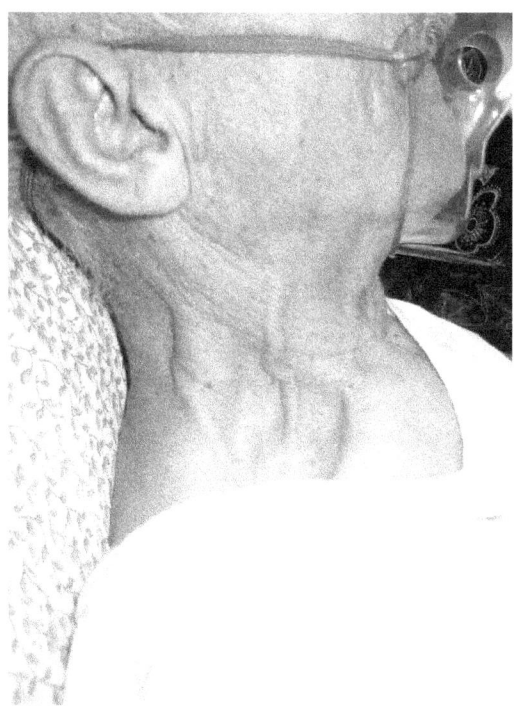

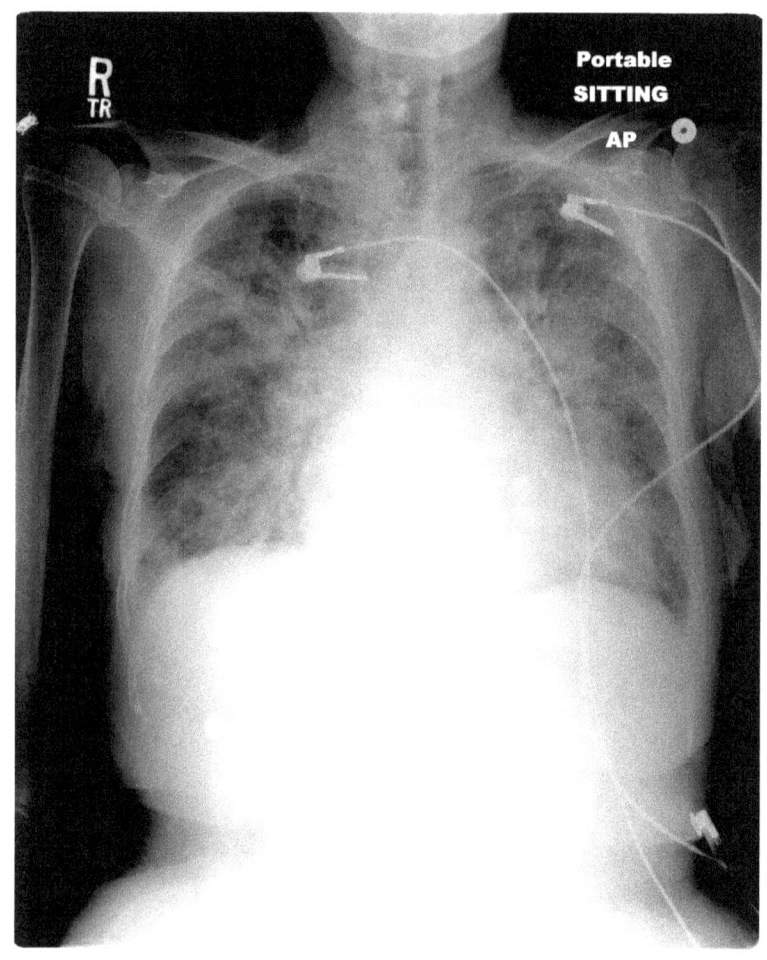

QUESTIONS

328. What is the likely diagnosis?
    a. Cardiogenic Pulmonary Edema
    b. Chronic Obstructive Pulmonary Disease
    c. Pneumonia
    d. Pulmonary Embolism
    e. Pulmonary Hypertension

329. Which of the following is the likely cause of this condition?

   a. Bacterial Infection
   b. Ischemic Heart Disease
   c. Hypercoagulable State
   d. Tobacco Abuse
   e. Viral Infection

330. Which of the following is the diagnostic standard for the diagnosis of this condition?

   a. Angiogram
   b. Blood Culture
   c. Echocardiogram
   d. Lung Biopsy
   e. Pulmonary Function Testing

331. Which of the following is included in the first line of treatment of this condition?

   a. Beta Agonist Inhalation
   b. Endothelin Receptor Antagonist
   c. IV Antibiotics
   d. Noninvasive Pressure-Support Ventilation
   e. Tissue Plasminogen Activator IV

ANSWERS

328. a

329. b

330. c

331. d

VISUAL STIMULUS REVIEW

The gross image shows significant jugular vein distention in this sitting upright patient. The chest radiogram shows cephalization of pulmonary vasculature and bilateral patchy alveolar infiltrates.

REFERENCES

- King M, Kingery J, Casey B. Diagnosis and evaluation of heart failure. Am Fam Physician. 2012 Jun 15;85(12):1161-8.
- Brown JR, Gottlieb SS. Acute decompensated heart failure. Cardiol Clin. 2012 Nov;30(4):665-71.

CASE #101: RASH AND WEIGHT LOSS

CASE

A 45-year-old man presents to his family doctor complaining of dark skin lesions that appeared over the last six months. He reports 30 lbs weight loss over the last 12 months.

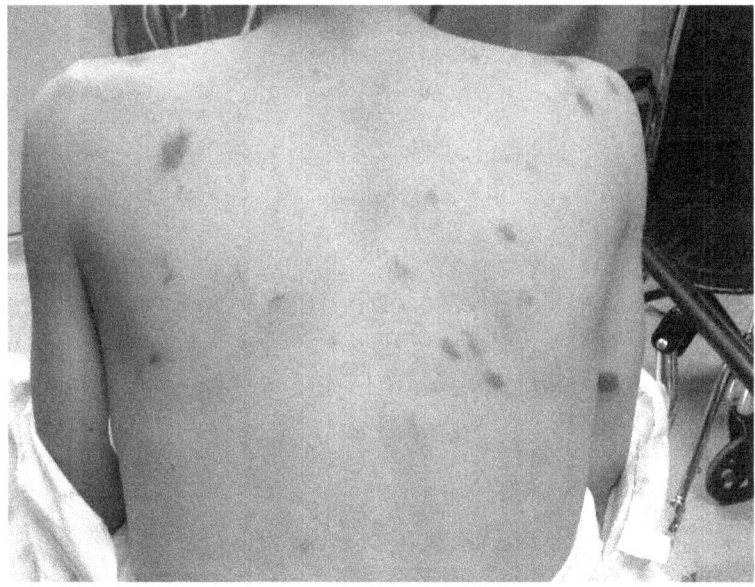

QUESTIONS

332. What is the likely diagnosis?
    a. Bacillary Angiomatosis
    b. Kaposi's Sarcoma
    c. Malignant Melanoma
    d. Port Wine Stains
    e. Squamous Cell Carcinoma

333. What is the likely cause of this condition?
    a. Bartonella Henselae
    b. Congenital Vascular Malformation
    c. Human Herpes Virus - 8
    d. Sun-Induced Malignant Transformation
    e. Platelet Dysfunction

334. Which of the following treatments can lead to remission of this condition?
    a. Antiretroviral Therapy
    b. Laser Therapy
    c. Local Chemotherapy
    d. Local Excision
    e. Radiation Therapy
    f. Systemic Chemotherapy

ANSWERS

332. b

333. c

334. a

VISUAL STIMULUS REVIEW

The patient has multiple brown- to violaceous-colored plaques that seem to follow the Langer lines.

REFERENCES

- Radu O, Pantanowitz L. Kaposi sarcoma. Arch Pathol Lab Med. 2013 Feb;137(2):289-94.

- Lacombe JM, Boue F, Grabar S, Viget N, Gazaignes S, et al. Risk of Kaposi sarcoma during the first months on combination antiretroviral therapy. AIDS. Feb 20 2013;27(4):635-643.

- Jacobson LP, Jenkins FJ, Springer G, et al. Interaction of human immunodeficiency virus type 1 and human herpesvirus type 8 infections on the incidence of Kaposi's sarcoma. J Infect Dis. Jun 2000;181(6):1940-9.

CASE #102: PAINFUL LUMP

CASE

A 37-year-old female patient presents to her family doctor's office complaining of a painful pruritic lesion that started growing six months earlier after she had her right ear pierced. She denies any fever or chills, recent trauma, or drainage from her ear. On exam the right ear mass is rubbery to palpation.

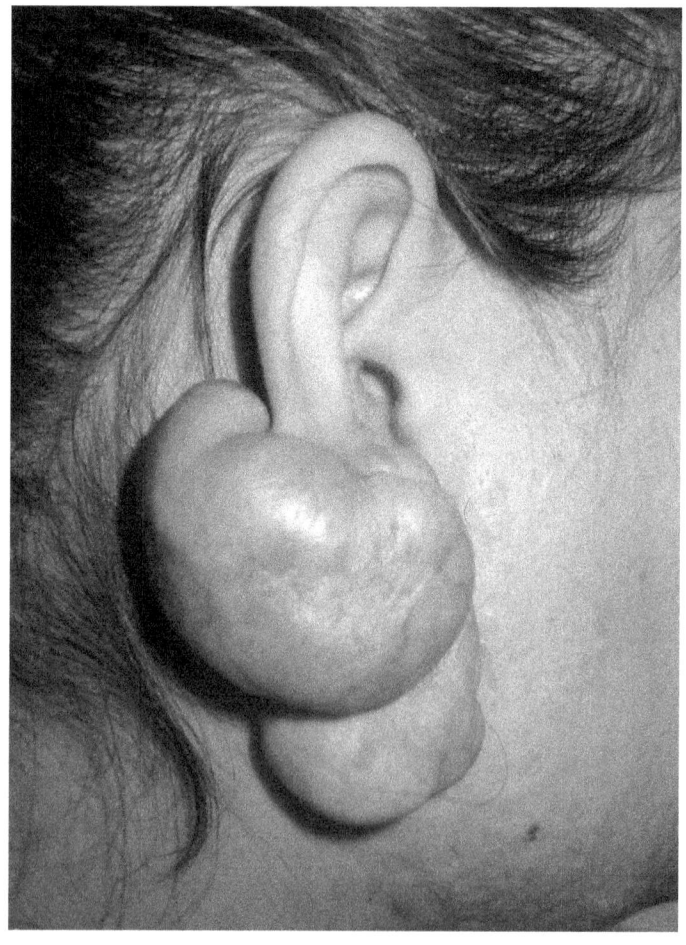

QUESTIONS

335. What is the likely diagnosis?

   a. Furuncular Myiasis

   b. Hypertrophic Scar

   c. Keloid

   d. Lipoma

   e. Squamous Cell Carcinoma

   f. Tuberculoma

336. Which of the following is a known risk factor for this condition?

   a. Botfly Exposure

   b. Chronic Inflammation

   c. Homelessness

   d. Hypertriglyceridemia

   e. Sun Exposure

337. Which of the following offers a reasonable chance of five years' cure for this condition?

   a. Antibiotic Therapy

   b. Local Excision

   c. Local Steroid Injection

   d. Intralesional Lidocaine Injection

   e. Wide Excision

   f. b and c

ANSWERS

335. c

336. b

337. f

VISUAL STIMULUS REVIEW

The image shows an erythematous mass to the right earlobe.

REFERENCES

- Profyris C, Tziotzios C, Do Vale I. Cutaneous scarring: Pathophysiology, molecular mechanisms, and scar reduction therapeutics Part I. The molecular basis of scar formation. J Am Acad Dermatol. 2012 Jan;66(1):1-10.

- Tziotzios C, Profyris C, Sterling J. Cutaneous scarring: Pathophysiology, molecular mechanisms, and scar reduction therapeutics Part II. Strategies to reduce scar formation after dermatologic procedures. J Am Acad Dermatol. 2012 Jan;66(1):13-24.

- Sidle DM, Kim H. Keloids: prevention and management. Facial Plast Surg Clin North Am. 2011 Aug;19(3):505-15.

- Viera MH, Caperton CV, Berman B. Advances in the treatment of keloids. Drugs Dermatol. 2011 May;10(5):468-80.

CASE #103: ABDOMINAL PAIN

CASE

A-70-year-old demented nursing home resident is brought to the emergency department by EMS for sudden onset abdominal pain and vomiting. The patient is complaining of diffuse cramping abdominal pain that started two hours before presentation. On physician examination, his vital signs are temp 99.2F (37.3C), heart rate 100/min, blood pressure 140/70 mmHg, and O_2Sat 97% on room air. His abdomen is markedly distended, tympanic, and diffusely tender.

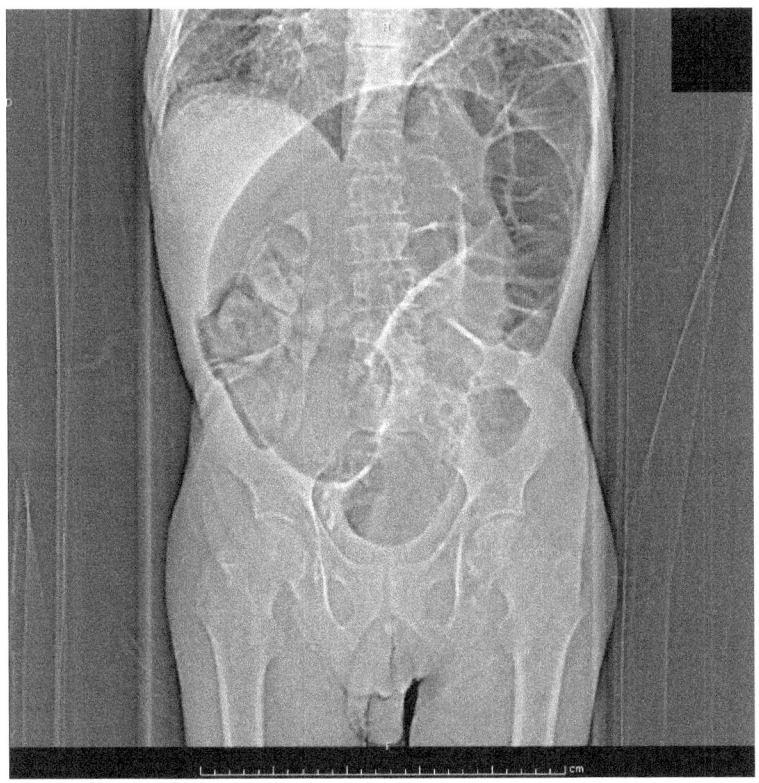

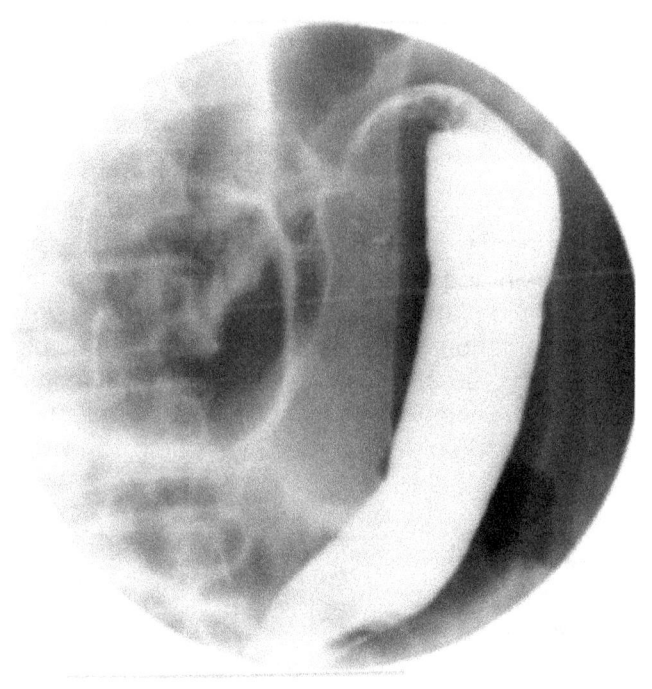

QUESTIONS

338. What is the likely diagnosis?
- a. Cecal Volvulus
- b. Complete Small Bowel Obstruction
- c. Ileus
- d. Partial Small Bowel Obstruction
- e. Mesenteric Artery Thrombosis

f. Sigmoid Volvulus

339. What is a known risk factor for this condition?
   a. Atrial Fibrillation
   b. Chronic Constipation
   c. History of Appendectomy
   d. Incomplete Dorsal Mesenteric Fixation of the Cecum
   e. Peripheral Vascular Disease

340. What is the first line therapy of this condition?
   a. Angiogram and SMA Stenting
   b. Decompression by Nasogastric Tube
   c. Detorsion by Colonoscopy
   d. Heparin IV
   e. Right Hemicolectomy
   f. Sigmoidectomy

341. Which of the following provides a definitive treatment for this condition?
   a. Right Hemicolectomy
   b. SMA Stenting
   c. Small Bowel Resection
   d. Sigmoidectomy
   e. Warfarin
   f. None of the above as spontaneous resolution is expected

ANSWERS

338. f

339. b

340. c

341. d

VISUAL STIMULUS REVIEW

The scout CT image shows a massively dilated loop of sigmoid colon extending to the diaphragm. The barium enema image shows a beaklike termination at the point of the sigmoid volvulus.

REFERENCES

- Osiro SB, Cunningham D, Shoja MM et al. The twisted colon: a review of sigmoid volvulus. Am Surg. 2012 Mar;78(3):271-9.
- Raveenthiran V, Madiba TE, Atamanalp SS, De U. Volvulus of the sigmoid colon. Colorectal Dis. 2010 Jul;12(7 Online):e1-17.

CASE #104: GROIN PAIN

CASE

A 20-year-old man presents to his family doctor complaining of a painful mass to his left groin for the last two weeks. He reports having unprotected sexual encounters with other men and recalls a painless ulcer to his glans penis about four weeks ago that completely resolved within a week. On physical examination, he has a painful fluctuant mass to his left groin and otherwise a normal genital and anorectal exam.

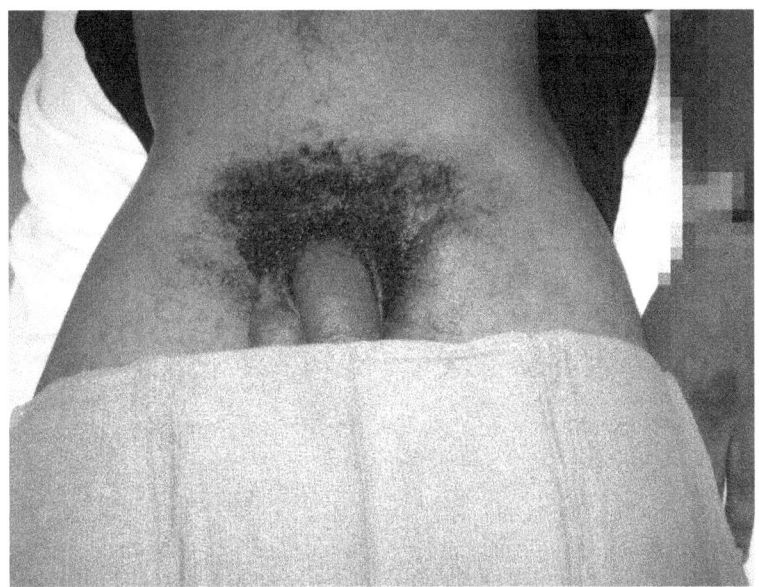

QUESTIONS

342. What is the likely diagnosis?
   a. Cat Scratch Disease
   b. Chancre

- c. Chancroid
- d. Granuloma Inguinalis
- e. Hodgkin's Lymphoma
- f. Lymphogranuloma Venereum

343. What is the likely cause of this condition
    - a. Bartonella Henselae
    - b. Chlamydia Trachomatis
    - c. Epstein Bar Virus
    - d. Haemophilus Ducreyi
    - e. Klebsiella Granulomatis
    - f. Treponema Pallidum

344. What is the common presentation of this condition in female patients?
    - a. Dysuria
    - b. Fever, Fatigue, and Weight Loss
    - c. Proctocolitis
    - d. Vulvar Ulcers
    - e. Vaginitis

345. Which of the following is part of the first line treatment of this condition?
    - a. Amoxicillin Clavulanate
    - b. Ceftriaxone
    - c. Doxycycline
    - d. Penicillin
    - e. Prednisone

ANSWERS

342. f

343. b

344. c

345. c

VISUAL STIMULUS REVIEW

The image shows a classic Bubo, which is a tender, purulent inguinal lymph node.

REFERENCES

- Roett MA, Mayor MT, Uduhiri KA. Diagnosis and management of genital ulcers. Am Fam Physician. 2012 Feb 1;85(3):254-62.

- White JA. Manifestations and management of lymphogranuloma venereum. Curr Opin Infect Dis. 2009 Feb;22(1):57-66.

CASE #105: ITCHY SCALP

CASE

A 5-year-old girl is brought to her pediatrician by her parents complaining of itching scalp for four days.

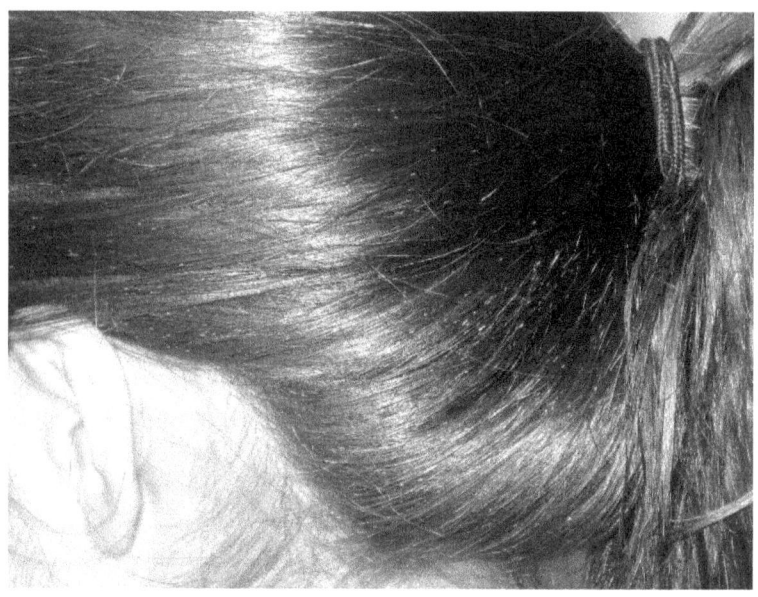

QUESTIONS

346. What is the likely diagnosis?
    a. Dandruff
    b. Pediculosis
    c. Psoriasis
    d. Seborrheic Dermatitis
    e. Scabies
    f. Tinea Capitis

347. What is the likely cause of this condition?
    a. Allergan Exposure
    b. Dermatophyte
    c. Lice
    d. Scabies Mites

348. How is this condition transmitted?
    a. Body Fluid
    b. Close Physical Contact and Fomites
    c. Direct Physical Contact
    d. Genetic
    e. None of the Above

349. Which of the following is recommended as a first line treatment for this condition?
    a. Ivermectin PO
    b. Scalp Shaving
    c. Steroid Lotion
    d. Permethrin Lotion
    e. Prednisone (PO)

ANSWERS

346. b

347. c

348. b

349. d

VISUAL STIMULUS REVIEW

The image shows hair nits.

REFERENCES

- Gunning K, Pippitt K, Kiraly B, Sayler M. Pediculosis and scabies: treatment update. Am Fam Physician. 2012 Sep 15;86(6):535-41.
- Feldmeier H. Pediculosis capitis: new insights into epidemiology, diagnosis and treatment. Eur J Clin Microbiol Infect Dis. 2012 Sep;31(9):2105-10.

CASE #106: EPIGASTRIC PAIN

CASE

A 20-year-old male patient presents to his family doctor complaining of recurrent epigastric pain and vomiting for the last six months. On exam he has mild suprapubic tenderness without guarding. His blood sample is shown in the image below.

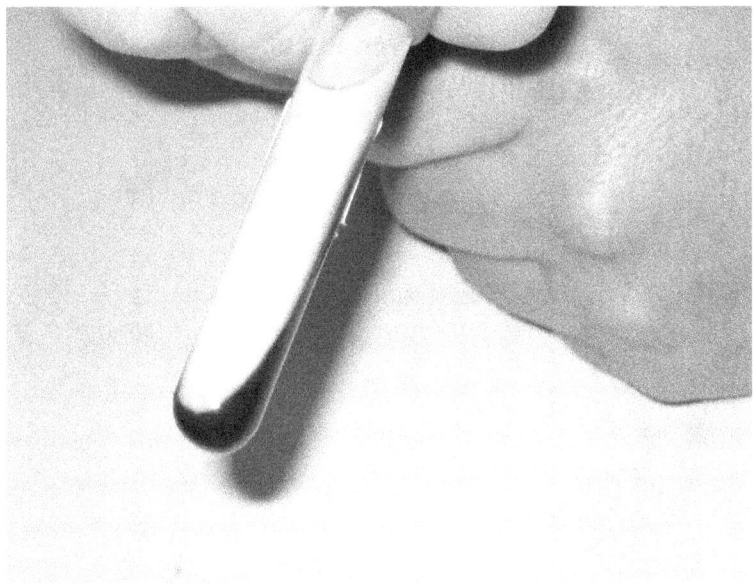

QUESTIONS

350. What is the likely diagnosis?
- a. Cryoglobulinemia
- b. Hyperbilirubinemia
- c. Hypercalcemia
- d. Hypertriglyceridemia
- e. Hypocalcemia

351. What is the likely cause of this patient's recurrent pain?

   a. Biliary Colic

   b. Cholecystitis

   c. Pancreatitis

   d. Renal Colic

352. Which of the following treatment is the first line treatment recommended in order to reduce the risk for recurrent pain?

   a. Acetyl Co-A Reductase Inhibitors

   b. Cholestyramine

   c. Fibrates

   d. Pancreatic Enzymes Supplementation

   e. Statins

353. Which of the following treatments is likely to improve the abnormality causing this condition in the fastest time?

   a. Fenofibrate

   b. Heparin Infusion

   c. Niacin

   d. Omega-3 Fatty Acids

   e. Plasma Pheresis

ANSWERS

350. d

351. c

352. c

353. e

VISUAL STIMULUS REVIEW

The image shows lipemic serum.

REFERENCES

- Berglund L, Brunzell JD, Goldberg AC. Evaluation and treatment of hypertriglyceridemia: an Endocrine Society clinical practice guideline. J Clin Endocrinol Metab. 2012 Sep;97(9):2969-89.

- Stefanutti C, Labbadia G, Morozzi C. Severe hypertriglyceridemia-related acute pancreatitis. Ther Apher Dial. 2013 Apr;17(2):130-7.

CASE #107: KNEE PAIN

CASE

A 24-year-old man who fell onto his flexed knee while roller blading presents to his family doctor complaining of severe right-knee pain. He is unable to bear weight on this leg because of severe pain.

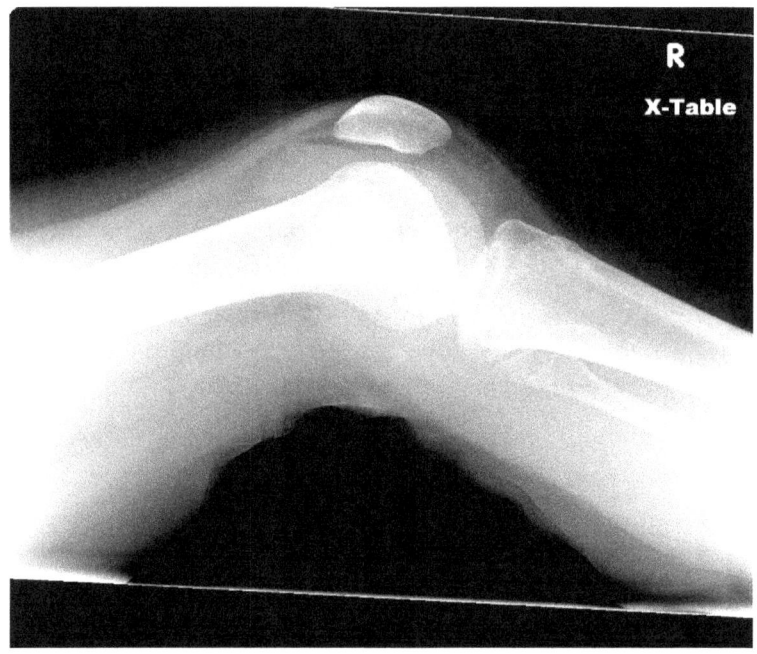

QUESTIONS

354. What is the likely diagnosis?
   a. Fibular Head Dislocation
   b. Intraarticular Fracture
   c. Knee Sprain
   d. Patellar Dislocation
   e. Tibial Shaft Fracture

355. What diagnostic finding is present in this plain film?
   a. Hemarthrosis
   b. Lipohemarthrosis
   c. Patella Alta
   d. Posterior Fibular Head Displacement
   e. Synovial Plica

356. Definitive management of this condition requires?
   a. Arthroscopic Ligament Tear Repair
   b. Aspiration Under Sterile Technique
   c. Close Reduction
   d. Knee Immobilizer with Early Remobilization
   e. Open Reduction and Internal Fixation

ANSWERS

354. b

355. b

356. e

VISUAL STIMULUS REVIEW

The radiograph shows intraarticular linear layering of fluid densities suggesting lipohemarthrosis.

REFERENCES

- Pallin DJ. Images in emergency medicine. Lipohemarthrosis. Ann Emerg Med. 2007 Aug;50(2):120, 135.

- SanDretto MA, Carrera GF. The double fat fluid level: lipohemarthrosis of the knee associated with suprapatellar plica Synovialis. Skeletal Radiol. 1983;10(1):30-3.

CASE #108: ABDOMINAL PAIN

CASE

A 60-year-old woman presents to the emergency department for recurrent episodes of right upper-quadrant pain for the last two weeks. She reports almost nightly fevers up to 103F (39.4C), chills that improve with Acetaminophen, and nausea. The pain became constant over the last two days. The patient has a temp of 103F (39.4), heart rate of 126/min, and blood pressure of 110/60 mmHg. She has severe RUQ tenderness to palpation with guarding and rebound over the right upper-quadrant. The patient's conjunctiva appears jaundiced. A CT of the abdomen is ordered.

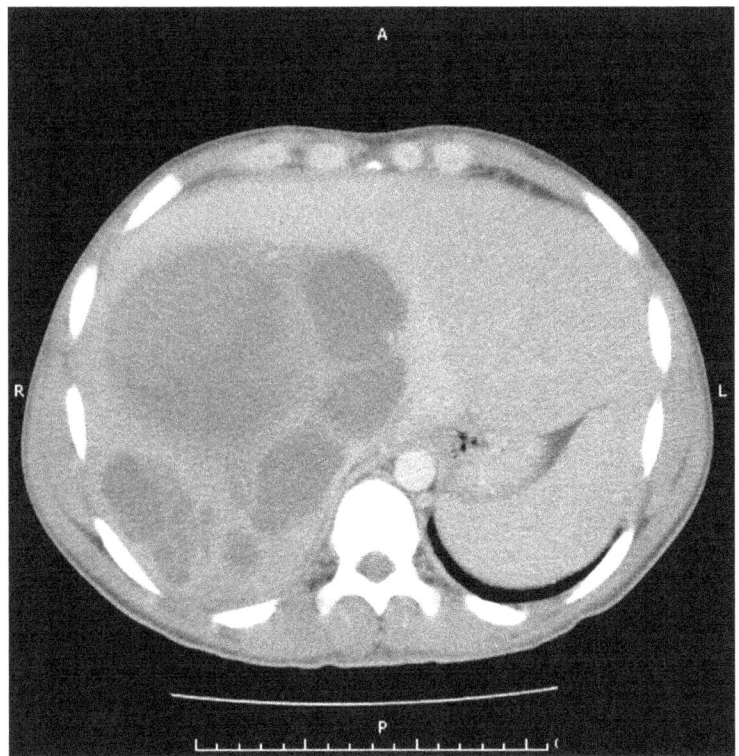

QUESTIONS

357. What is the likely diagnosis?
    a. Biliary Colic
    b. Amebic Liver Abscess
    c. Fungal Liver Abscess
    d. Hepatocellular Carcinoma
    e. Hydatid Cysts
    f. Pyogenic Liver Abscess

358. What is the likely etiology of this condition?
    a. Appendicitis
    b. Biliary Process
    c. Cryptogenic
    d. Endocarditis
    e. Pyelonephritis

359. What is the likely cause of this condition?
    a. Candida Albicans
    b. Entamoeba Histolytica
    c. Escherichia Colic
    d. Polymicrobial
    e. Toxin-Induced Malignant Transformation

360. Which of the following is a risk factor for this condition in infants?
    a. Advanced-Aged Mother
    b. Low Birth Weight
    c. Neonatal Jaundice Treated with Phototherapy
    d. Umbilical Vein Catheterization

ANSWERS

357. d

358. b

359. d

360. d

VISUAL STIMULUS REVIEW

The CT image shows a multiseptated liver mass, which is hypodense to the surrounding parenchyma.

REFERENCES

- Reid-Lombardo KM, Khan S, Sclabas G. Hepatic cysts and liver abscess. Surg Clin North Am. 2010 Aug;90(4):679-97.

- Mishra K, Basu S, Roychoudhury S, Kumar P. Liver abscess in children: an overview. World J Pediatr. 2010 Aug;6(3):210-6.

CASE #109: SORE THROAT

CASE

A 19-year-old woman presents to the emergency department for worsening throat for three days. She reports no past medical history, with difficulty swallowing solids and liquids over the last couple of days. She is able to swallow her own saliva. On physical examination, she is toxic-appearing with a tender and hard floor of mouth. She is unable to open her mouth wider than 2 cm.

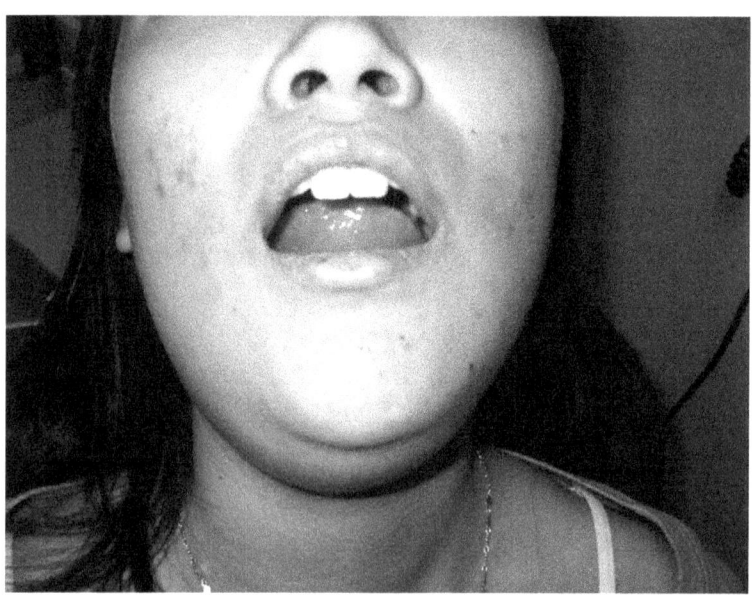

QUESTIONS

361. What is the likely diagnosis?
    a. Epiglottitis
    b. Laryngitis
    c. Lemierre's Syndrome
    d. Ludwig's Angina
    e. Retropharyngeal Abscesses

362. What is the likely cause of this condition?
    a. Actinomyces
    b. Bacteroides
    c. Prevotella
    d. Streptococcus Viridans
    e. Mixed Flora

363. Which of the following conditions is likely to predispose to this condition?
    a. Dental Infection
    b. Endocarditis
    c. Partially Treated Pharyngitis
    d. Untreated Pharyngitis

364. Further evaluation of this patient's condition will require which of the following tests?
    a. Complete Blood Count
    b. Computerized Tomography of the Neck
    c. Direct Laryngoscopy
    d. Indirect Laryngoscopy
    e. Lateral Neck X-Ray
    f. Ultrasound of the Neck

ANSWERS

361. c

362. e

363. a

364. b

VISUAL STIMULUS REVIEW

The image shows trismus with protruding swollen tongue and elevation of the floor of the mouth. The image also shows swelling to the submandibular tissue.

REFERENCES

- Derber CJ, Troy SB. Head and neck emergencies: bacterial meningitis, encephalitis, brain abscess, upper airway obstruction, and jugular septic thrombophlebitis. Med Clin North Am. 2012 Nov;96(6):1107-26.

- Reynolds SC, Chow AW. Severe soft tissue infections of the head and neck: a primer for critical care physicians. Lung. 2009 Sep-Oct;187(5):271-9.

- Vieira F, Allen SM, Stocks RM, Thompson JW. Deep neck infection. Otolaryngol Clin North Am. 2008 Jun;41(3):459-83

CASE #110: PRODUCTIVE COUGH

CASE

A 70-year-old man is brought his family doctor by his daughter for two weeks of productive cough and fever. The patient reports fevers and night sweats as well as weight loss over the last two to three weeks with some blood mixed in his sputum that started the day before. The patient mentioned that the sputum is brownish-yellow with a bad taste and foul smell.

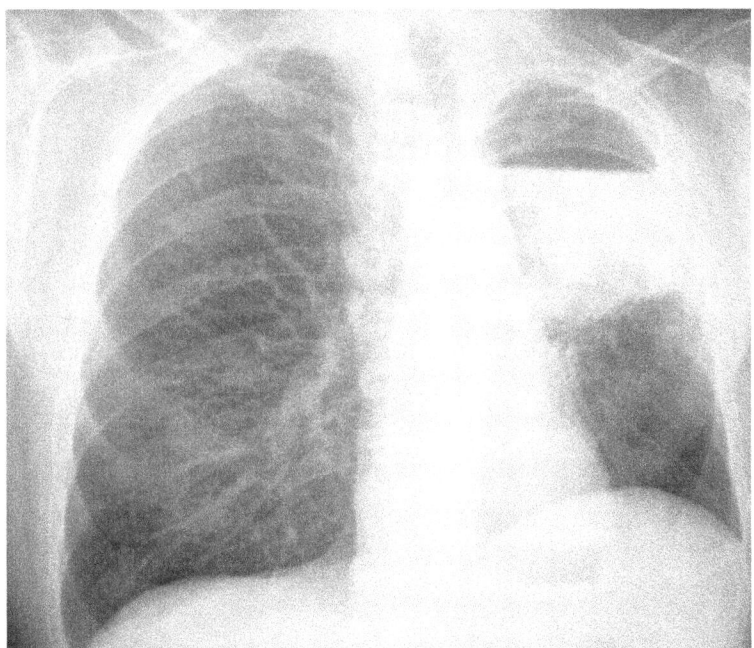

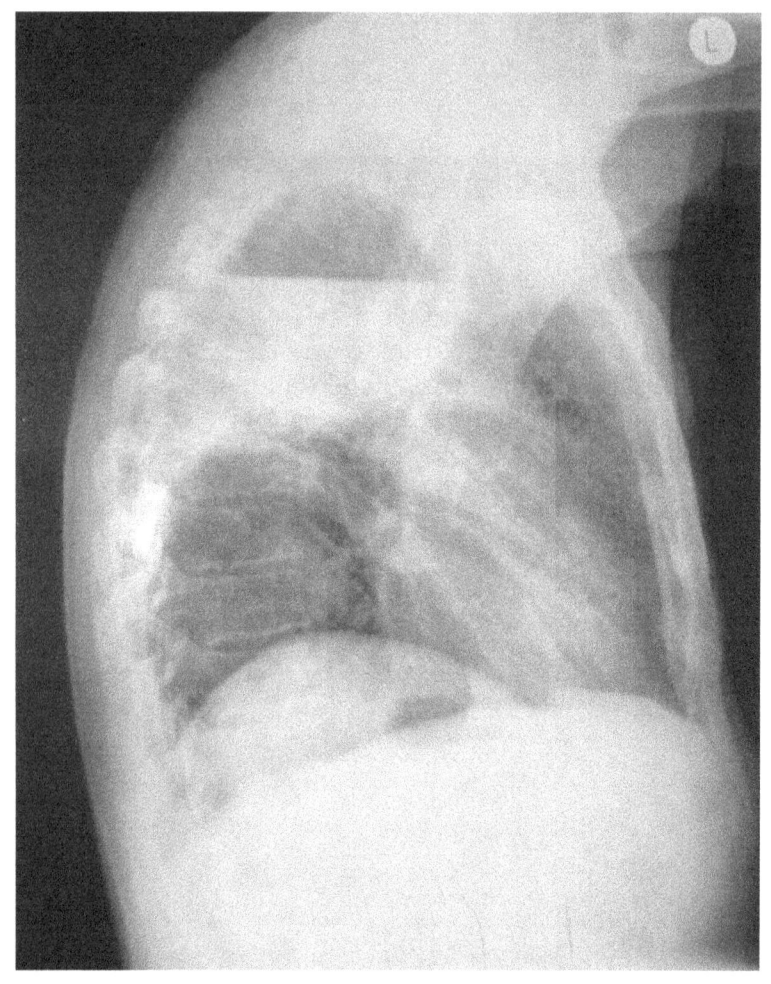

QUESTIONS

365. What is the likely diagnosis?
    a. Bronchogenic Carcinoma
    b. Empyema
    c. Hydatid Cysts
    d. Lung Abscess
    e. Pneumonia

366. What is the most common cause of this condition?
    a. Aspiration Pneumonia
    b. Community Acquired Pneumonia
    c. Eating Raw Meat
    d. Homelessness
    e. Smoking

367. Which of the following findings is more expected in this patient?
    a. Clubbing of Fingers
    b. Gingivitis
    c. Oral Thrush
    d. Osler Nodes
    e. Splinter Hemorrhages

368. Which of the following is the recommended first line treatment for this condition?
    a. Chest Tube Insertion
    b. IV Antibiotics
    c. Lobectomy
    d. Oral Antibiotics
    e. Pneumonectomy

ANSWERS

365. d

366. a

367. b

368. b

VISUAL STIMULUS REVIEW

- The radiograms show an air-fluid level inside an irregularly shaped cavity.

REFERENCES

- Desai H, Agrawal A. Pulmonary emergencies: pneumonia, acute respiratory distress syndrome, lung abscess, and empyema. Med Clin North Am. 2012 Nov;96(6):1127-48.

- Mansharamani NG, Koziel H. Chronic lung sepsis: lung abscess, bronchiectasis, and empyema. Curr Opin Pulm Med. 2003 May;9(3):181-5.

CASE #111: RASH AND FEVER

CASE

A 25-year-old man presents to his family doctor complaining of fever, fatigue, and myalgias for three days. His physical examination is unremarkable except for the finding visible in the image below.

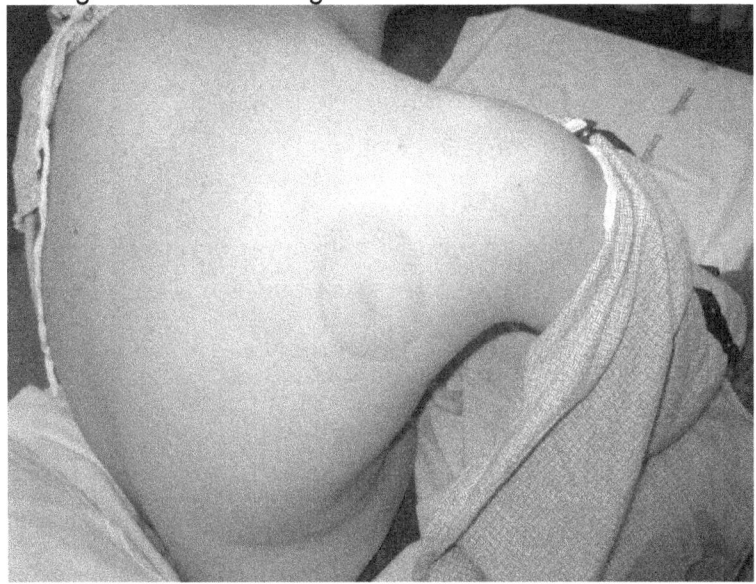

QUESTIONS

369. What is the likely diagnosis?

    a. Babesiosis

    b. Human Granulocytic Anaplasmosis

    c. Lyme Disease

    d. Rheumatic Fever

    e. Syphilis

    f. Tinea Corporis

370. What is the name of the visible sign in the image?
- a. Erythema Annulare Centrifugum
- b. Erythema Marginatum
- c. Erythema Migrans
- d. Erythema Multiforme

371. What is the likely cause of this condition?
- a. Contact with an Infected Fly
- b. Droplet Transmission
- c. Mosquito Bite
- d. Skin to Skin Contact
- e. Tick Bite

372. What is the likely causative organism of this condition?
- a. Babesia Microti
- b. Borrelia Burgdorferi
- c. Streptococus Pyogenes
- d. Treponema Pallidum
- e. Trichophyton Rubrum

373. What is the first line treatment for this condition in this patient?
- a. Amoxicillin PO
- b. Ceftriaxone IV
- c. Doxycycline PO
- d. Penicillin G IM
- e. Penicillin VK PO
- f. Terbinafine PO

ANSWERS

369. c

370. c

371. e

372. b

373. c

VISUAL STIMULUS REVIEW

The image shows a flat bull's-eye target-like erythematous lesion with central clearing.

REFERENCES

- Halperin JJ, Baker P, Wormser GP. Common misconceptions about Lyme disease. Am J Med. 2013 Mar;126(3):264.e1-7.

- Wright WF, Riedel DJ, Talwani R, Gilliam BL. Diagnosis and management of Lyme disease. Am Fam Physician. 2012 Jun 1;85(11):1086-93.

CASE #112: FEVER AND WEIGHT LOSS

CASE

A 20-year-old man presents to his family doctor for fever, weight loss, fatigue, and drenching night sweats for the last three months. He reports one to weeks of daily fevers up to 103F (39.4) followed by about a week of normal temperature. He denies cough, diarrhea, sore throat, headache, or travel out of the United States.

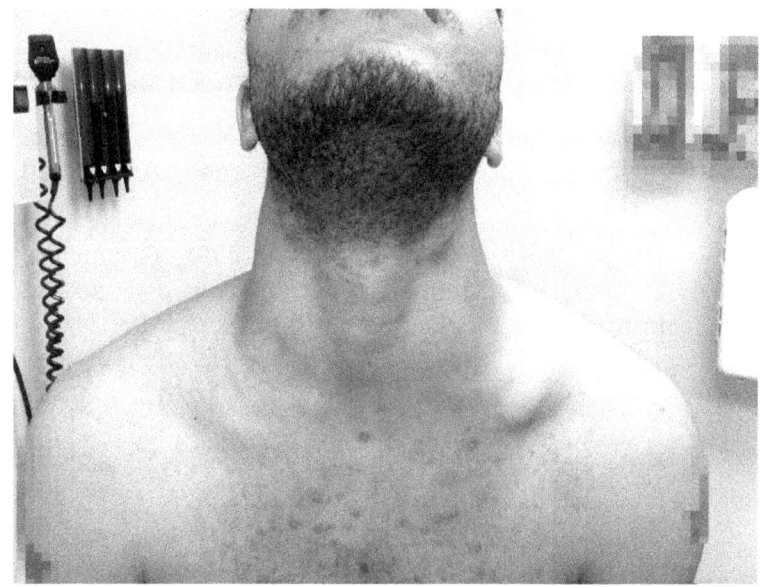

QUESTIONS

374. What is the likely diagnosis?
    a. Cat Scratch Disease
    b. Hodgkins Lymphoma
    c. Infectious Mononucleosis
    d. Malaria
    e. Tuberculosis

375. Which of the following is a known risk factor for this condition?
    a. Asian Ethnicity
    b. Diabetes Mellitus
    c. EBV Exposure
    d. Female Gender
    e. Homelessness
    f. Travel to Endemic Area

376. Which of the following is required for definitive diagnosis of this condition?
    a. Antibody Titer Testing
    b. Blood Cultures
    c. Fine Needle Aspiration
    d. HIV PCR
    e. Lymph Node Excision

ANSWERS

374. b

375. c

376. e

VISUAL STIMULUS REVIEW

The image shows diffuse lymphadenopathy, specifically bilateral anterior cervical and supraclavicular

REFERENCES

- Ansell SM. Hodgkin lymphoma: 2012 update on diagnosis, risk-stratification, and management. Am J Hematol. 2012 Dec;87(12):1096-103.
- Townsend W, Linch D. Hodgkin's lymphoma in adults. Lancet. 2012 Sep 1;380(9844):836-47.

CASE #113: FEVER AND MUSCLE ACHES

CASE

A 30-year-old man is brought to the emergency department by his wife for headache, fever, and confusion. The wife reports that the patient returned from a trip to South Africa about two weeks prior, and that a week after his return he started to complain of fever, headache muscle aches, shaking, chills, and joint pains. She reports that the fever resolved the day before and that he felt better over nights. That morning he woke up with high fever and shaking chills and decided to stay in bed. When she returned home around noon, she found him confused. The patient is lethargic with a supple neck. The rest of his physical examination shows normal bilateral breath sounds, tachycardia without any murmurs, and a soft and non-tender abdomen. He opens his eyes and localizes pain but is unable to follow commands and speaks in incomprehensible words. The following laboratory is performed.

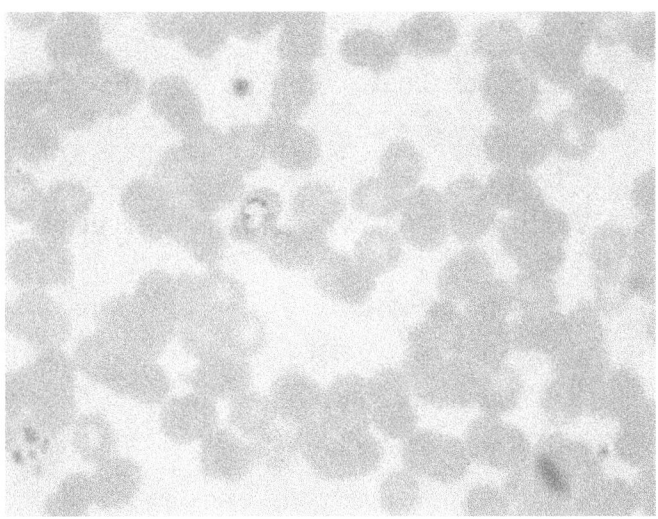

QUESTIONS

377. What is the likely diagnosis?
    a. Babesiosis
    b. Bacterial Meningitis
    c. Ehrlichiosis
    d. Malaria
    e. Viral Encephalitis

378. What is the likely causative organism of this condition?
    a. Anaplasma
    b. Babesia Microti
    c. Herpes Simplex Virus
    d. Plasmodium Malaria
    e. Neisseria Meningitis

379. Definitive diagnosis of this condition requires which of the following studies?
    a. Antibody Titers
    b. Blood Culture
    c. CSF Culture
    d. Thick Smear
    e. Thin Smear
    f. CSF PCR

380. Which of the following findings is expected to be present in this patient?
    a. Leukocytosis
    b. Purpura
    c. Splenomegaly
    d. Unequal Pupils

ANSWERS

377. d

378. d

379. e

380. c

VISUAL STIMULUS REVIEW

The thin blood smear image shows a ring-form malaria parasite.

REFERENCES

- Centers for Disease Control and Prevention. Malaria. Available at http://www.cdc.gov/malaria. Accessed Jun 9, 2013.

- Fox TG, Manaloor JJ, Christenson JC. Travel-related infections in children. Pediatr Clin North Am. 2013 Apr;60(2):507-27.

- Akinosoglou KS, Solomou EE, Gogos CA. Malaria: a haematological disease. Hematology. 2012 Mar;17(2):106-14.

CASE #114: BREAST PAIN

CASE

A 34-year-old woman presents to her family doctor complaining of right breast pain for three days. She is three weeks postpartum and is breast-feeding from both breasts. On exam she is febrile to 102.4F (39.1C) and tachycardic to 106/min; her right breast is swollen, indurated, and tender. There is no palpable fluctuance.

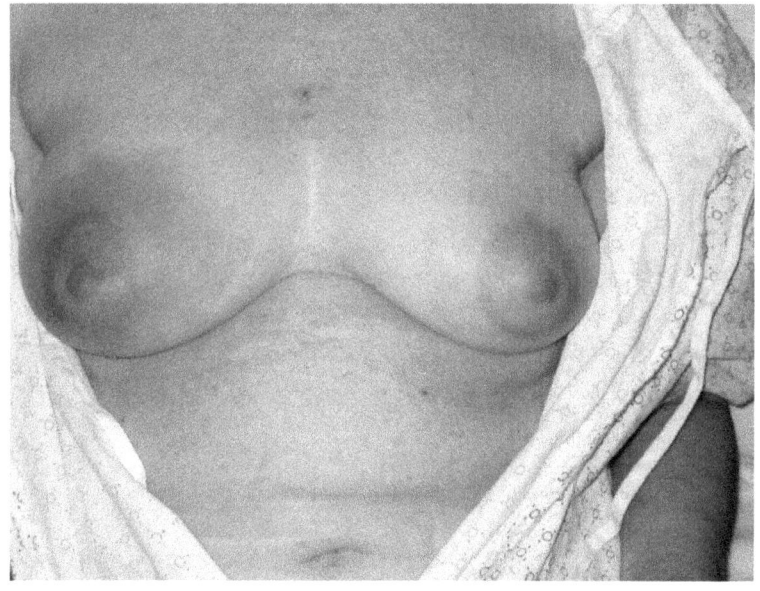

QUESTIONS

381. What is the likely diagnosis?
    a. Breast Abscess
    b. Breast Cellulitis
    c. Inflammatory Breast Carcinoma
    d. Mastitis

382. Which of the following is the likely cause of this condition?

    a. Candida Albicans

    b. Mechanical Inflammation

    c. Staphylococcus Aureus

    d. Staphylococcus Epidermidis

    e. Streptococcus Pyogenes

383. Which of the following therapies should be recommended?

    a. Continue breast-feeding from both breasts.

    b. Continue breast-feeding only from left breast but stop from right.

    c. Continue breast-feeding only from right breast but stop from left.

    d. Continue breast-feeding from left but pump out of right.

    e. Stop breast-feeding but pump out of both breasts.

    f. a, c, or e

384. Which of the following antibiotics is recommended for this condition?

    a. Amoxicillin

    b. Ciprofloxacin

    c. Clindamycin

    d. Doxycycline

    e. Penicillin VK

ANSWERS

381. d

382. c

383. f

384. c

VISUAL STIMULUS REVIEW

The image shows an erythematous and swollen right breast.

REFERENCES

- Jahanfar S, Ng CJ, Teng CL. Antibiotics for mastitis in breastfeeding women. Cochrane Database Syst Rev. 2013 Feb 28;2:CD005458.

- Dixon JM, Khan LR. Treatment of breast infection. BMJ. 2011 Feb 11;342:d396.

- Spencer JP. Management of mastitis in breastfeeding women. Am Fam Physician. 2008 Sep 15;78(6):727-31.

CASE #115:   EARACHE

CASE

A 43-year-old man presents to his family doctor complaining of left earache for two weeks. He reports that he was seen by another doctor 10 days ago and is still taking Amoxicillin 500 mg PO three times daily. Despite his treatment, he reports ongoing daily fevers, worsening of the pain that now also progressed to behind his ear as well as drainage of pus from the ear that started three days ago. On physical examination, he has tenderness and fluctuance behind his left ear.

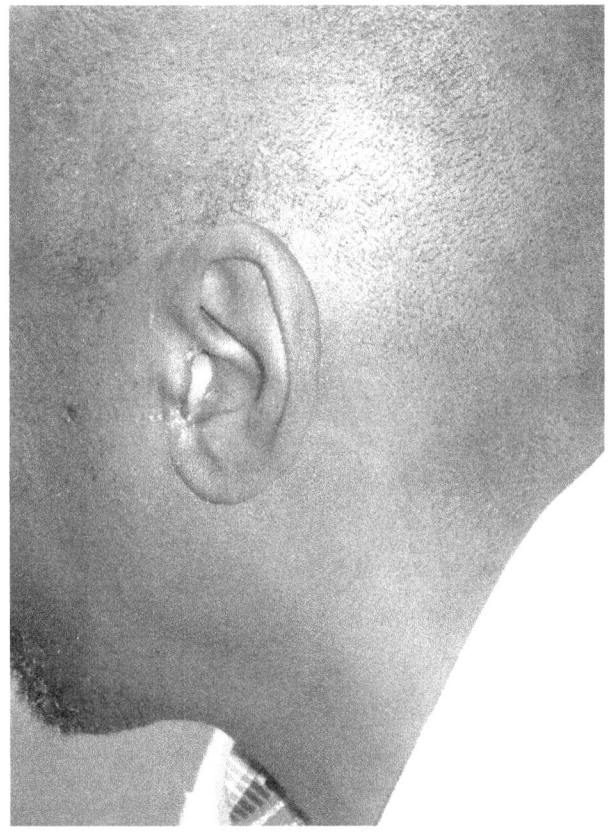

QUESTIONS

385. What is the likely diagnosis?
    a. Acute Otitis Media
    b. Acute Otitis Media with Tympanic Membrane Perforation
    c. Malignant Otitis Externa
    d. Mastoiditis
    e. Retroauricular Lymphadenitis

386. What is the likely cause of this condition?
    a. Group A Beta-Hemolytic Streptococci
    b. Haemophilus Influenzae
    c. Pseudomonas Aeruginosa
    d. Staphylococcus Aureus
    e. Streptococcus Pneumoniae

387. Which of the following will provide definitive management of this condition?
    a. Amoxicillin PO
    b. Amoxicillin Clavulanic PO
    c. Ceftriaxone IV
    d. Mastoidectomy and Intravenous Antibiotics
    e. Vancomycin IV

388. Which of the following is an expected complication of this condition?
    a. Epidural Abscess
    b. Facial Nerve Palsy
    c. Meningitis
    d. Sigmoid Sinus Thrombosis
    e. Any of the above

ANSWERS

385. d

386. e

387. d

388. e

VISUAL STIMULUS REVIEW

The image shows erythema and swelling over the left mastoid bone and purulent discharge from the left external ear canal.

REFERENCES

- Toll EC, Nunez DA. Diagnosis and treatment of acute otitis media: review. J Laryngol Otol. 2012 Oct;126(10):976-83.

- Osborn AJ, Blaser S, Papsin BC. Decisions regarding intracranial complications from acute mastoiditis in children. Curr Opin Otolaryngol Head Neck Surg. 2011 Dec;19(6):478-85.

CASE #116:   FEVER

CASE

A 4-year-old boy, fully vaccinated to date, with no known past medical history is brought to the emergency department by EMS for a new onset seizure. The mother reports that he was diagnosed with pharyngitis a couple of days before and started on Amoxicillin. He had continued fevers. He became more confused during the day, developed a rash, and had a single generalized seizure that lasted three minutes just before she called the ambulance. The patient's vital signs are temp 104.5F (40.3C), heart rate 148/min, blood pressure 80/50 mmHg, and O₂Sat 96% on room air. On exam the patient is lethargic, localizes to pain, and follows one-step commands. His throat exam shows minimal erythema and no exudates. His lung sounds are clear bilaterally; his abdomen is soft and non-tender. His rash as seen in the image is non-blanching.

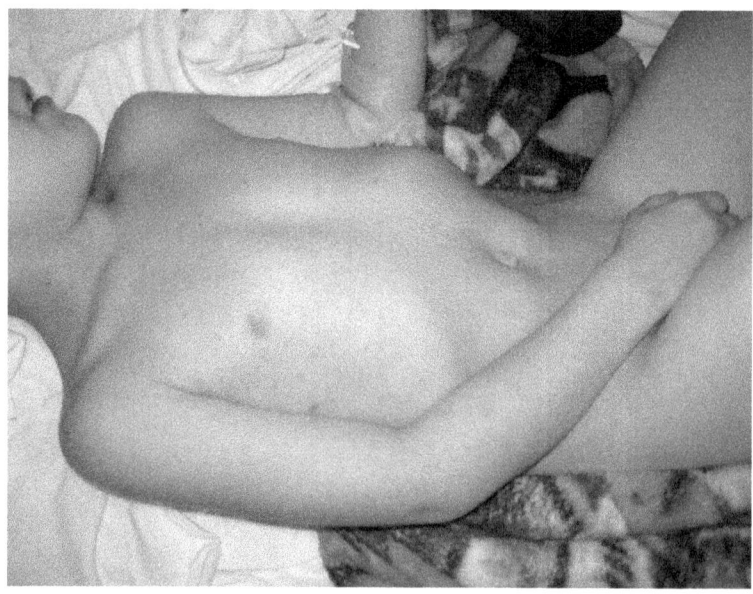

QUESTIONS

389. What is the likely diagnosis?
    a. Disseminated Intravascular Coagulation
    b. Encephalitis
    c. Febrile Seizures
    d. Influenza Related Sepsis
    e. Meningitis

390. What is the likely cause of this condition?
    a. Haemophilus Influenza
    b. Neisseria Meningitidis
    c. Streptococus Epidermidis
    d. Streptococcus Pneumonia
    e. Streptococus Pyogenes

391. Which of the following laboratory findings is expected in this patient?
    a. High CSF Glucose
    b. High CSF Protein
    c. High Serum Glucose
    d. Low CSF Absolute Neutrophil Count
    e. Low Serum Lactate

392. Which of the following is indicated as a first line therapy in the management of this patient?
    a. Ceftriaxone IV
    b. Ampicillin IV
    c. Clindamycin IV
    d. Norepinephrine IV
    e. Oseltamivir PO
    f. Valacyclovir IV

ANSWERS

389. e

390. b

391. b

392. a

VISUAL STIMULUS REVIEW

The image shows diffuse petechial rash.

REFERENCES

- van de Beek D, Brouwer MC, Thwaites GE, Tunkel AR. Advances in treatment of bacterial meningitis. Lancet. 2012 Nov 10;380(9854):1693-702.

- Gaieski DF, Nathan BR, Weingart SD, Smith WS. Emergency neurologic life support: meningitis and encephalitis. Neurocrit Care. 2012 Sep;17 Suppl 1:S66-72.

- Agrawal S, Nadel S. Acute bacterial meningitis in infants and children: epidemiology and management. Expert Rev Anti Infect Ther. 2011 Nov;9(11):1053-65.

- Curtis S, Stobart K, Vandermeer B, Simel DL, Klassen T. Clinical features suggestive of meningitis in children: a systematic review of prospective data. Pediatrics. 2010 Nov;126(5):952-60.

CASE #117: FEVER AND FATIGUE

CASE

A 16-year-old previously healthy girl presents to her family doctor complaining of extreme fatigue and sore throat for the last seven days. She reports daily fevers up to 102.2F (39C) and anorexia with some nausea as well. She also complains of sore throat but is able to tolerate liquids and solids with no dysphagia. Her voice is normal, and she denies any cough. She reports a fine non-pruritic erythematous rash that resolved three days ago. On exam, she has bilateral enlarged and tender anterior and posterior cervical lymph nodes.

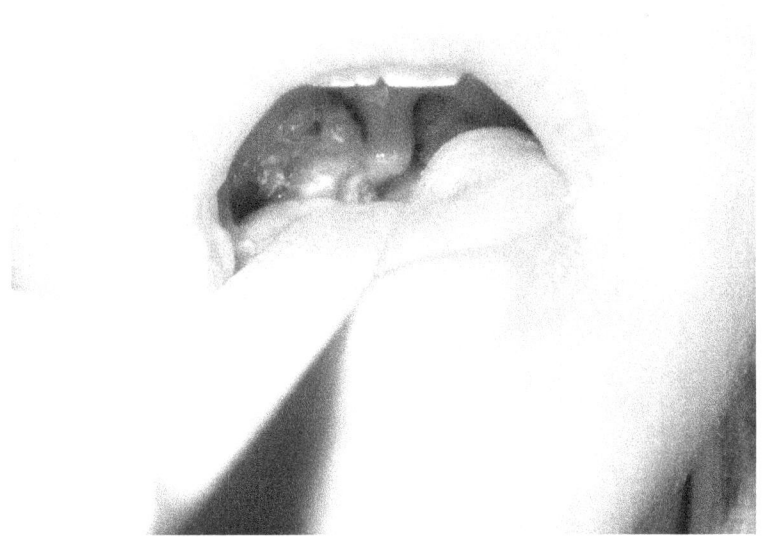

QUESTIONS

393. What is the likely diagnosis?
    a. Bacterial Tonsillitis
    b. Infectious Mononucleosis
    c. Pertussis
    d. Viral Laryngitis

394. What is the likely cause of this condition?
    a. Bartonella
    b. Cytomegalovirus
    c. Epstein Bar Virus
    d. Streptococcus Group A
    e. Streptococcus Group B

395. How is the condition transmitted?
    a. Blood Transfusion
    b. Cervical Secretions
    c. Oral Secretions
    d. Uterine Secretions
    e. All of the above

396. What is the most common presentation of this condition?
    a. Arthralgia
    b. Asymptomatic Seroconversion
    c. Fatigue
    d. Myalgia
    e. Pharyngitis

ANSWERS

393. b

394. c

395. e

396. b

VISUAL STIMULUS REVIEW

The gross image shows tonsillar enlargement, erythema, and exudates as well as uvular edema (rare sign but almost pathognomonic for EBV pharyngitis).

REFERENCES

- Vouloumanou EK, Rafailidis PI, Falagas ME. Current diagnosis and management of infectious mononucleosis. Curr Opin Hematol. 2012 Jan;19(1):14-20.

- Luzuriaga K, Sullivan JL. Infectious mononucleosis. N Engl J Med. 2010 May 27;362(21):1993-2000.

CASE #118: AGITATION

CASE

A 53-year-old man is brought to the emergency department for severe agitation after alleged drug use. The patient is medicated with Haloperidol and Lorazepam for severe agitation and placed in restraints for his agitation. His vital signs are temp 100.3F (37.9C), heart rate 130/min, blood pressure 210/120 mmHg, and O_2Sat 98% on room air. He has no signs of external trauma on physical exam and is moving all four extremities.

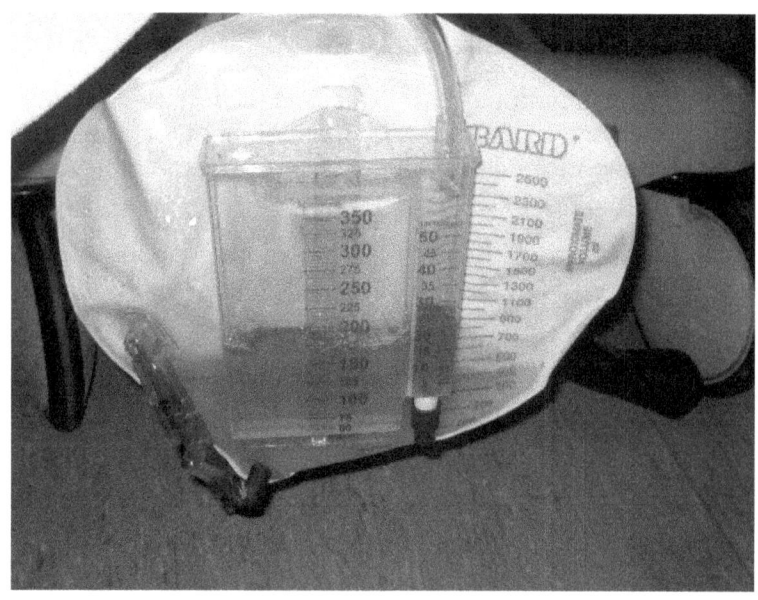

QUESTIONS

397. What is the likely diagnosis?

    a. Alcohol Withdrawal

    b. Hemorrhagic Cystitis

    c. Malignant Hyperthermia

    d. Rhabdomyolysis

    e. Viral Encephalitis

398. What is the likely cause of this condition?

    a. Alcohol Addiction

    b. Cocaine Intoxication

    c. Escherichia Colli

    d. Herpes Simplex

    e. Opiate Intoxication

399. Which of the following findings is expected in this condition?

    a. Serum Creatine Phosphokinase 300 U/L

    b. Serum Glucose 450 mg/dl

    c. Serum Potassium 2.7 mEq/L

    d. Serum Sodium 110 mEq/L

    e. Urine RBC: 3 per low-field power

400. Which of the following is an expected complication of this condition?

    a. Acute Renal Failure

    b. Acute Respiratory Failure

    c. Korsakoff Syndrome

    d. Seizure Disorder

    e. Stroke

ANSWERS

397. d

398. b

399. e

400. a

VISUAL STIMULUS REVIEW

The image shows erythematous urine.

REFERENCES

- Parekh R, Care DA, Tainter CR. Rhabdomyolysis: advances in diagnosis and treatment. Emerg Med Pract. 2012 Mar;14(3):1-15.

- Al-Ismaili Z, Piccioni M, Zappitelli M. Rhabdomyolysis: pathogenesis of renal injury and management. Pediatr Nephrol. 2011 Oct;26(10):1781-8.

- Cervellin G, Comelli I, Lippi G. Rhabdomyolysis: historical background, clinical, diagnostic and therapeutic features. Clin Chem Lab Med. 2010 Jun;48(6):749-56.

CASE #119: FACE PAIN

CASE

A 73-year-old woman presents to her family doctor complaining of progressive pain and swelling to the left side of her face. She has a history of diabetes mellitus type 2, hypertension, and depression that are all well controlled on medical therapy. The patient reports that the pain to her face gets worse when she eats. On physical examination, her temp is 101.7F (38.7C), heart rate of 104/min, and blood pressure of 140/80 mmHg. The left side of her face and mostly around the left mandibular angle is exquisitely tender to palpation but without any mass or fluctuation.

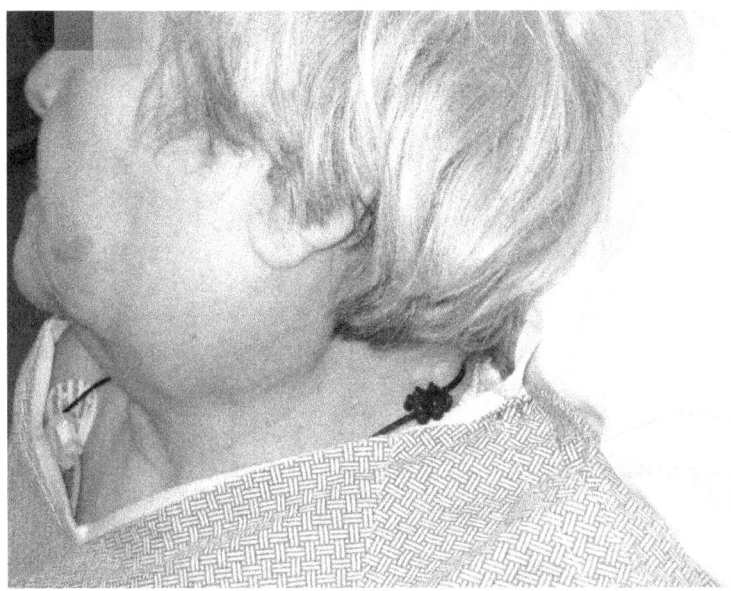

QUESTIONS

401. What is the likely diagnosis?
    a. Facial Abscess
    b. Facial Cellulitis
    c. Mastoiditis
    d. Mikulicz disease
    e. Parotitis
    f. Submandibular Carcinoma

402. What is the likely cause of this condition?
    a. Human Immunodeficiency Virus
    b. Measles Virus
    c. Mumps Virus
    d. Squamous Cell Carcinoma
    e. Staphylococcus Aureus
    f. Streptococcus Viridans

403. Which of the following is a risk factor for this condition?
    a. Anticholinergic Medications
    b. Chewing Tobacco
    c. Male Gender
    d. Skipping the MMR vaccine
    e. Smoking Tobacco

404. Which of the following is part of the first line treatment of this condition?
    a. Amoxicillin
    b. Antiretrovirals
    c. Fine Needle Aspiration
    d. Incision and Drainage
    e. Sialo-Endoscopy
    f. Trimethoprim-Sulfamethoxazole

ANSWERS

401. e

402. e

403. a

404. f

VISUAL STIMULUS REVIEW

The image shows swelling and erythema overlying the left parotid gland.

REFERENCES

- Cascarini L, McGurk M. Epidemiology of salivary gland infections. Oral Maxillofac Surg Clin North Am. 2009 Aug;21(3):353-7.

- Brook I. The bacteriology of salivary gland infections. Oral Maxillofac Surg Clin North Am. 2009 Aug;21(3):269-74.

- Fattahi TT, Lyu PE, Van Sickels JE. Management of acute suppurative parotitis. J Oral Maxillofac Surg. 2002 Apr;60(4):446-8.

CASE #120: SWOLLEN EYE

CASE

A 14-month-old boy is brought to the pediatrician for evaluation of a swollen eye that has progressed over the last eight weeks. The parents just moved into town and report normal vaginal delivery and no known medical history. On physical examination, the child has limited extraocular movement on the right and a palpable abdominal mass. A CT scan is ordered.

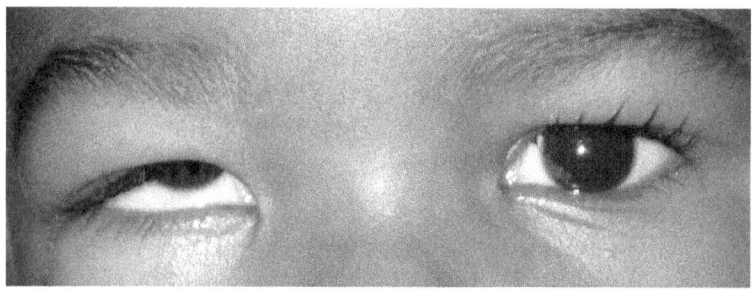

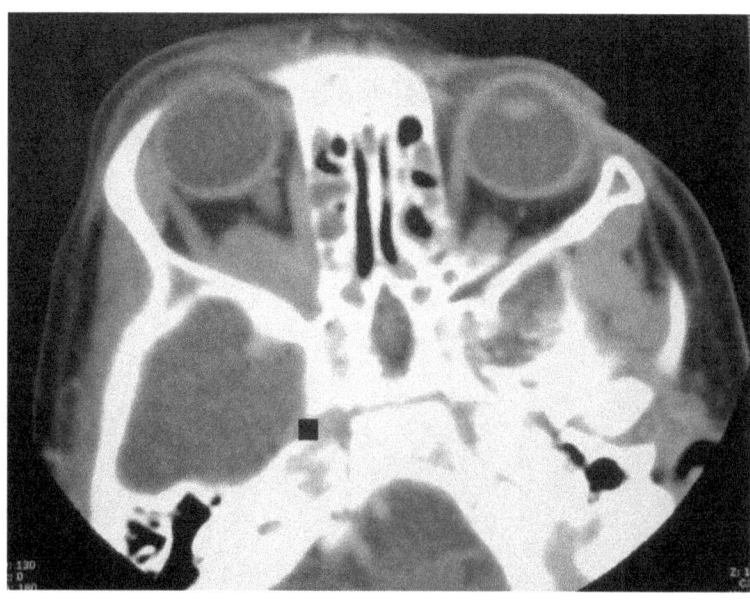

QUESTIONS

405. What is the likely diagnosis?
    a. Neuroblastoma
    b. Orbital Abscess
    c. Orbital Cellulitis
    d. Renal Cell Carcinoma
    e. Retinoblastoma
    f. Wilms Tumor

406. Which of the following studies yield a result that is specific for this condition?
    a. Blood Culture
    b. Erythrocyte Sedimentation Rate
    c. Liver Function Tests
    d. Urinalysis
    e. Urine Collection for Catecholamines

407. Which of the following treatment modalities demonstrated efficacy in the treatment of this condition?
    a. Bone Marrow Transplant
    b. IV Antibiotics
    c. Multi-Agent Chemotherapy
    d. Radiation Therapy
    e. Surgical Excision
    f. a, c, d, and e

ANSWERS

405. a

406. e

407. f

VISUAL STIMULUS REVIEW

The gross image shows a proptotic right eye with an upward gaze. The CT image shows a soft tissue density to the right orbit that does not seem to origin from the eye globe and is in close relationship with the proximal extraocular muscles.

REFERENCES

- Davenport KP, Blanco FC, Sandler AD. Pediatric malignancies: neuroblastoma, Wilm's tumor, hepatoblastoma, rhabdomyosarcoma, and sacroccygeal teratoma. Surg Clin North Am. 2012 Jun;92(3):745-67.

- Zage PE, Louis CU, Cohn SL. New aspects of neuroblastoma treatment: ASPHO 2011 symposium review. Pediatr Blood Cancer. 2012 Jul 1;58(7):1099-105.

- Davidoff AM. Neuroblastoma. Semin Pediatr Surg. 2012 Feb;21(1):2-14.

CASE #121:   SEIZURES

CASE

A 30-year-old man with no known medical history is brought to the emergency department for generalized seizure. He is awake and alert with normal vital signs and physical exam at this time. His wife reports that he was watching TV on the sofa when he suddenly had a generalized seizure. He slowly recovered en route to the hospital and is now back to his normal self. He recalls occasional headaches over the last two months. A CT of his head is ordered.

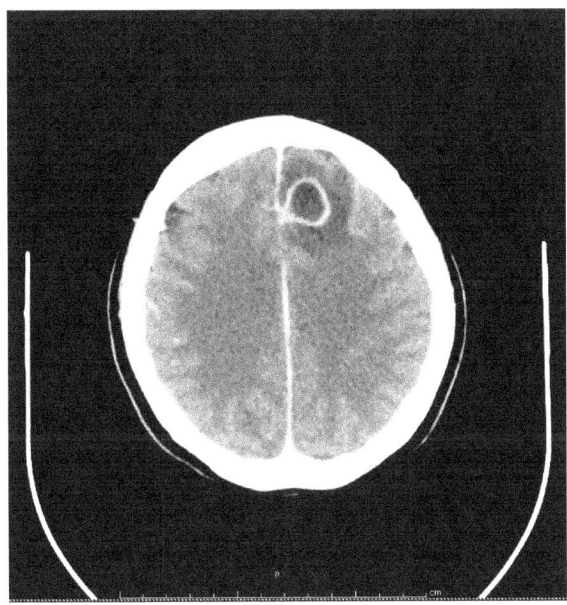

QUESTIONS

408. What is the likely diagnosis?
    a. Brain Abscess
    b. Cryptococcosis
    c. Glioblastoma Multiforme
    d. Meningioma
    e. Neurocysticercosis

409. What is the likely cause of this condition?
    a. Cryptococcus Neoformans
    b. Estrogen Exposure
    c. Malignant Transformation
    d. Staphylococcus Aureus
    e. Taenia Solium

410. What is the likely etiology of this condition
    a. Ingestion of Agent
    b. Inhalation of Agent
    c. Transmucosal Contact with Body Fluid
    d. Malignant Transformation

411. Which of the following is a risk factor for this condition?
    a. Caucasian Ethnicity
    b. History of Stroke
    c. Immigrants from Latin Countries
    d. Obesity
    e. Underweight

412. Which of the following should be included in the initial treatment plan for this condition?

  a. Albendazole
  b. Antiepileptic Agent
  c. IV Antibiotics
  d. Prednisone
  e. Ventriculoperitoneal Shunt
  f. a, b, and d

ANSWERS

408. e

409. e

410. a

411. c

412. f

VISUAL STIMULUS REVIEW

The CT image (post IV contrast) shows a hypodense lesion in the left frontal lobe with peripheral enhancement and perilesional edema.

REFERENCES

- Baird RA, Wiebe S, Zunt JR et al. Evidence-based guideline: treatment of parenchymal neurocysticercosis: report of the Guideline Development Subcommittee of the American Academy of Neurology. Neurology. 2013 Apr 9;80(15):1424-9.

- Lerner A, Shiroishi MS, Zee CS, Law M, Go JL. Imaging of neurocysticercosis. Neuroimaging Clin N Am. 2012 Nov;22(4):659-76.

CASE #122: ELBOW SWELLING

CASE

A 64-year-old man with no past medical history presents to his family doctor with swelling over his posterior right elbow. He first noticed the swelling about five weeks prior. He took daily ibuprofen for the past three weeks with no improvement in symptoms. He denies any trauma to the elbow, and on examination had a full and painless range of motion of his right elbow. On palpation over his right olecranon, there is a mildly tender and fluctuant mass.

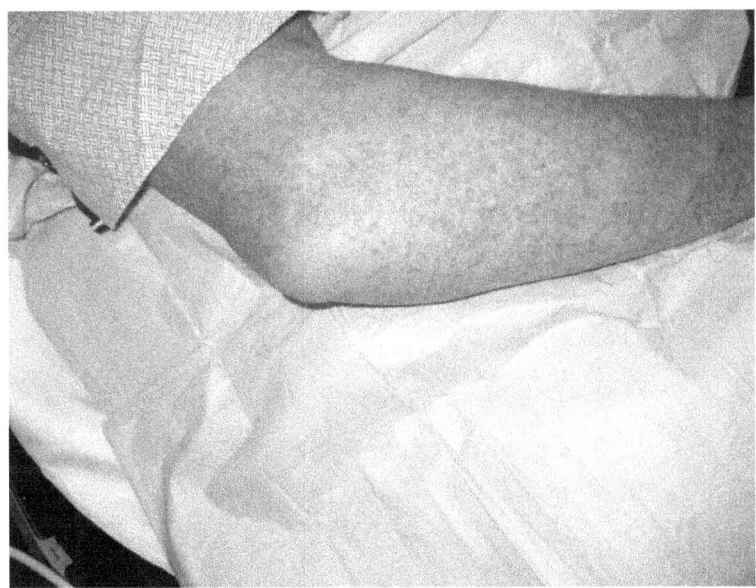

QUESTIONS

413. What is the likely diagnosis?

   a. Gout

   b. Olecranon Bursitis

   c. Olecranon Fracture

   d. Rheumatoid Arthritis

   e. Septic Arthritis

   f. Tennis Elbow

414. What is the most common cause of this condition?

   a. Staphylococcus Aureus

   b. Streptococus Pyogenes

   c. Repetitive Microtrauma

   d. Uremia

415. What is the recommended treatment for this condition?

   a. Continue NSAIDs

   b. Endoscopic Bursal Resection

   c. Needle Aspiration and Drainage

   d. Open Reduction Internal Fixation

   e. Oral Antibiotics

ANSWERS

413. b

414. c

415. c

VISUAL STIMULUS REVIEW

The gross image shows an erythematous soft tissue mass over the right olecranon.

REFERENCES

- Del Buono A, Franceschi F, Palumbo A, Diagnosis and management of olecranon bursitis. Surgeon. 2012 Oct;10(5):297-300.

- Herrera FA, Meals RA. Chronic olecranon bursitis. J Hand Surg Am. 2011 Apr;36(4):708-9.

- McFarland EG, Mamanee P, Queale WS, Cosgarea AJ. Olecranon and prepatellar bursitis: treating acute, chronic, and inflamed. Phys Sportsmed. 2000 Mar;28(3):40-52.

CASE #123: UMBILICAL DISCHARGE

CASE

A 7-day-old baby boy is brought to his pediatrician for foul smelly discharge from his umbilicus. This is a full-term (40 weeks) and normal spontaneous vaginal delivery baby that has no medical conditions to date. The parents report that they followed the umbilical cord stump instructions they were given at the hospital and that the baby has goo PO intake (breast-feeding) and is making wet diapers every two to three hours. On physical examination, the baby has normal vital signs and is not irritable. His abdomen is soft and not tender, but he does have tenderness to his umbilical area. He has foul-smelling discharge from the umbilical cord stump.

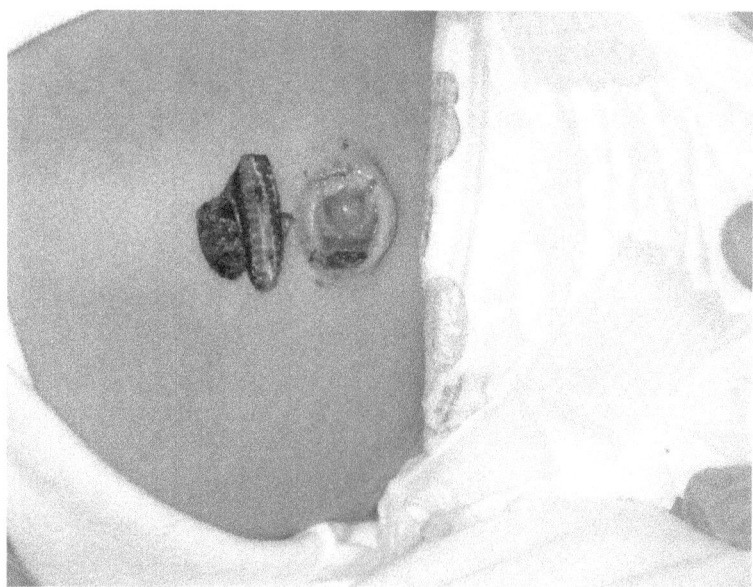

QUESTIONS

416. What is the likely diagnosis?
    a. Abdominal Wall Cellulitis
    b. Fournier's Gangrene
    c. Normal Degenerated Umbilical Cord Stump
    d. Omphalitis
    e. Urachal Cyst

417. What is the most common cause of this condition?
    a. Bacteroides Fragilis
    b. Escherichia Colli
    c. Fat Necrosis
    d. Polymicrobial
    e. Staphylococcus Aureus
    f. Streptococcus Group B

418. Which of the following studies may help determine need for surgical intervention?
    a. Abdominal Wall Ultrasound
    b. Complete Blood Count
    c. C-Reactive Protein
    d. Gram Stain
    e. Surgical Intervention is not indicated in this condition.

419. Which of the following treatments is part of the first line treatment of this condition in this specific patient?
    a. Chlorhexidine Body Wash
    b. Dry Stump Care
    c. Hyperbaric Oxygen
    d. Intravenous Antibiotics
    e. Oral Antibiotics

ANSWERS

416. d

417. d

418. a

419. d

VISUAL STIMULUS REVIEW

The image shows necrotic stump that already separated from the umbilicus as well as purulent discharge from the umbilicus with surrounding abdominal wall erythema and localized swelling to the umbilicus.

REFERENCES

- Brook I. Anaerobic infections in children. Adv Exp Med Biol. 2011;697:117-52.
- Fraser N, Davies BW, Cusack J. Neonatal omphalitis: a review of its serious complications. Acta Paediatr. 2006 May;95(5):519-22.
- Manikoth P, George M, Vaishnav A, Sajwani MJ. Omphalitis. Lancet. 2004 Oct 23-29.

CASE #124: EYE PAIN

CASE

A 23-year-old man presents to the emergency department after he was punched in his face four hours prior. He reports pain to his right eye and denies any other injuries. On physical examination, he has right periorbital swelling with tenderness around his eye. His vision is 20/20 OS, OD, and OU, and he has a normal slit lamp examination. The eye is not proptotic. He reports binocular diplopia on upward gaze, and he seems to have minimally limited right eye upward gaze.

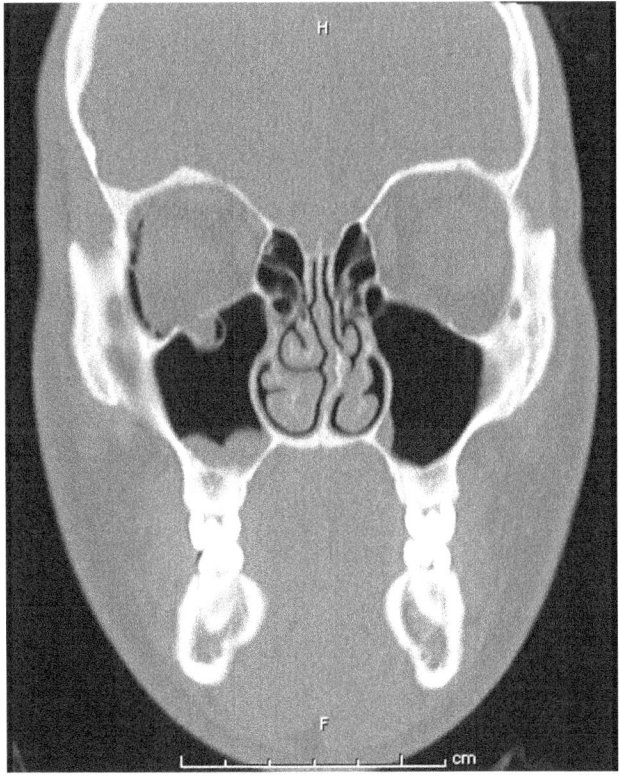

QUESTIONS

420. What is the likely diagnosis?

   a. Hyphema

   b. Lens Dislocation

   c. Orbital Floor Fracture

   d. Retrobulbar Hematoma

   e. Traumatic Iritis

421. Which of the following structures is likely to be affected in this type of injury?

   a. Inferior Rectus Muscle

   b. Lateral Cantus

   c. Macula

   d. Medial Cantus

   e. Superior Rectus Muscle

422. Which of the following is an indication for surgical repair of this condition?

   a. Associated Nondisplaced Fracture of the Medial Orbital Wall

   b. Double Vision On Lateral End Gaze

   c. Entrapment of an Extraocular Muscles

   d. Exophthalmus

   e. Hyphema >20%

ANSWERS

420. c

421. a

422. c

VISUAL STIMULUS REVIEW

The image shows right orbital floor fracture with air in the right orbit as well as a small amount of blood in the right maxillary sinus.

REFERENCES

- Ellis E 3rd. Orbital trauma. Oral Maxillofac Surg Clin North Am. 2012 Nov;24(4):629-48.
- Kubal WS. Imaging of orbital trauma. Radiographics. 2008 Oct;28(6):1729-39.
- Ceallaigh PO, Ekanaykaee K, Beirne CJ, Patton DW. Diagnosis and management of common maxillofacial injuries in the emergency department. Part 4: orbital floor and midface fractures. Emerg Med J. 2007 Apr;24(4):292-3.

CASE #125: TESTICULAR PAIN

CASE

A 45-year-old man presents to his family doctor complaining of right testicular pain for three days. He is a sexually active male with one long-term female partner and is not using condoms. He denies any history of STDs. He is afebrile, and his vital signs are within normal limits. On exam his right testicle is exquisitely tender including over its posterior border. There is no penile discharge.

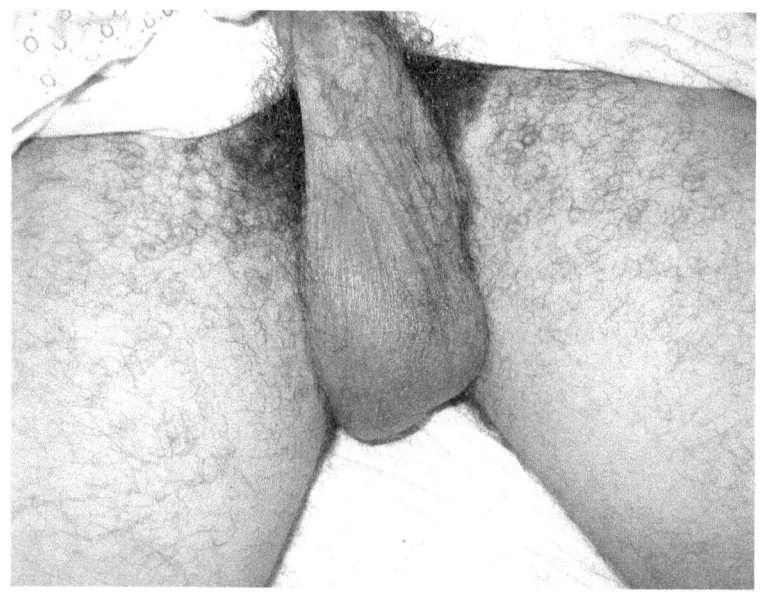

QUESTIONS

423. What is the likely diagnosis?
    a. Epididymo-Orchitis
    b. Inguinal Hernia
    c. Orchitis
    d. Testicular Torsion

424. What is the likely cause of this condition?
    a. Abdominal Wall Weakness
    b. Chlamydia
    c. Escherichia Colli
    d. Mumps
    e. Neisseria Gonorrhea
    f. Vascular Ischemia

425. What is the first line treatment for this condition?
    a. Azithromycin 1 g PO
    b. Ceftriaxone 250 mg IM
    c. Doxycycline 100 mg PO BID x 14 days
    d. Emergent Exploration and Detorsion
    e. Levofloxacin 500 mg PO BID x 14 days
    f. b + (a or c)

ANSWERS

423. a

424. c

425. e

VISUAL STIMULUS REVIEW

- The image shows an enlarged right hemiscrotum and erythematous scrotal skin.

REFERENCES

- Trojian TH, Lishnak TS, Heiman D. Epididymitis and orchitis: an overview. Am Fam Physician. 2009 Apr 1;79(7):583-7.

- Tracy CR, Steers WD, Costabile R. Diagnosis and management of epididymitis. Urol Clin North Am. 2008 Feb;35(1):101-8.

CASE #126: ALTERED MENTAL STATUS

CASE

A 53-year-old man is brought to the emergency department by EMS. The paramedic reports the patient was found confused on the floor of his apartment. The neighbors report that he lives alone and is known to be an alcoholic. The patient is lethargic and stuporous; he is moving all four extremities but mumbles in response to questions.

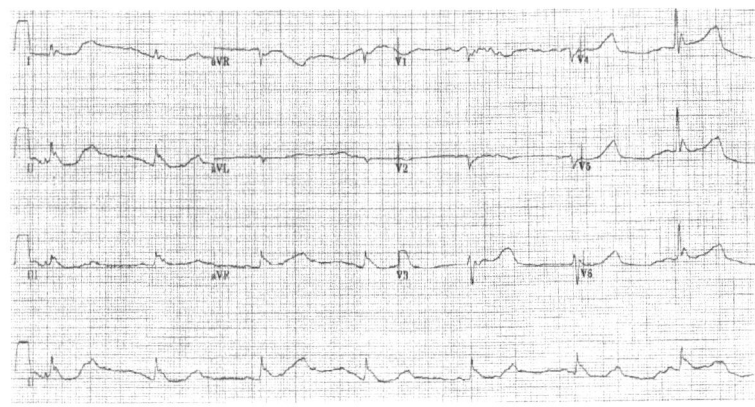

QUESTIONS

426. What is the likely diagnosis?

   a. Hypocalcemia

   b. Hypokalemia

   c. Hypomagnesemia

   d. Hyponatremia

   e. Hypothermia

427. What finding is visible on the EKG tracing?

   a. Deep Q Waves

   b. Osborne (J) Waves

   c. Picked T Waves

   d. U Waves

428. Which of the following findings is expected in this patient?

   a. Ca^{+2} 3 mEq/l

   b. K 2 mEq/l

   c. Mg 1.1 mg/dl

   d. Na 105 mEq/l

   e. Temp 86F (30C)

ANSWERS

426. e

427. b

428. e

VISUAL STIMULUS REVIEW

The EKG shows marked bradycardia with wide QRS and QT intervals as well as Osborne (J) waves.

REFERENCES

- Brown DJ, Brugger H, Boyd J, Paal P. Accidental hypothermia. N Engl J Med. 2012 Nov 15;367(20):1930-8.
- Ravi K. Mareedu, Naga P. et al. Classic EKG Changes of Hypothermia. Clin Med Res. 2008 December; 6(3-4): 107–108.

CASE #127: KNEE PAIN

CASE

A 13-year-old boy is brought to his pediatrician for right knee pain progressively getting worse over the last week. He is an active child and plays basketball almost daily. He is able to ambulate with mild to moderate pain, but the pain gets worth when he plays basketball, runs, or climbs up or downstairs. On exam he has point tenderness to palpation to the right tibial tubercle.

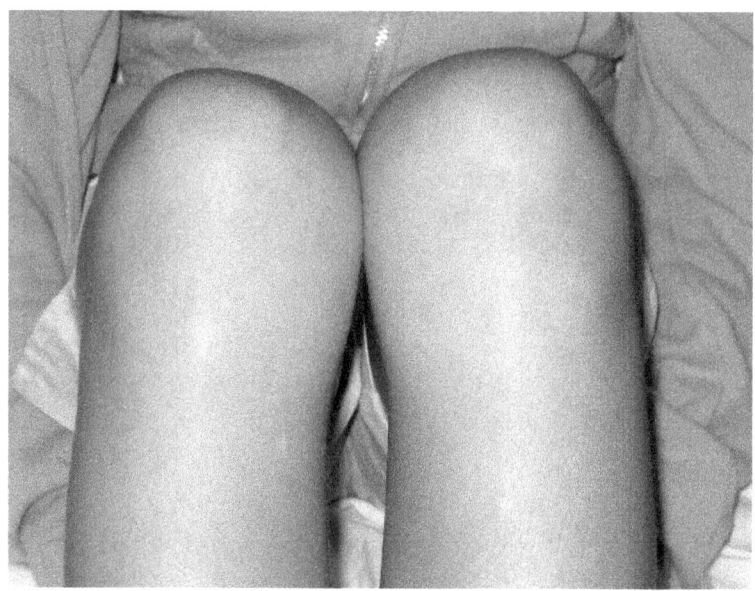

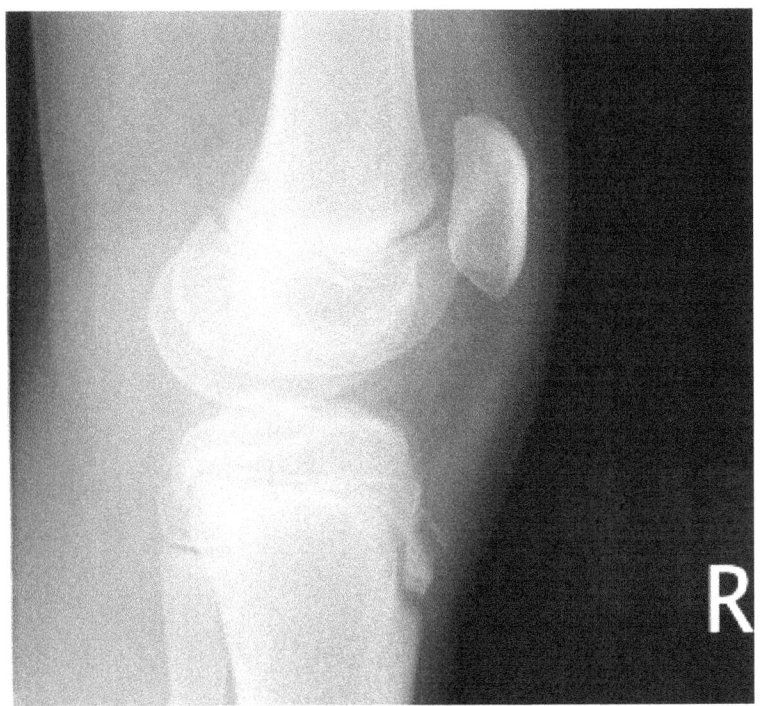

QUESTIONS

429. What is the likely diagnosis?

    a. Avulsion Fracture

    b. Knee Osteochondritis Dissecans

    c. Jumper's Knee

    d. Osgood Schlatter Syndrome

    e. Patellar Tendonitis

430. What is the recommended therapy for this condition?
    a. Avoid Pain-Producing Activities
    b. Knee Immobilizer
    c. Long Posterior Leg Splint
    d. Ossicle Excision
    e. Short Posterior Leg Splint
    f. Steroid Injections

ANSWERS

429. d

430. a

VISUAL STIMULUS REVIEW

The gross image shows swelling to the right knee tibial tubercle. The radiogram shows an elongated and fragmented tibial tubercle in this skeletally immature patient.

REFERENCES

- Gholve PA, Scher DM, Khakharia S et al. Osgood Schlatter syndrome. Curr Opin Pediatr. 2007 Feb;19(1):44-50.
- Krause BL, Williams JP, Catterall A. Natural history of Osgood-Schlatter disease. J Pediatr Orthop. Jan-Feb 1990;10(1):65-8.

CASE #128: BACK PAIN

CASE

A 30-year-old woman presents to her family doctor complaining of bilateral hearing loss over the last six months. She has a medical history of kyphosis and scoliosis as well as chronic back pain.

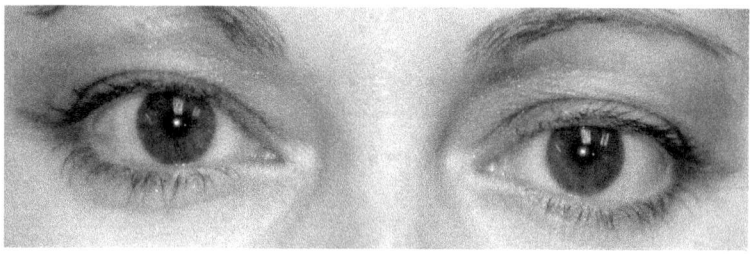

QUESTIONS

431. What is the likely diagnosis?

    a. Achondroplasia
    b. Hypochondroplasia
    c. Maffucci Syndrome
    d. Osteogenesis Imperfecta
    e. Rickets

432. What is the cause of this condition?

    a. Abnormal Protein Synthesis
    b. Primary Hormonal Deficiency
    c. Renal Losses
    d. Vitamin A Deficiency
    e. Vitamin D Deficiency
    f. Vitamin D Deficiency

433. What is the most common presentation of this condition?

    a. Bleeding Gums
    b. Repeated Fractures After Minor Trauma
    c. Skin Nodules
    d. Short and Deformed Bones

ANSWERS

431. d

432. a

433. b

VISUAL STIMULUS REVIEW

The image shows blue sclera.

REFERENCES

- Zhao X, Yan SG. Recent progress in osteogenesis imperfecta. Orthop Surg. 2011 May;3(2):127-30.
- Shapiro JR, Sponsellor PD. Osteogenesis imperfecta: questions and answers. Curr Opin Pediatr. 2009 Dec;21(6):709-16.

CASE #129: BACK PAIN

CASE

A 50-year-old man presents to the emergency department for worsening lower back pain and right leg weakness over the last two weeks. He has a medical history of IV drug abuse and chronic back pain. His vital signs show temp 100.9F (38.3C), heart rate 98/min, and blood pressure of 150/75 mmHg. Physical examination reveals midline tenderness to L2-L4 area and normal strength and sensation to bilateral lower extremities.

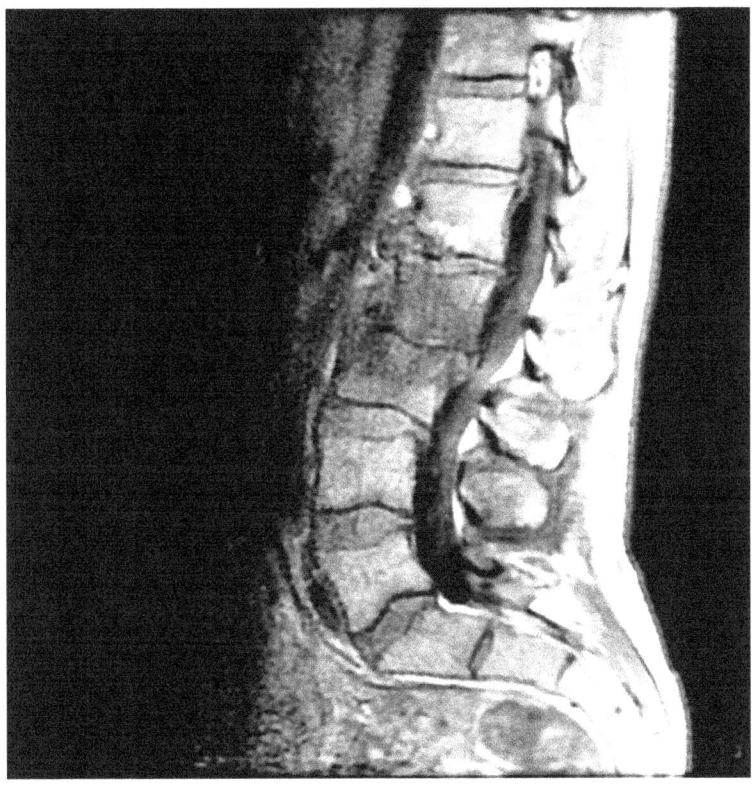

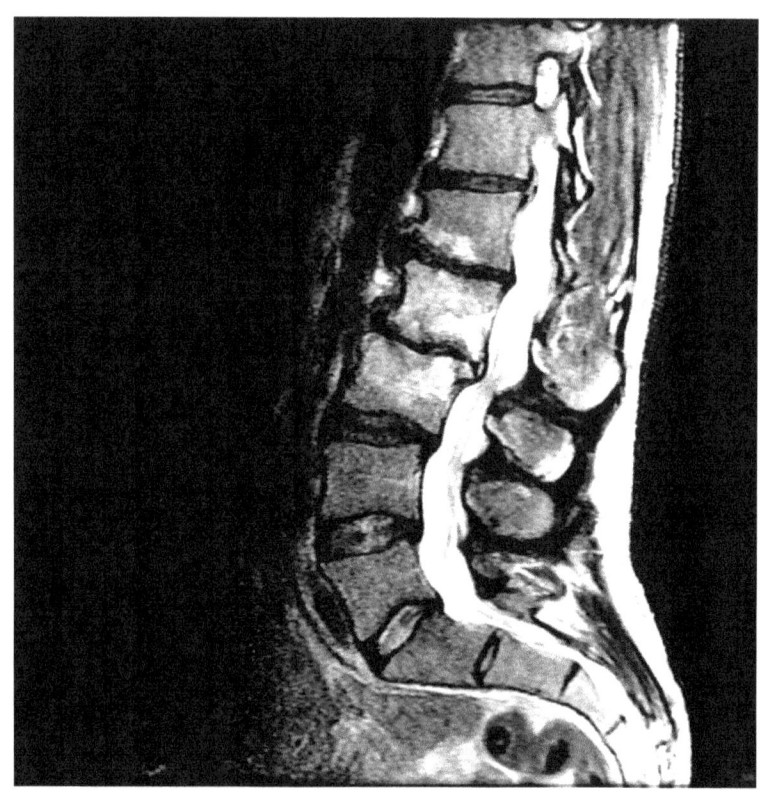

QUESTIONS

434. What is the likely diagnosis?
    a. Discitis
    b. Disc Herniation
    c. Epidural Abscess
    d. Epidural Metastases
    e. Osteomyelitis
    f. Sciatica

435. What is the likely cause of this condition?
    a. Age-Related Disc Degeneration
    b. Colon Cancer
    c. Endocarditis
    d. Irritation of a Nerve Root
    e. Urinary Tract Infection

436. What is the likely etiology of this condition?
    a. Enterobacteriaceae
    b. Staphylococcus Aureus
    c. Streptococcus Pneumonia
    d. Streptococus Pyogenes
    e. Tuberculosis

437. Which of the following findings is expected in this patient?
    a. Cellulitis
    b. Decreased Rectal Tone
    c. Elevated C-Reactive Protein
    d. Occult Blood Positive Stool
    e. Positive Straight Leg Raising Test

ANSWERS

434. e

435. c

436. b

437. c

VISUAL STIMULUS REVIEW

The T1 weighted MRI image shows decreased signal intensity in the L2 and L3 vertebral bodies and disk as well as inability to discern a margin between the disk and the adjacent vertebral bodies.

The T2 weighted MRI image shows increased signal intensity in L1-L3 vertebral bodies and absence of the intranuclear cleft.

REFERENCES

- Mylona E, Samarkos M, Kakalou E et al. Pyogenic vertebral osteomyelitis: a systematic review of clinical characteristics. Semin Arthritis Rheum. 2009 Aug;39(1):10-7.

- Bamberger DM. Diagnosis and treatment of osteomyelitis. Compr Ther. Summer 2000;26(2):89-95.

CASE #130: SHOULDER PAIN

CASE

A 72-year-old woman presents to the emergency department for right shoulder pain after a ground-level fall.

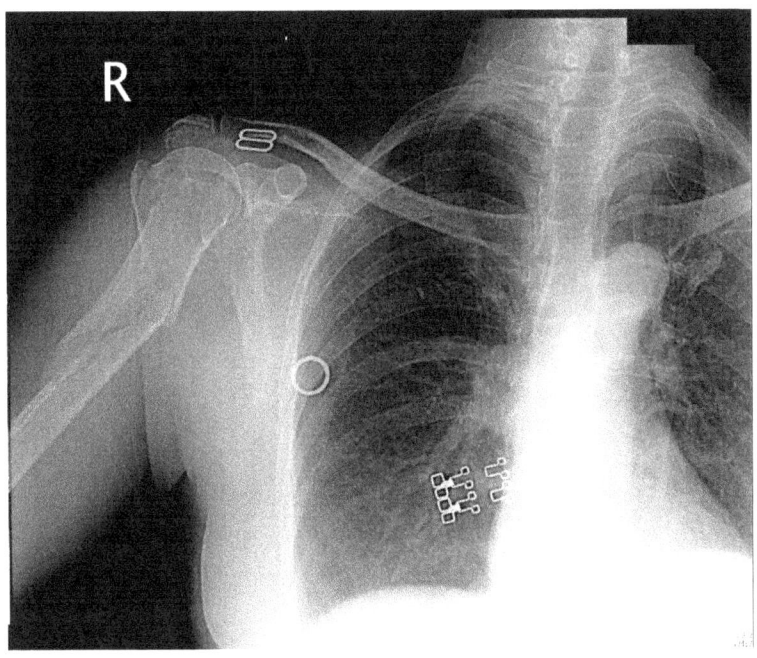

QUESTIONS

438. What is the likely diagnosis?

    a. Clavicle Fracture

    b. Humerus Fracture

    c. Scapular Fracture

    d. Shoulder Dislocation

439. What is the likely cause of this condition?

    a. Bone Metastasis

    b. Hypocalcemia

    c. Osteopetrosis

    d. Osteoporosis

    e. Vitamin D Deficiency

440. Which of the following studies can assess the severity of the condition that caused this presentation?

    a. 25-Hydroxyvitamin D

    b. Bone Marrow Biopsy

    c. Dual-Energy X-Ray Absorptiometry

    d. Intact PTH

    e. Technetium-99m Bone Scan

ANSWERS

438. b

439. d

440. c

VISUAL STIMULUS REVIEW

The radiogram shows severe osteopenia and a comminuted fracture of the right proximal humerus.

REFERENCES

- Warriner AH, Saag KG. Osteoporosis diagnosis and medical treatment. Orthop Clin North Am. 2013 Apr;44(2):125-35.

- Mazziotti G, Bilezikian J, Canalis E et al. New understanding and treatments for osteoporosis. Endocrine. 2012 Feb;41(1):58-69.

CASE #131:   EARACHE

CASE

A 72-year-old man with a history of diabetes mellitus presents to his family doctor complaining of severe right earache and swelling for three days. His vital signs are temp 103.2F (39.5C), heart rate 116/min, and blood pressure 150/70 mmHg. On physical examination, he has severe tenderness to his right ear as well as the soft tissue between his right mandible ramus to the mastoid tubercle.

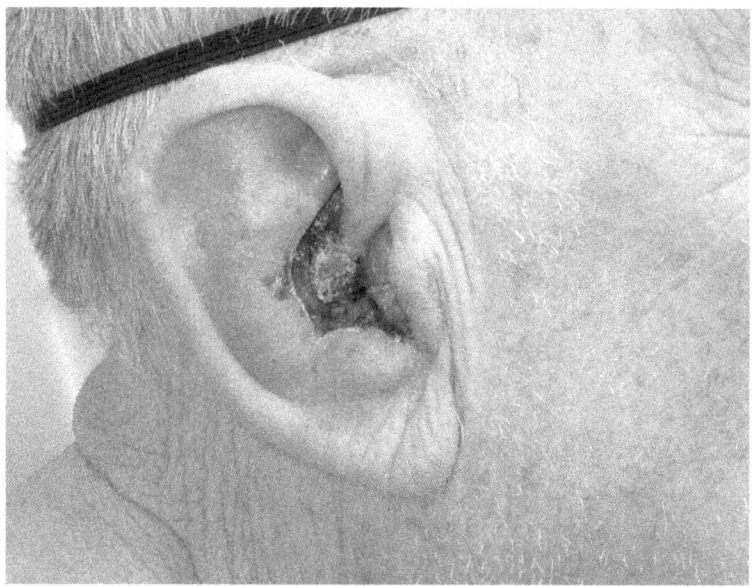

QUESTIONS

441. What is the likely diagnosis?

   a. Costochondritis

   b. External Ear Canal Carcinoma

   c. Malignant Otitis Externa

   d. Paget's Disease

   e. Otitis Externa Herpetica

442. What is the likely cause of this condition?

   a. Aspergillus Fumigatus

   b. Pseudomonal Aeruginosa

   c. Staphylococcus Aureus

   d. Staphylococcus Epidermidis

   e. Streptococus Pyogenes

443. Which of the following is a common risk factor for development of this condition?

   a. Aural Irrigation

   b. Hyperglycemia

   c. Swimming in a Freshwater Lake

   d. Tympanic Membrane Perforation

444. Which of the following cranial nerves is most commonly involved in advanced cases of this condition?

   a. CN III

   b. CN V

   c. CN VII

   d. CN IX

ANSWERS

441. c

442. b

443. a

444. c

VISUAL STIMULUS REVIEW

The image shows erythema and swelling to the helix and antihelix with necrotic (black) and granulation tissue covering the concha and the external auditory meatus.

REFERENCES

- Hollis S, Evans K. Management of malignant (necrotising) otitis externa. J Laryngol Otol. 2011 Dec;125(12):1212-7.

- Carfrae MJ, Kesser BW. Malignant otitis externa. Otolaryngol Clin North Am. 2008 Jun;41(3):537-49.

CASE #132: PELVIC PAIN

CASE

A 27-year-old woman presents to the emergency department for severe sudden-onset right-sided pelvic pain that started while she was jogging about an hour ago. She had three paroxysms of such pain over the last hour, each lasting about 10 minutes. The pain has been constant since her arrival. The pain is sharp and stabbing and is radiating to her back. She reports nausea and vomiting. On physical examination, she has normal vital signs and moderate tenderness over her right lower quadrant. On pelvic examination, she has moderate tenderness over her right adnexa. An ultrasound is performed.

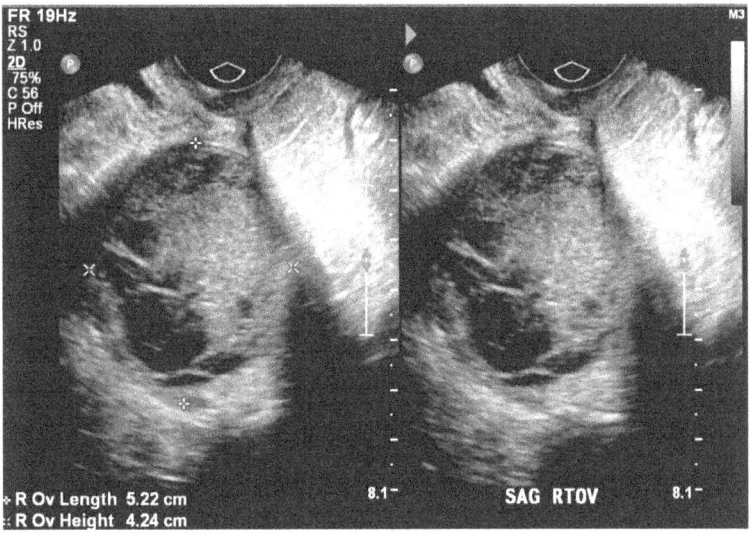

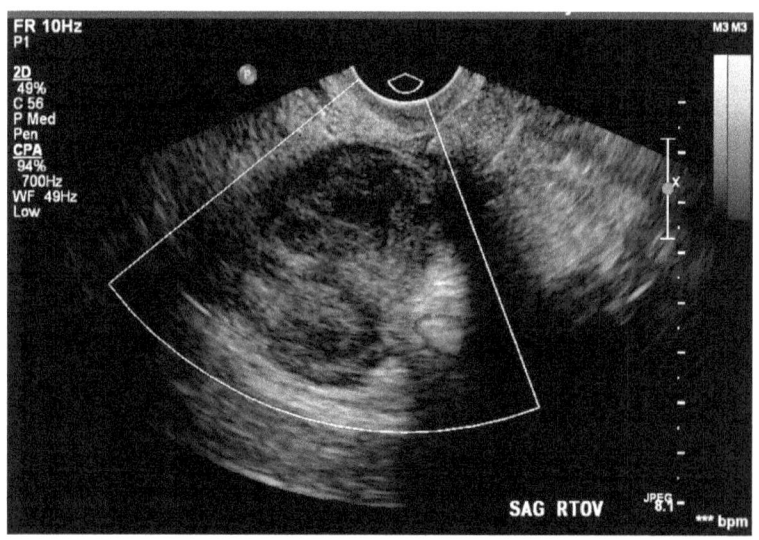

QUESTIONS

445. What is the likely diagnosis?

    a. Acute Appendicitis

    b. Ectopic Pregnancy

    c. Nephrolithiasis

    d. Ovarian Torsion

    e. Small Bowel Obstruction

446. What is the likely cause of this condition?

    a. Intraabdominal Scars

    b. Obstructing Appendicolith

    c. Obstructing Urethral Stone

    d. Ovarian Cyst

    e. Rupture of Ectopic Pregnancy

447. What is the first line treatment for this condition?
   a. Intravenous Antibiotics
   b. Laparoscopy
   c. Laparotomy
   d. Methotrexate
   e. Nasogastric Tube
   f. Nephrostomy Tube

ANSWERS

445. d

446. d

447. b

VISUAL STIMULUS REVIEW

The ultrasound images show a mildly enlarged right ovary with multiple follicles and no Doppler flow signals.

REFERENCES

- Huchon C, Fauconnier A. Adnexal torsion: a literature review. Eur J Obstet Gynecol Reprod Biol. 2010 May;150(1):8-12.

- McWilliams GD, Hill MJ, Dietrich CS 3rd. Gynecologic emergencies. Surg Clin North Am. 2008 Apr;88(2):265-83.

CASE #133:   EPIGASTRIC PAIN

CASE

A 45-year-old man presents to the emergency department for gradual onset abdominal pain, nausea, and vomiting over the past two days. The pain is described as epigastric and radiating to the back in a belt-like fashion. His vital signs are temp of 100.9F (382.C), heart rate 118/min, blood pressure of 170/90 mmHg. On physical examination, the patient has epigastric tenderness with moderate guarding.

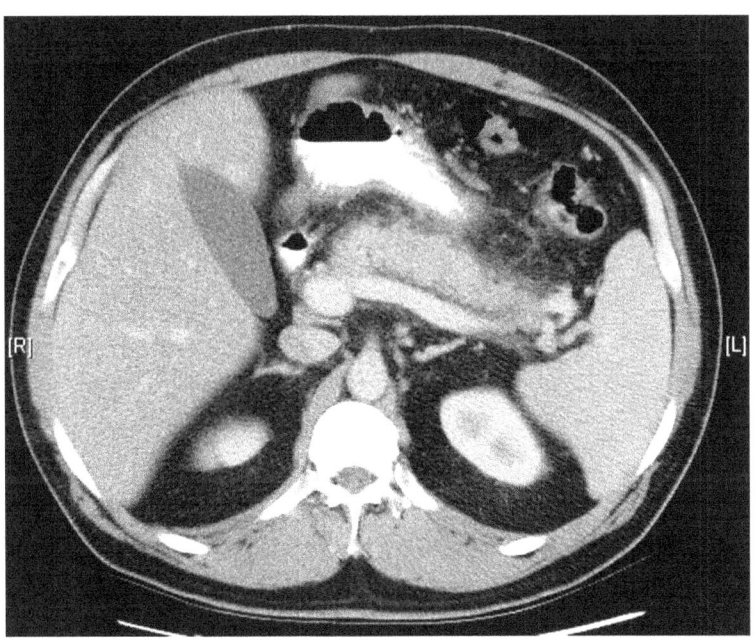

QUESTIONS

448. What is the likely diagnosis?

    a. Acute Appendicitis

    b. Acute Cholecystitis

    c. Acute Gastritis

    d. Acute Pancreatitis

    e. Aortic Dissection

449. What is the most common cause of this condition in the United States?

    a. Biliary Tract Disease

    b. Binge Alcohol Drinking

    c. Chronic Dehydration

    d. Infectious

    e. Hypertension

    f. Malnutrition

450. Which of the following abnormalities may cause this condition?

    a. Hypercalcemia

    b. Hyperkalemia

    c. Hypernatremia

    d. Hypocalcemia

    e. Hypokalemia

    f. Hyponatremia

451. Which of the following correlates with disease severity of this condition?

    a. ALT Level

    b. C-reactive Protein Level

c. Lactic Acid Level
d. Lipase Level
e. Neutrophil-Lymphocyte Ratio
f. All of the above

ANSWERS

448. d

449. a

450. a

451. f

VISUAL STIMULUS REVIEW

The CT image shows diffuse enlargement of the pancreas and diffuse haziness on the scan.

REFERENCES

- Suppiah A, Malde D, Arab T, Hamed M, Allgar V, Smith AM, et al. The Prognostic Value of the Neutrophil-Lymphocyte Ratio (NLR) in Acute Pancreatitis: Identification of an Optimal NLR. J Gastrointest Surg. 2013 Apr;17(4):675-81.

- Sah RP, Garg P, Saluja AK. Pathogenic mechanisms of acute pancreatitis. Curr Opin Gastroenterol. 2012 Sep;28(5):507-15.

- O'Connor OJ, McWilliams S, Maher MM. Imaging of acute pancreatitis. AJR Am J Roentgenol. 2011 Aug;197(2):W221-5.

CASE #134: DIFFICULTY URINATING

CASE

A 6-year-old boy is brought to his pediatrician for penile pain and difficulty urinating for one day. The patient is an uncircumcised boy who reports waking up with a painful and swollen penis. He was able to urinate with no difficulty before he went to sleep but is unable to since this morning.

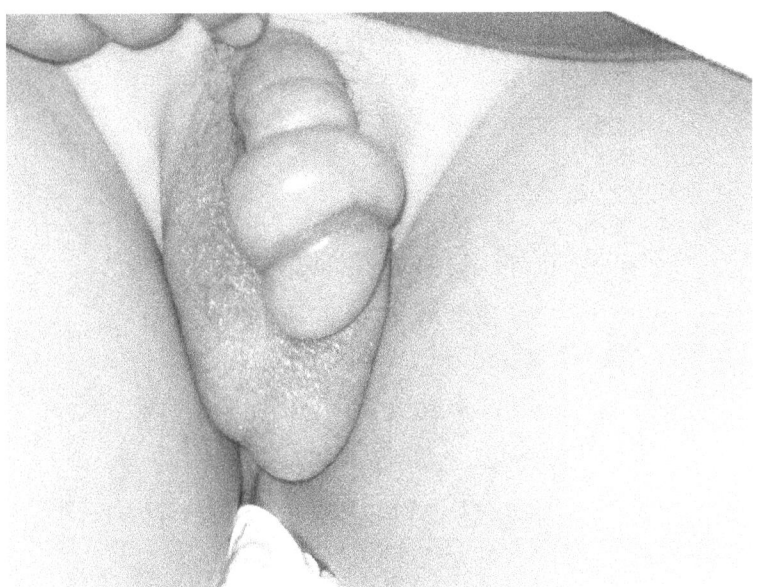

QUESTIONS

452. What is the likely diagnosis?
    a. Foreskin Angioedema
    b. Hair Tourniquet
    c. Paraphimosis
    d. Phimosis

453. What is the most common cause of this condition?
    a. Allergic Reaction
    b. Care Giver's Hair
    c. Iatrogenic
    d. Poor Hygiene
    e. Self-Inflicted

454. Which of the following describes first line management of this condition?
    a. Emergent Circumcision
    b. Incision of Constricting Band
    c. Manual Reduction
    d. Needle Aspiration
    e. Topical Steroid Ointment Application

ANSWERS

452. c

453. c

454. c

VISUAL STIMULUS REVIEW

The image shows a swollen glans penis with a collar of a retracted edematous foreskin.

REFERENCES

- Dubin J, Davis JE. Penile emergencies. Emerg Med Clin North Am. 2011 Aug;29(3):485-99.
- Choe JM. Paraphimosis: current treatment options. Am Fam Physician. 2000 Dec 15;62(12):2623-6.

CASE #135: FINGER PAIN

CASE

A 47-year-old female with no past medical history presents to her family doctor's office complaining of swelling to her right middle finger that has been worsening over the previous three days.

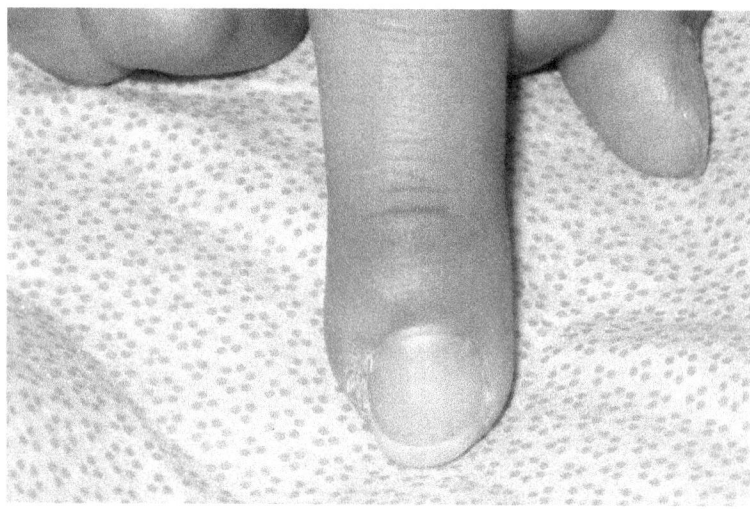

QUESTIONS

455. What is the likely diagnosis?

   a. Felon

   b. Herpetic Whitlow

   c. Onychomycosis

   d. Paronychia

   e. Psoriasis

456. What is the most common cause of an acute presentation of this condition?

   a. Candida Albicans

   b. Herpes Simplex Virus

   c. Pseudomonas Aeruginosa

   d. Staphylococcus Aurous

   e. Streptococus Pyogenes

457. What is the most common cause of a chronic or recurrent presentation of this condition?

   a. Candida Albicans

   b. Herpes Simplex Virus

   c. Pseudomonas Aeruginosa

   d. Staphylococcus Aurous

   e. Streptococus Pyogenes

ANSWERS

455. d

456. d

457. a

VISUAL STIMULUS REVIEW

The image shows erythema, swelling, and purulence along the lateral nail fold.

REFERENCES

- Ritting AW, O'Malley MP, Rodner CM. Acute paronychia. J Hand Surg Am. 2012 May;37(5):1068-70.

- McDonald LS, Bavaro MF, Hofmeister EP, Kroonen LT. Hand infections. J Hand Surg Am. 2011 Aug;36(8):1403-12.

- Clark DC. Common acute hand infections. Am Fam Physician. 2003 Dec 1;68(11):2167-76.

CASE #136: SHORTNESS OF BREATH

CASE

A 34-year-old man with no past medical history and who is not a smoker presents to his family doctor complaining of five weeks of dyspnea on exertion, dry cough, weight loss, fever, and chills. His vital signs are temp 101.9F (38.8C), heart rate 116/min, respiratory rate 36/min, blood pressure 120/70 mmHg, and O_2Sat of 88% on room air. On physical examination, the patient has clear bilateral lung sounds.

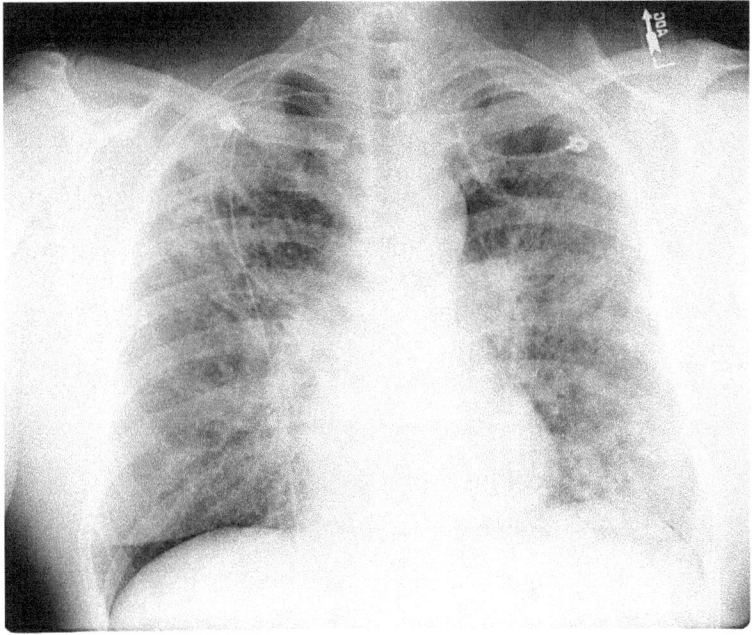

QUESTIONS

458. What is the likely diagnosis?

   a. ARDS

   b. Pneumonia

   c. Pulmonary Edema

   d. Pulmonary Embolus

   e. Pulmonary Fibrosis

459. What is the likely cause of this condition?

   a. Aspergillosis

   b. Hypercoagulable State

   c. Mycoplasma Pneumonia

   d. Pneumocystis Jiroveci

   e. Staphylococcus Aureus

   f. Streptococus Pneumonia

460. Which of the following risk factors is most commonly found in patients with this condition?

   a. AIDS

   b. Diabetes Mellitus Type 1

   c. Prolonged Immobilization

   d. Post Influenza

   e. Smoking

   f. Solid Organ Transplant

461. Which of the following findings is likely to be present in this condition?

   a. Elevated D-Dimers

   b. Elevated LDH

   c. Elevated Platelet Count

d. Elevated White Blood Cell Count
e. Low Platelet Count
f. Low Sodium

462. Which of the following is part of the first line treatment of this condition?

   a. Amphotericin B
   b. Ceftriaxone
   c. Heparin
   d. Trimethoprim-Sulfamethoxazole
   e. Vancomycin

ANSWERS

458. b

459. d

460. a

461. b

462. d

VISUAL STIMULUS REVIEW

The chest radiogram shows diffuse bilateral infiltrate that extend from the perihilar regions.

REFERENCES

- Gilroy SA, Bennett NJ. Pneumocystis pneumonia. Semin Respir Crit Care Med. 2011 Dec;32(6):775-82.

- Carmona EM, Limper AH. Update on the diagnosis and treatment of Pneumocystis pneumonia. Ther Adv Respir Dis. 2011 Feb;5(1):41-59.

- Catherinot E, Lanternier F, Bougnoux ME et al. Pneumocystis jirovecii Pneumonia. Infect Dis Clin North Am. 2010 Mar;24(1):107-38.

CASE #137: FEVER AND CONFUSION

CASE

A 57-year-old man is brought to the hospital by EMS for altered mental status and generalized seizures. EMS reports that he has a history of alcoholism and that he was found by bystanders after he fell and had a seizure. On exam the patient is lethargic, nonverbal, and localizes to pain in all extremities. His temp is 102.5F (39.2C), heart rate 120/min, respirations 20/min, blood pressure 100/60 mmHg, and O_2Sat 97%.

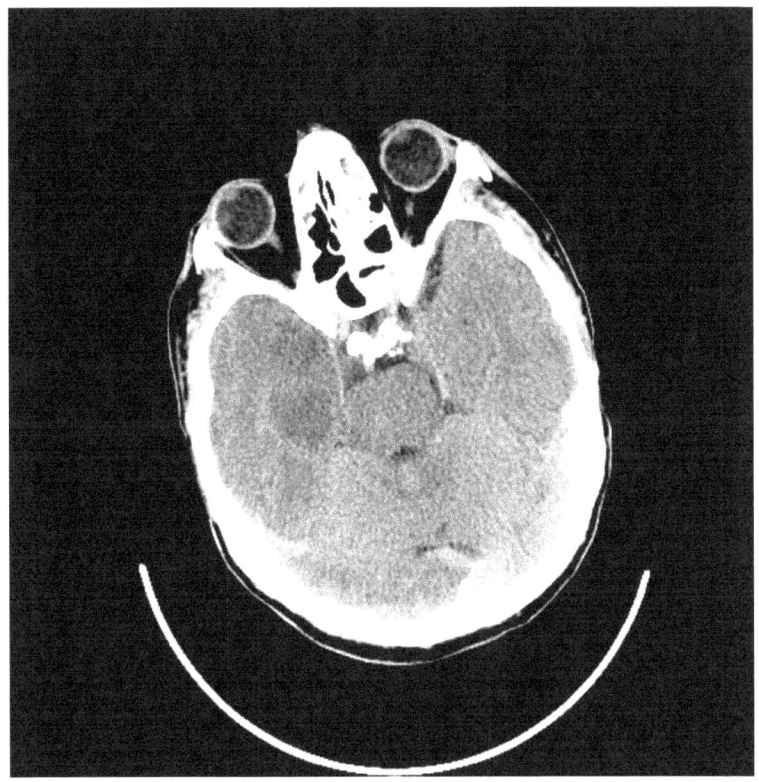

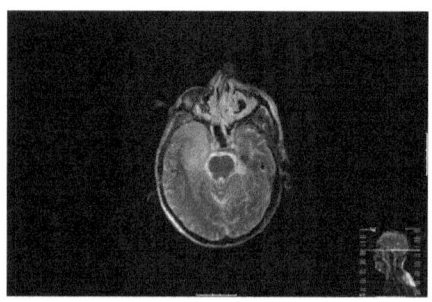
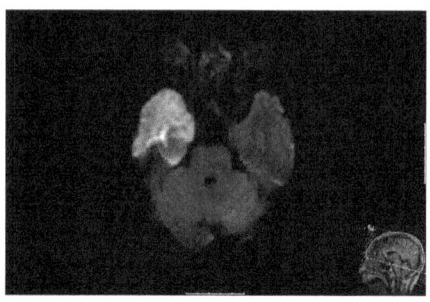

QUESTIONS

463. What is the likely diagnosis?
    a. Alcohol Withdrawal Seizures
    b. Glioblastoma Multiforme
    c. Herpes Simplex Encephalitis
    d. Pneumococcal Meningitis
    e. West Nile Virus Encephalitis

464. CSF analysis is likely to yield which of the following findings?
    a. WBCs 2/µl, Normal Protein
    b. WBCs 100/µl, Elevated Protein
    c. WBCs 100/µl, Normal Protein
    d. WBCs 6000/µl, Elevated Protein
    e. WBCs 6000/µl, Normal Protein

465. First line treatment of this condition includes which of the following?

   a. Acyclovir IV
   b. Ceftriaxone IV
   c. Methyl-Prednisolone IV
   d. Thiamin IV

466. What is the estimated mortality of this condition if left untreated?

   a. 1%
   b. 25%
   c. 50%
   d. 75%

ANSWERS

463. c

464. b

465. a

466. d

VISUAL STIMULUS REVIEW

The CT image shows low-density changes in the right temporal lobe. The MRI brain images show areas of hyperintensity signals in the right temporal lobe corresponding to the edematous changes seen on CT.

REFERENCES

- Sabah M, Mulcahy J, Zeman A. Herpes simplex encephalitis. BMJ. 2012 Jun 6;344:e3166.
- Skelly MJ, Burger AA, Adekola O. Herpes simplex virus-1 encephalitis: a review of current disease management with three case reports. Antivir Chem Chemother. 2012 Sep 25;23(1):13-8.

CASE #138: PAINFUL RASH

CASE

A 54-year-old man with no past medical history presents to his family doctor for painful skin blistering for five days. He reports painful mouth sores that started about three month ago and resolving spontaneously before reappearing and new blisters to his forearms, legs, and upper chest and back that appeared more recently. Some of the early blisters have healed without scarring. He denies taking any prescription medications and has been taking acetaminophen (OTC) for his pain. On physical examination, firm sliding (lateral) pressure on normal-appearing skin produces a blister.

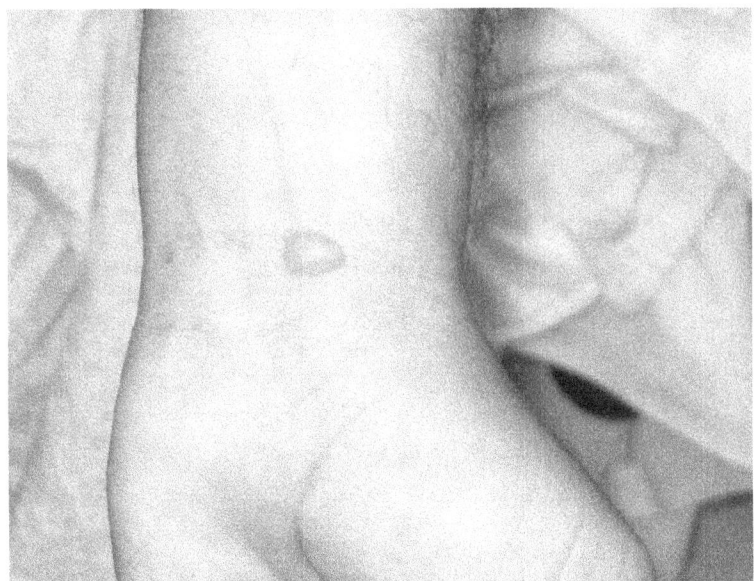

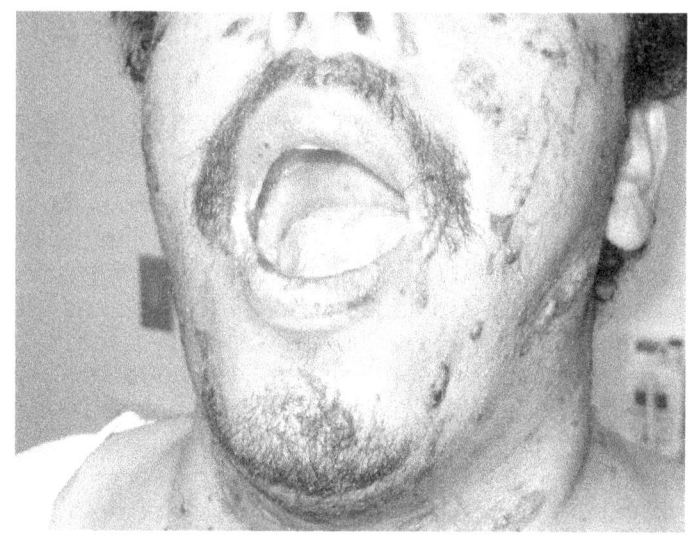

QUESTIONS

467. What is the likely diagnosis?
    a. Bullous Pemphigoid
    b. Erythema Multiforme
    c. Pemphigus Vulgaris
    d. Photosensitivity Reaction
    e. Porphyria Cutanea Tarda
    f. Toxic Epidermal Necrolysis

468. Which of the following findings is commonly seen in this condition?
    a. Auspitz Sign
    b. Cullen's Sign
    c. Darier's Sign
    d. Hutchinson's Sign
    e. Nikolsky's Sign

ANSWERS

467. c

468. e

VISUAL STIMULUS REVIEW

The first image shows intact thin-walled clear fluid-filled blisters surrounded by healthy-appearing skin to the left forearm.

The second image shows multiple erosions to the skin of the face and neck as well oral mucosal erosions to the buccal and palatine surfaces.

REFERENCES

- Tsuruta D, Ishii N, Hashimoto T. Diagnosis and treatment of pemphigus. Immunotherapy. 2012 Jul;4(7):735-45.
- Venugopal SS, Murrell DF. Diagnosis and clinical features of pemphigus vulgaris. Immunol Allergy Clin North Am. 2012 May;32(2):233-43

CASE #139: SHORTNESS OF BREATH

CASE

A 34-year-old man with no past medical history presents to the emergency department complaining of constant chest pain for the last three days as well as shortness of breath. He describes the chest pain as retrosternal with radiation to the neck, upper back, and left arm that is worse when taking a deep breath and laying supine and slightly improved when leaning forward. He reports worsening dyspnea on exertion over the last couple of days. His vital signs are temp 100.5F (38C), heart rate 150/min regular, respirations 24/min, blood pressure 130/70 mmHg, and O_2Sat 97% on room air. On physical exam, he seems to be in mild distress; his lung sounds are clear bilaterally; his heart sounds are distant, tachycardic, and regular with a systolic friction rub. His radial, femoral, and dorsalis pedis pulses are strong and symmetric. He does not have pedal edema.

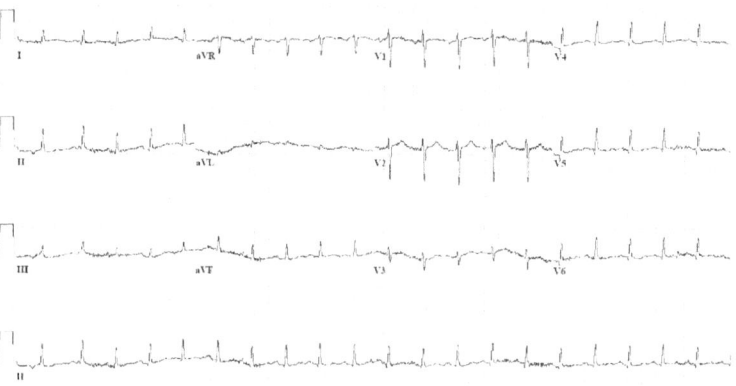

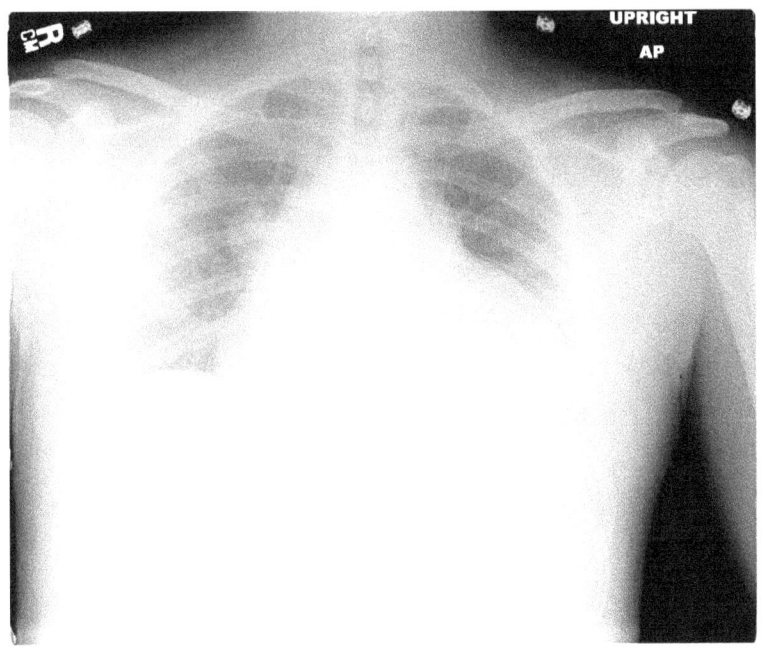

QUESTIONS

469. What is the likely diagnosis?

    a. Acute Myocardial Infarction

    b. Aortic Dissection

    c. Pericarditis

    d. Pneumothorax

    e. Pulmonary Edema

470. What finding(s) are visible on the chest radiogram?
    a. Alveolar Fluid
    b. Enlarged Cardiac Silhouette
    c. Extra-Pulmonary Air
    d. Pulmonary Artery Congestion
    e. Wide Mediastinum

471. What is the most common cause of this condition?
    a. Coxsackie Virus B
    b. Coronary Artery Thrombosis
    c. Systemic Lupus Erythematosus
    d. Syphilis
    e. Tuberculosis

472. Definitive diagnosis of this condition requires which of the following?
    a. Arteriogram
    b. CT Angiogram
    c. Inspiratory + Expiratory Chest X-Ray
    d. Echocardiogram
    e. Serum Beta Natriuretic Peptide Measurement

473. Which of the following is part of the first line treatment of this condition?
    a. Aortic Repair
    b. Ceftriaxone IV
    c. Coronary Angiography and Stenting
    d. Furosemide IV
    e. Heparin IV

f. Indomethacin

474. As you examine the patient, he becomes diaphoretic and faints. His heart rate is now 170/min, blood pressure 60/40 mmHg, and O_2Sat 97% on room air. What happened to this patient?

    a. Cardiac Tamponade

    b. Massive Pulmonary Edema

    c. Rupture of Thoracic Aorta

    d. Rupture of Mitral Valve

    e. Tension Pneumothorax

    f. Ventricular Tachycardia

475. What treatment is indicated at this time?

    a. Cardioversion

    b. Chest Tube Insertion

    c. Defibrillation

    d. Norepinephrine

    e. Pericardiocentesis

    f. Tissue Plasminogen Activator IV

ANSWERS

469. c

470. b

471. a

472. d

473. f

474. a

475. e

VISUAL STIMULUS REVIEW

The ECG tracing shows sinus tachycardia and very low voltage.

The chest radiogram shows an enlarged cardiac silhouette.

REFERENCES

- McConaghy JR, Oza RS. Outpatient diagnosis of acute chest pain in adults. Am Fam Physician. 2013 Feb 1;87(3):177-82.

- Htwe TH, Khardori NM. Cardiac emergencies: infective endocarditis, pericarditis, and myocarditis. Med Clin North Am. 2012 Nov;96(6):1149-69.

CASE #140: EYE SWELLING

CASE

A 4-year-old boy is brought to his pediatrician for left eye swelling for two days. The patient is up to date on his vaccinations and has no past medical history. The parents report a recent history of dry cough and runny nose over the last five days. The vitals are temp 101.9F (38.8C), heart rate 110/min, blood pressure 100/60 mmHg, and O_2Sat 99% on room air. On exam the left eyelid is swollen, the eye is closed shut, and there is no resistance to retropulsion. On eyelid opening, the patient has no proptosis, normal pupillary exam, and no pain or limitation of extra ocular movement. The left side of his face is warm to palpation.

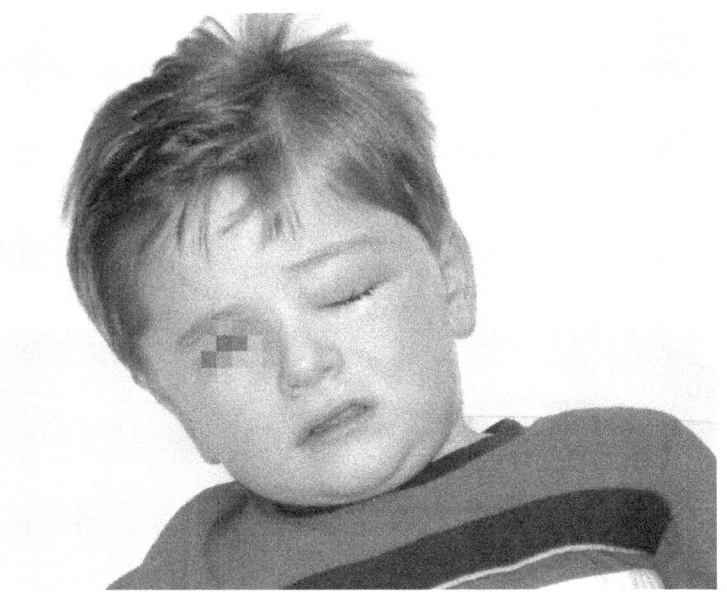

QUESTIONS

476. What is the likely diagnosis?
    a. Allergic Reaction
    b. Cavernous Sinus Thrombosis
    c. Insect Bite
    d. Orbital Cellulitis
    e. Periorbital Cellulitis
    f. Sinusitis

477. What is the likely cause of this condition?
    a. Conjunctivitis
    b. Haemophilus Influenza
    c. Staphylococcus Aureus
    d. Staphylococcus Epidermidis
    e. Streptococus Viridans

478. Which of the following findings is an indication for emergent surgical intervention?
    a. Afferent Pupillary Defect
    b. Diplopia
    c. Vision Acuity 20/80
    d. Limited Extra Ocular Movement

479. Which of the following studies can help achieve a definitive diagnosis?
    a. CT Orbits
    b. CT Venogram
    c. Complete Blood Count with Differential
    d. Retropulsion Test
    e. Sedimentation Rate
    f. Sinus X-Ray

ANSWERS

476. e

477. c

478. a

479. a

VISUAL STIMULUS REVIEW

The image shows a swollen left upper eyelid with periorbital erythema.

REFERENCES

- Baring DE, Hilmi OJ. An evidence based review of periorbital cellulitis. Clin Otolaryngol. 2011 Feb;36(1):57-64.
- Givner LB. Periorbital versus orbital cellulitis. Pediatr Infect Dis J. 2002 Dec;21(12):1157-8.

CASE #141: SORE THROAT

CASE

A 34-year-old man presents to the emergency department complaining of sore throat and difficulty swallowing. He has no past medical history, is a smoker, and is not taking any chronic medications. The patient reports a three-day history of sore throat with one day of severe pain to the right side of his throat, difficulty swallowing liquids and fluids as well as fever. His vital signs are temp of 102.0F (38.9C), heart rate 116/min, respiratory rate 18/min, blood pressure 130/75 mmHg, O_2Sat 99% on room air. On physical examination, his uvula is deviated to the right, and the superior pole of the right tonsil is displaced downward.

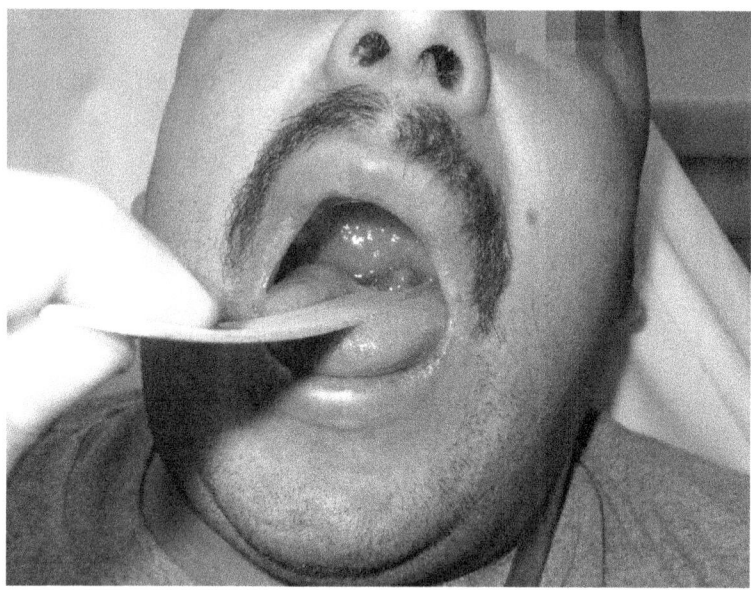

QUESTIONS

480. What is the likely diagnosis?
    a. Acute Tonsillitis
    b. Actinomycosis
    c. Ludwig's Angina
    d. Peritonsillar Abscess
    e. Retropharyngeal Abscess
    f. Tonsillar Abscess

481. What is the likely cause of this condition?
    a. Treated Tonsillitis
    b. Untreated Tonsillitis
    c. Hematogenous Seeding
    d. a and b

482. What is the most common etiology of this condition?
    a. Actinomyces
    b. Epstein Bar Virus
    c. Haemophilus Influenza
    d. Staphylococcus Aureus
    e. Streptococcus Group A
    f. Streptococcus Pneumonia

483. What is the first line treatment of this condition?
    a. Incision and Drainage
    b. IV Antibiotics
    c. Needle Aspiration
    d. Oral Antibiotics
    e. a and c

ANSWERS

480. d

481. d

482. e

483. e

VISUAL STIMULUS REVIEW

The image shows pharyngeal erythema with fullness to the right peritonsillar area.

REFERENCES

- Tagliareni JM, Clarkson EI. Tonsillitis, peritonsillar and lateral pharyngeal abscesses. Oral Maxillofac Surg Clin North Am. 2012 May;24(2):197-204

- Powell J, Wilson JA. An evidence-based review of peritonsillar abscess. Clin Otolaryngol. 2012 Apr;37(2):136-45.

CASE #142: PELVIC PAIN

CASE

A 24-year-old woman who has an IUD presents to the emergency department complaining of pelvic pain and vaginal discharge for three days. She reports two sexual partners and not using condoms with either one. On further history she also reports fever and chills over the last couple of days and yellow vaginal discharge. Her vital signs are temp of 102.0F (38.9C), heart rate 116/min, respiratory rate 18/min, blood pressure 130/75 mmHg, O_2Sat 99% on room air. On pelvic examination, she has cervical motion tenderness and severe tenderness on palpation of the uterus and the right adnexa.

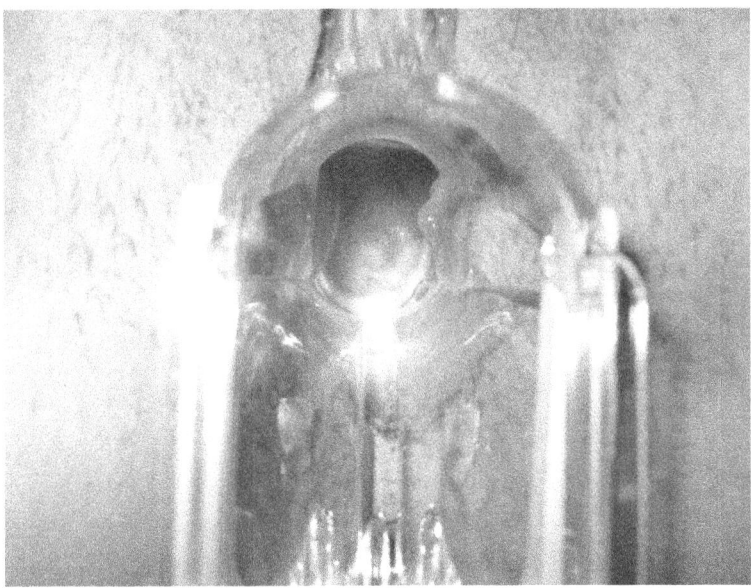

QUESTIONS

484. What is the likely diagnosis?
    a. Appendicitis
    b. Cervicitis
    c. Endometritis
    d. Ovarian Torsion
    e. Pelvic Inflammatory Disease
    f. Vaginitis

485. What is the most common cause of this condition?
    a. Bacteroides Fragilis
    b. Chlamydia trachomatis
    c. Escherichieae Colli
    d. Gardnerella Vaginalis
    e. Neisseria Gonorrhoeae
    f. Streptococcus Agalactiae

486. What condition is likely present if this patient also has right upper-quadrant tenderness?
    a. Acalculous Cholecystitis
    b. Acute Cholecystitis
    c. Fitz-Hugh-Curtis Syndrome
    d. Pancreatitis
    e. Pyelonephritis

ANSWERS

484. e

485. b

486. c

VISUAL STIMULUS REVIEW

The image shows a mucopurulent cervical discharge. The external os of the cervix does not appear erythematous.

REFERENCES

- Chappell CA, Wiesenfeld HC. Pathogenesis, diagnosis, and management of severe pelvic inflammatory disease and tubo-ovarian abscess. Clin Obstet Gynecol. 2012 Dec;55(4):893-903.

- Gradison M. Pelvic inflammatory disease. Am Fam Physician. 2012 Apr 15;85(8):791-6.

CASE #143: DRAINING LUMP

CASE

A 19-year-old male patient presents to the emergency department complaining of painful swelling and drainage to his lower back that progressively increased over the past week. He is afebrile, and his vital signs are within normal limits. He has no past medical history and denies history of trauma or other skin infections.

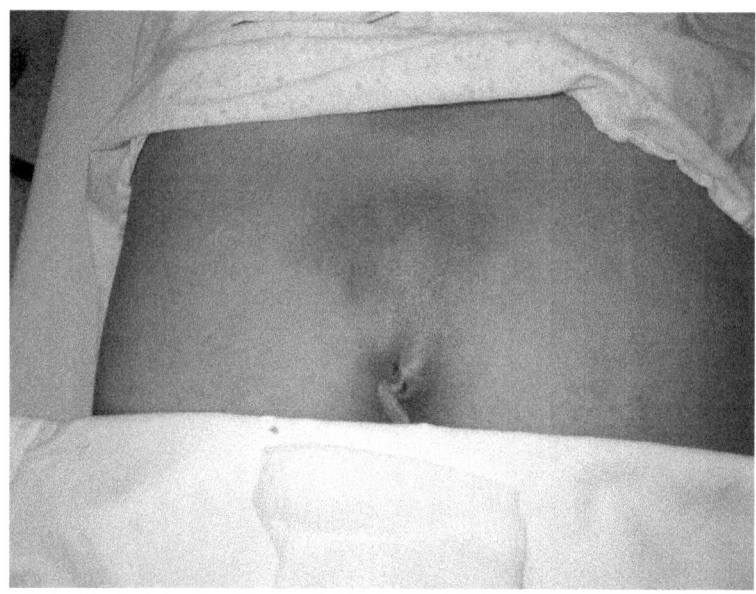

QUESTIONS

487. What is the likely diagnosis?
    a. Hidradenitis Suppurativa
    b. Pilonidal Abscess
    c. Rectocutaneous Fistula
    d. Sacral Cellulitis

488. What is the likely cause of this condition?
    a. Congenital
    b. Crohn's Complication
    c. Ingrown Hair
    d. Localized Trauma

489. Which of the following is a risk factor for this condition?
    a. Deep Natal Cleft
    b. Hirsutism
    c. Male Gender
    d. Obesity
    e. Sedentary Lifestyle
    f. All of the above

490. What is the first line therapy of this condition?
    a. Incision and Drainage
    b. IV Antibiotics
    c. Oral Antibiotics
    d. Sitz Baths

ANSWERS

487. b

488. c

489. f

490. a

VISUAL STIMULUS REVIEW

The image shows erythema and swelling to the sacrococcygeal area with pus draining out of a sinus tract.

REFERENCES

- Humphries AE, Duncan JE. Evaluation and management of pilonidal disease. Surg Clin North Am. 2010 Feb;90(1):113-24.

- Kitchen P. Pilonidal sinus — management in the primary care setting. Aust Fam Physician. 2010 Jun;39(6):372-5.

- Velasco AL, Dunlap WW. Pilonidal disease and hidradenitis. G Clin North Am. 2009 Jun;89(3):689-701.

CASE #144: DIFFICULTY SLEEPING

CASE

A 5-year-old girl is brought to her pediatrician for restless sleeping for the last two weeks. The parents report that this healthy girl started crying at night and early morning complaining that she can't sleep. They also noticed that she itches around her buttocks and perineum but were unable to see any wounds or rashes to that area. They deny any weight loss, vomiting, or diarrhea. On physical exam, her vital signs are within normal limits, and her abdomen is soft and not tender.

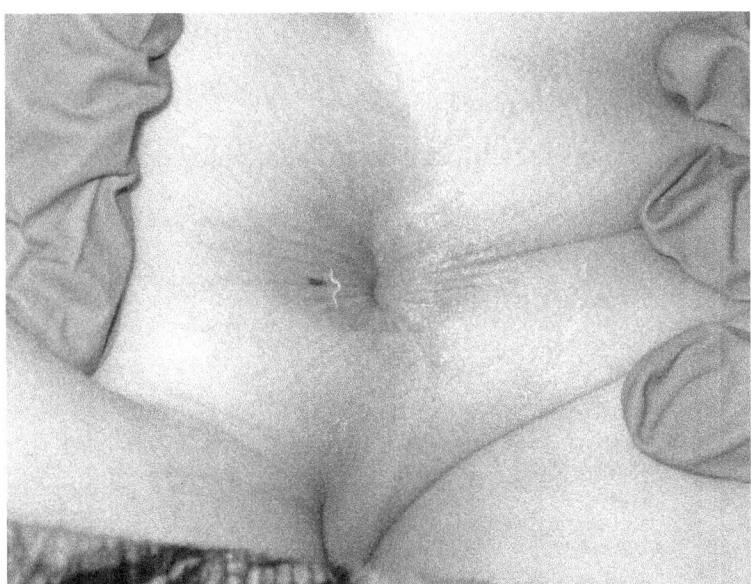

QUESTIONS

491. What is the likely diagnosis?

   a. Anusitis
   b. Crohn's Disease
   c. Pinworm
   d. Tapeworm
   e. Proctitis
   f. Pruritus Ani

492. What is the likely cause of this condition?

   a. Ascaris Lumbricoides
   b. Echinococcus
   c. Enterobius Vermicularis
   d. Schistosomiasis
   e. Trichinella

493. What is the transmission route of this condition?

   a. Direct Skin Penetration
   b. Fecal, Oral
   c. Fomite, Oral
   d. Mosquito Bite
   e. b and c

494. What anatomic part serves as the main reservoir for the cause of this condition?

   a. Anus
   b. Ascending Colon
   c. Descending Colon
   d. Ileocecum
   e. Rectum
   f. Sigmoid Colon

495. Which of the following statement is correct?
    a. Mebendazole is an effective agent for treatment of this condition.
    b. At least three doses separated by three weeks are usually needed to successfully treat this condition.
    c. All household members should be treated simultaneously.
    d. All bedding, gowns, chairs, and stretchers that patients with this condition have been in contact with must be washed and cleaned before used for further patient care.
    e. All of the above
    f. Only a and c

ANSWERS

491. c

492. c

493. e

494. d

495. e

VISUAL STIMULUS REVIEW

The image shows a pinworm next to the anus.

REFERENCES

- Stermer E, Sukhotnic I, Shaoul R. Pruritus ani: an approach to an itching condition. J Pediatr Gastroenterol Nutr. 2009 May;48(5):513-6.

- Kucik CJ, Martin GL, Sortor BV. Common intestinal parasites. Am Fam Physician. 2004 Mar 1;69(5):1161-8.

CASE #145: ITCHY RASH

CASE

A 4-year-old boy is brought to his pediatrician for an itchy rash. The parents report a single lesion to his left chest that appeared about 10 days ago with multiple lesions that followed about 10 days later. The parents deny any medical history, medications, recent travel, or exposure to people with similar lesions. There are no lesions to the hands or feet.

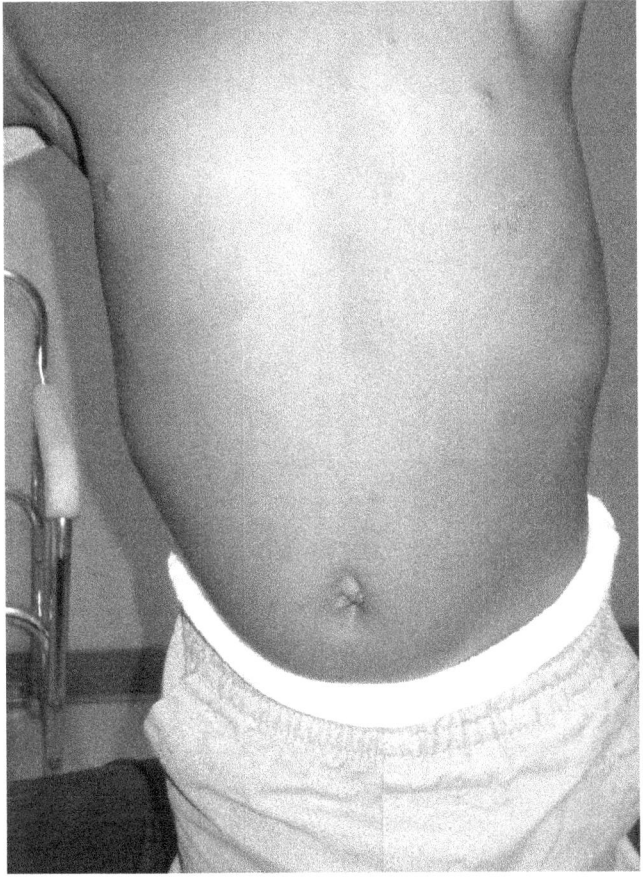

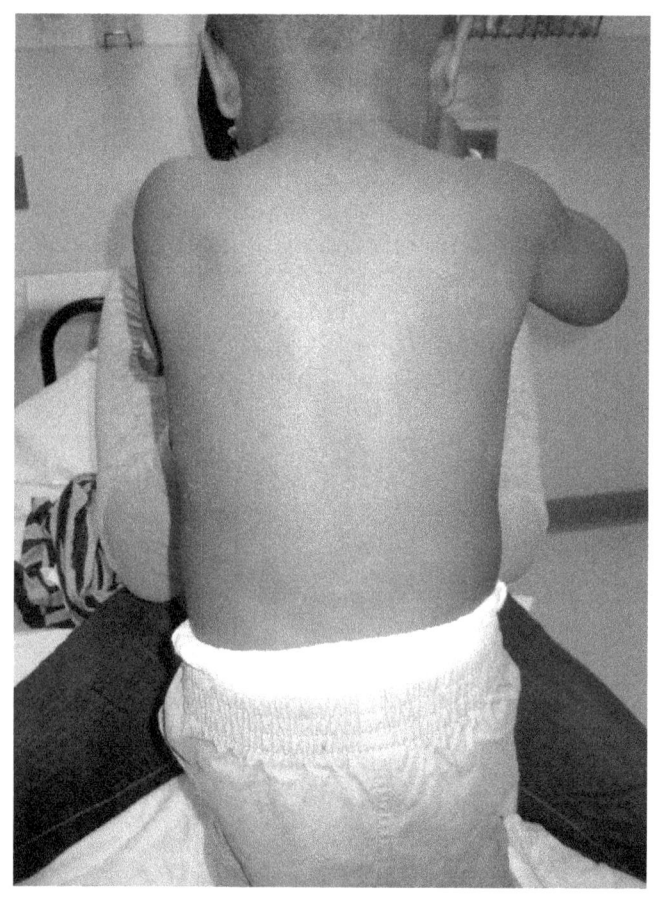

QUESTIONS

496. What is the likely diagnosis?
   a. Erythema Multiforme
   b. Pityriasis Rosea
   c. Psoriasis
   d. Scabies
   e. Syphilis
   f. Tinea Versicolor

497. What finding is present in this patient?
   a. Auspitz Sign
   b. Cullen's Sign
   c. Darier's Sign
   d. Herald Patch
   e. Nikolsky's Sign

498. Which of the following is a first line therapy for this condition?
   a. Betamethasone Ointment
   b. Penicillin IM
   c. Prednisone PO
   d. Terbinafine Body Wash
   e. Zinc Oxide Ointment

ANSWERS

496. b

497. d

498. e

VISUAL STIMULUS REVIEW

The first image shows an oval plaque with fine scales.

The second image shows multiple macules and papules with scaling diffusely distributed parallel to skin tension lines.

REFERENCES

- Drago F, Broccolo F, Rebora A. Pityriasis rosea: an update with a critical appraisal of its possible herpesviral etiology. J Am Acad Dermatol. 2009 Aug;61(2):303-18.

- Stulberg DL, Wolfrey J. Pityriasis rosea. Am Fam Physician. 2004 Jan 1;69(1):87-91.

CASE #146: ITCHY RASH

CASE

A 25-year-old woman presents to her family doctor complaining of intense pruritus and rash for two days. She reports no past medical history, no medications, and no known exposure or history of similar rash. She was walking through a friend's yard a couple of days before the onset of the rash, helping her move yard furniture. On examination, the patient has diffuse lesions as seen below mostly on bilateral upper and lower extremities.

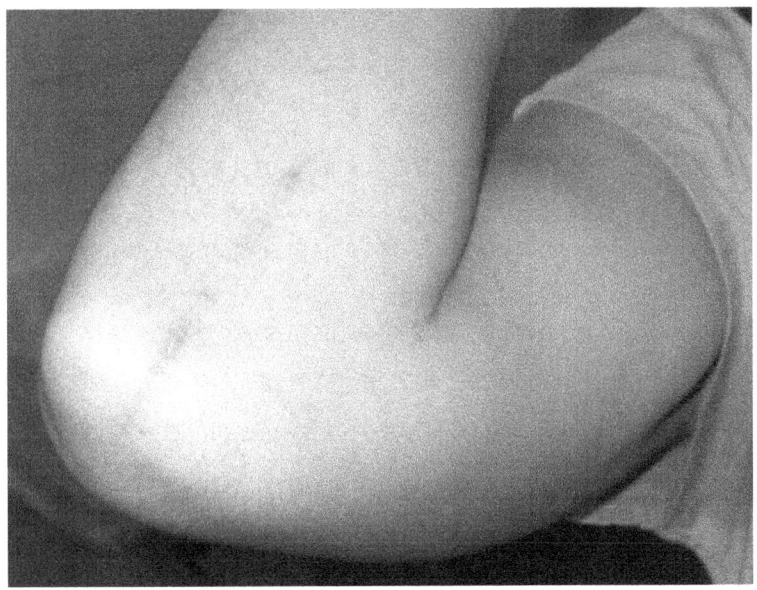

QUESTIONS

499. What is the likely diagnosis?

    a. Allergic Contact Dermatitis

    b. Irritant Contact Dermatitis

    c. Eczema

    d. Tinea Corporis

500. What is the likely cause of this condition?

    a. Chemical Irritant

    b. Direct Mechanical Trauma

    c. Trichophyton Rubrum

    d. Type I Allergic Reaction

    e. Type IV Allergic Reaction

501. Which of the following statement is true?

    a. This condition is likely to improve with a short course of topical antifungal ointment.

    b. This condition is likely to improve with a short course of topical steroid ointment.

    c. This condition is more prevalent in males.

    d. This condition requires skin breakdown to develop.

    e. This is likely at least the second time this patient has been exposed to the causative substance.

ANSWERS

499. a

500. e

501. e

VISUAL STIMULUS REVIEW

The image shows a linear streak to the right forearm that includes papules and vesicles on an erythematous base.

REFERENCES

- Martin SF. Allergic contact dermatitis: xenoinflammation of the skin. Curr Opin Immunol. 2012 Dec;24(6):720-9.

- Usatine RP, Riojas M. Diagnosis and management of contact dermatitis. Am Fam Physician. 2010 Aug 1;82(3):249-55.

- Sasseville D. Clinical patterns of phytodermatitis. Dermatol Clin. 2009 Jul;27(3):299-308.

CASE #147: DOUBLE VISION

CASE

A 30-year-old woman presents to her family doctor complaining of worsening diplopia and fatigue over the past month. She has no past medical history and is not taking any medications but reports a recent dry cough and sore throat that are improving. She reports double vision and generalized weakness, mostly to her arms, that is getting worth as the day progress. Her vital signs are within normal limits. The patient has a normal sensory and deep reflexes exam.

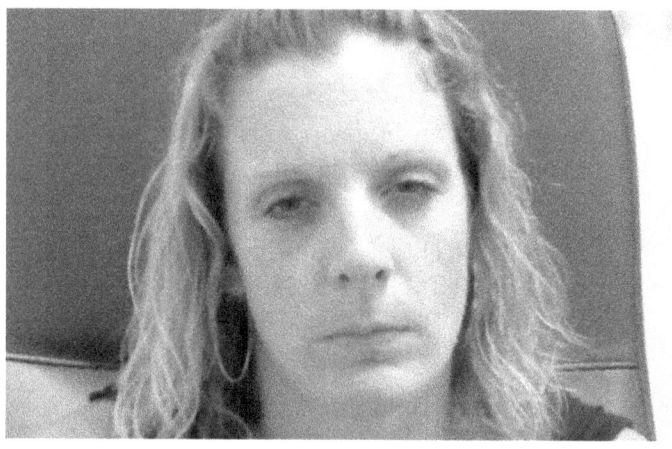

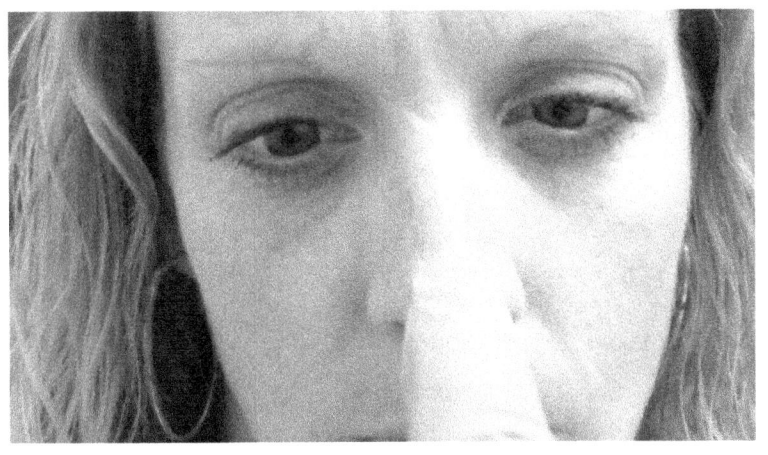
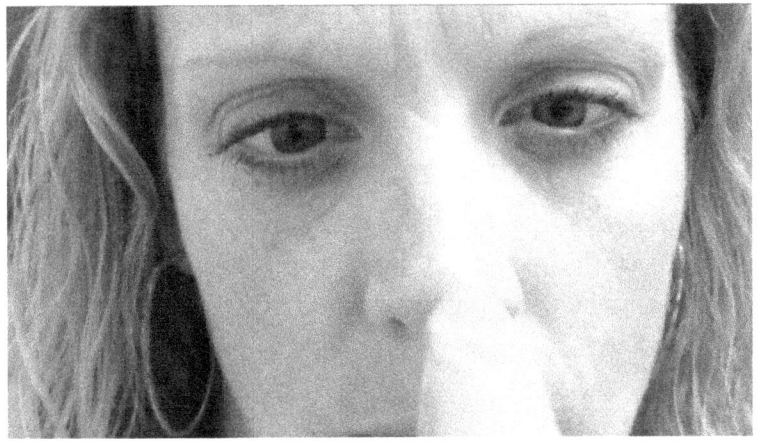

QUESTIONS

502. What is the likely diagnosis?
- a. Botulism
- b. Cavernous Sinus Thrombosis
- c. Lambert-Eaton Myasthenic Syndrome
- d. Multiple Sclerosis
- e. Myasthenia Gravis
- f. Tolosa-Hunt Syndrome

503. What is the likely cause of this condition?
- a. Binding of Synaptic Acetylcholine
- b. Blocked Acetylcholine Receptors
- c. Demyelination
- d. Impaired Presynaptic Acetylcholine Release
- e. Increase in Intracranial Pressure

504. Which of the following is a common co-morbidity in patients with this condition?
- a. Acute Gastroenteritis
- b. Sinusitis
- c. Small Cell Lung Cancer
- d. Thymoma

ANSWERS

502. e
503. b
504. d

VISUAL STIMULUS REVIEW

The first image shows a mask-like face with ptosis and a horizontal smile.

The second and third images show delayed adduction of the right eye during convergence.

REFERENCES

- Spillane J, Higham E, Kullmann DM. Myasthenia gravis. BMJ. 2012 Dec 21;345:e8497
- Silvestri NJ, Wolfe GI. Myasthenia gravis. Semin Neurol. 2012 Jul;32(3):215-26.

CASE #148:   EARACHE

CASE

A 45-year-old woman presents to her family doctor complaining of right ear pain and swelling for five days. She has a history of left-ear deformity that she developed about five years ago and is not taking any medications. She denies any trauma to the right ear. On physical exam, she has no mastoid process tenderness but has severe tenderness to palpation to the right auricle but no tenderness to the lobule.

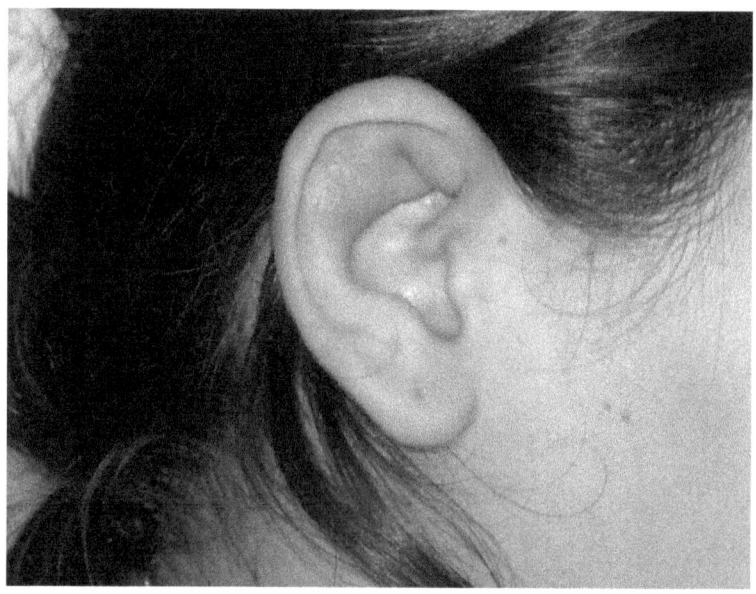

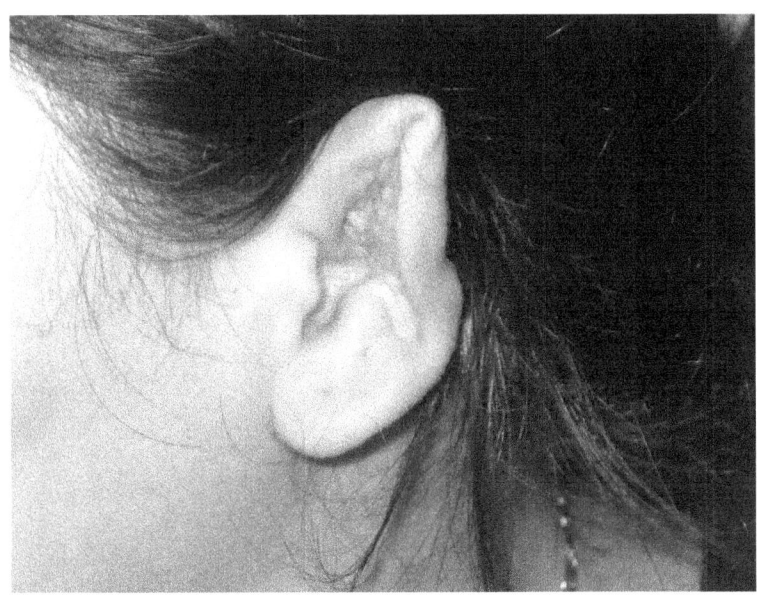

QUESTIONS

505. What is the likely diagnosis?
   a. Auricular Cellulitis
   b. Auricular Hematoma
   c. Relapsing Polychondritis
   d. Rheumatoid Arthritis
   e. Wegener Granulomatosis

506. What is the likely cause of this condition?
   a. Avascular Necrosis of the Auricular Cartilage
   b. Bacterial Infection
   c. Cartilage Specific Antibodies
   d. Granulomatous Inflammation

507. Which of the following findings is common in patients with this condition?

   a. Boutonniere Deformity
   b. Mastoid Process Tenderness
   c. Nasal Chondritis
   d. Splinter Hemorrhages
   e. Strawberry Gingival Hyperplasia

ANSWERS

505. c

506. c

507. c

VISUAL STIMULUS REVIEW

The first image shows swelling and erythema of the right auricle with sparing of the lobule.

The second image shows a forward collapsed left ear with diffuse nodularity.

REFERENCES

- Yoo JH, Chodosh J, Dana R. Relapsing polychondritis: systemic and ocular manifestations, differential diagnosis, management, and prognosis. Semin Ophthalmol. 2011 Jul-Sep;26(4-5):261-9.

- Rapini RP, Warner NB. Relapsing polychondritis. Clin Dermatol. 2006 Nov-Dec;24(6):482-5.

CASE #149: SKIN DISCOLORATION

CASE

A 19-year-old woman presents to her family doctor complaining of skin discoloration to her neck that developed over the past 12 months. She has no known past medical history and is not taking any medications. This is her first visit to this doctor. She reports irregular menstrual periods since menarche with no more than five periods a year.

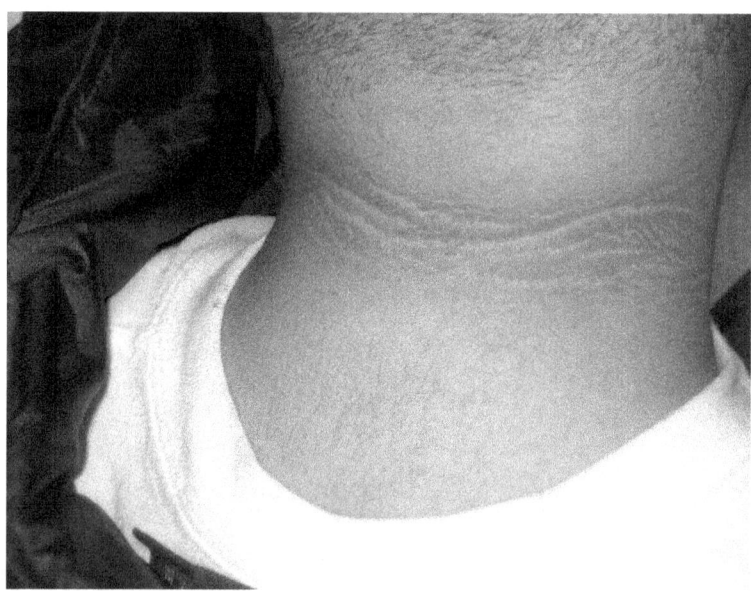

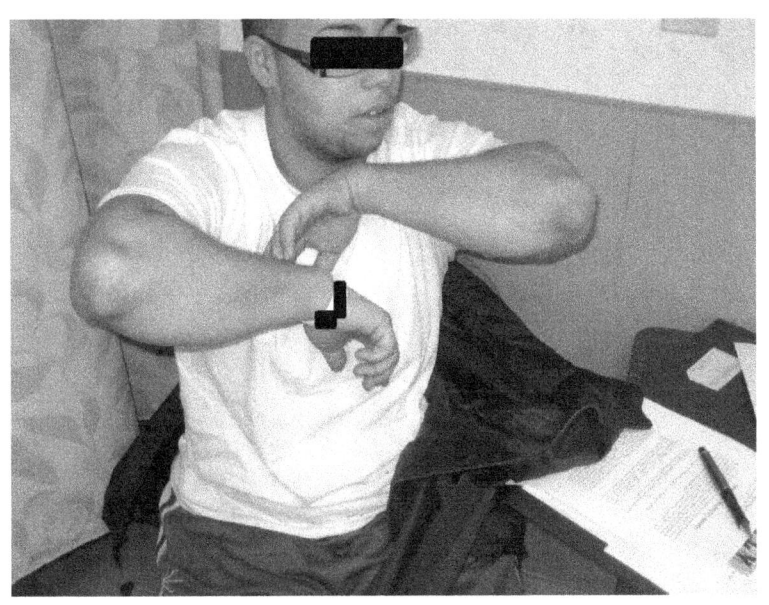
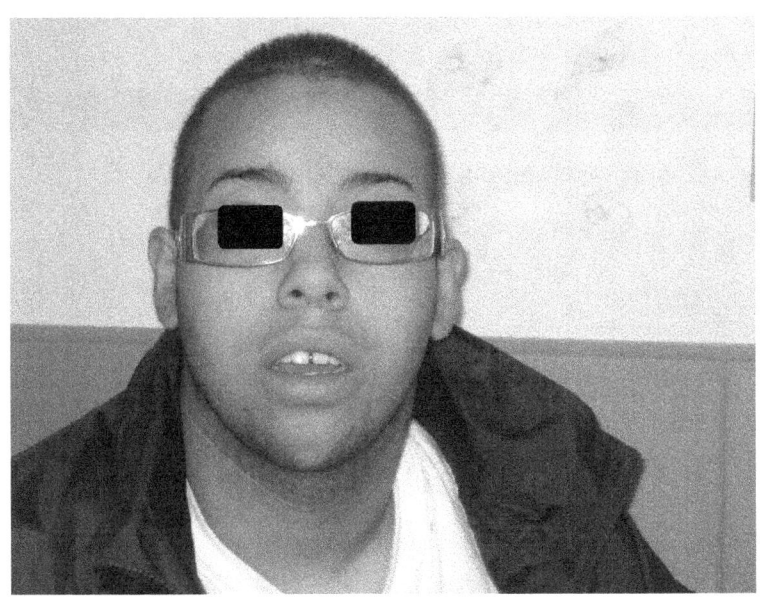

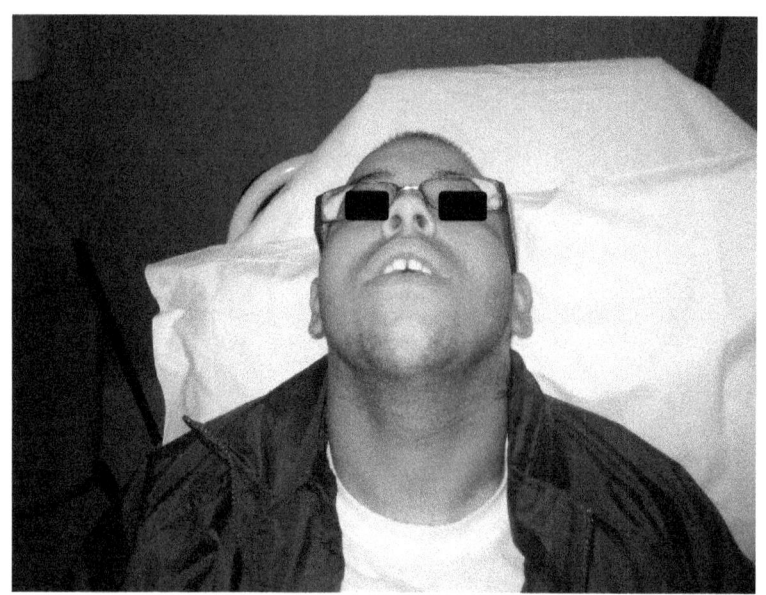

QUESTIONS

508. What finding is seen on this patient's neck?
    a. Acanthosis Nigricans
    b. Elephantiasis
    c. Lichenification
    d. Linear Hypopigmentation

509. What is the likely diagnosis?
    a. Acromegaly
    b. Adrenal Tumor
    c. Cushing syndrome
    d. Hypothyroidism
    e. Pellagra
    f. Polycystic Ovary Syndrome

510. Which of the following is included in the first line treatment of this condition?

    a. Adrenalectomy

    b. Androgen Blocking Agents

    c. Clomiphene Citrate

    d. Combination Oral Contraceptive

    e. Niacin

    f. Levothyroxine

ANSWERS

508. a

509. f

510. d

VISUAL STIMULUS REVIEW

The first image shows darkening and thickening of the nape of her neck and hirsutism.

The following images show excess body hair in a male distribution pattern and increased muscle mass.

REFERENCES

- Nicandri KF, Hoeger K. Diagnosis and treatment of polycystic ovarian syndrome in adolescents. Curr Opin Endocrinol Diabetes Obes. 2012 Dec;19(6):497-504.

- Rackow BW. Polycystic ovary syndrome in adolescents. Curr Opin Obstet Gynecol. 2012 Oct;24(5):281-7.

- Bode D, Seehusen DA, Baird D. Hirsutism in women. Am Fam Physician. 2012 Feb 15;85(4):373-80.

CASE #150:   KNEE PAIN

CASE

A 24-year-old carpenter presents to his family doctor complaining of left knee pain and redness. He has no past medical history, and he works as a carpet layer. He reports that his pain gets worse with ambulation or kneeling and improves with rest. He denies any trauma or fevers. On physical exam, his vital signs are within normal limits, and he has near full painless range of motion of his left knee with mildly limited maximal flexion secondary to pain. There are no other joint or skin abnormalities. Palpation of the patella reveals mild tenderness and fluctuant edema over the lower pole of the patella and no skin breakdown.

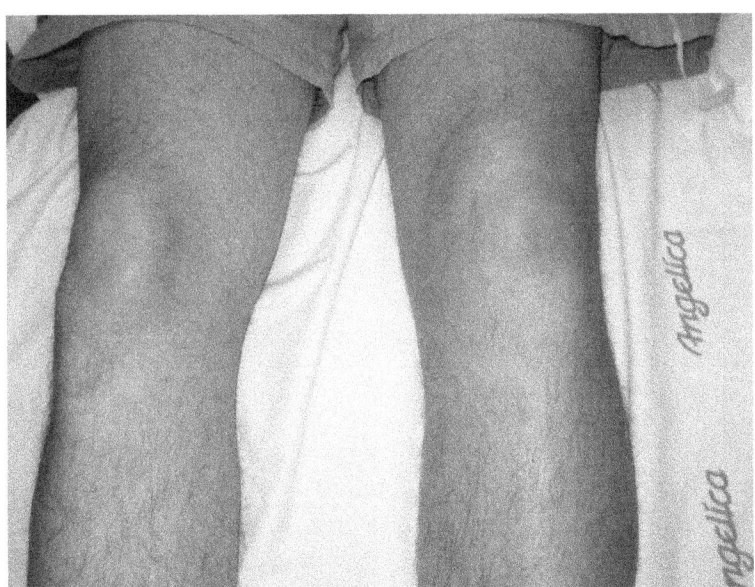

QUESTIONS

511. What is the likely diagnosis?
    a. Knee Cellulitis
    b. Osteoarthritis
    c. Prepatellar Bursitis
    d. Rheumatoid Arthritis
    e. Septic Knee

512. What is the likely cause of this condition?
    a. Chronic Synovitis
    b. Degenerative Alterations
    c. Hematogenous Seeding
    d. Repeated Microtrauma

513. Which of the following is indicated in order to determine proper management of this condition?
    a. Arthrocentesis
    b. Bursal Fluid Aspiration
    c. Knee MRI
    d. Knee X-Ray
    e. None of the above

ANSWERS

511. c

512. d

513. b

VISUAL STIMULUS REVIEW

The image shows erythema and skin edema to the prepatellar area.

REFERENCES

- Aaron DL, Patel A, Kayiaros S, Calfee R. Four common types of bursitis: diagnosis and management. J Am Acad Orthop Surg. 2011 Jun;19(6):359-67.

- Butcher JD, Salzman KL, Lillegard WA. Lower extremity bursitis. Am Fam Physician. 1996 May 15;53(7):2317-24.

- McAfee JH, Smith DL. Olecranon and prepatellar bursitis. Diagnosis and treatment. West J Med. 1988 Nov;149(5):607-10.

CASE #151: ANAL PAIN

CASE

A 28-year-old man presents to the emergency department complaining of severe rectal pain and pruritus. He has no past medical history and reports an unprotected anal receptive sexual encounter about 10 days prior to his visit. He complains of constant rectal pain that gets worse with defecation, passage of mucous, and frequent small volume diarrhea as well a constant need to have a bowel movement. On physical exam, the patient has normal vital signs and a soft non-tender abdomen with no inguinal lymphadenopathy and no perianal vesicles or induration.

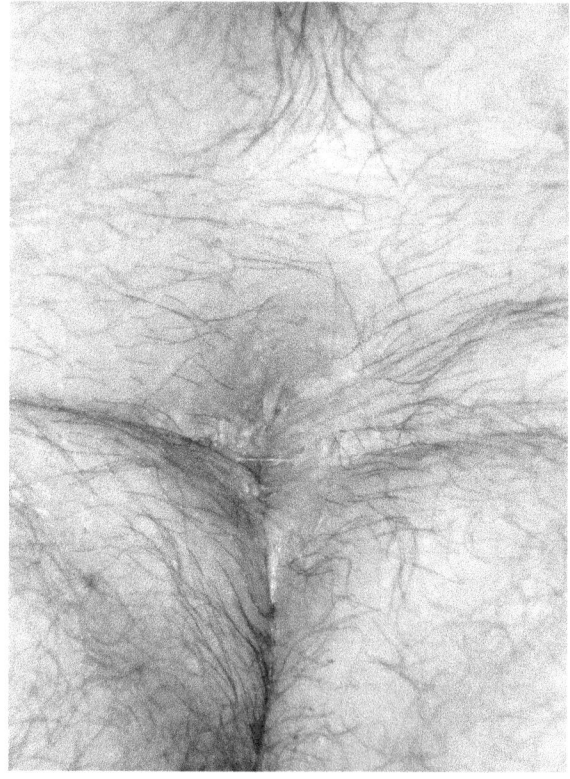

QUESTIONS

514. What is the likely diagnosis?
    a. Anal Fissure
    b. Diverticulitis
    c. Inflammatory Bowel Disease
    d. Perirectal Abscess
    e. Proctitis

515. What is the likely cause of this condition?
    a. Autoimmune Process
    b. Chlamydia Trachomatis
    c. Clostridium Difficile
    d. Direct Trauma
    e. Neisseria Gonorrhea
    f. HSV 2

516. Which of the following treatments should be offered to the patient?
    a. Acyclovir PO
    b. Ceftriaxone IM
    c. Ciprofloxacin PO
    d. Doxycycline PO
    e. Metronidazole PO
    f. b and d

ANSWERS

514. e

515. e

516. f

VISUAL STIMULUS REVIEW

The image shows perianal erythema with purulent anal discharge.

REFERENCES

- Hoentjen F, Rubin DT. Infectious proctitis: when to suspect it is not inflammatory bowel disease. Dig Dis Sci. 2012 Feb;57(2):269-73.
- Felt-Bersma RJ, Bartelsman JF. Haemorrhoids, rectal prolapse, anal fissure, peri-anal fistulae and sexually transmitted diseases. Best Pract Res Clin Gastroenterol. 2009;23(4):575-92.

CASE #152: ITCHY RASH

CASE

A 30-year-old man with no past medical history presents to his family doctor complaining of pruritic rash to his legs that progressed over the last couple of weeks. He denies any trauma, arthralgias, recent illness, or history of same.

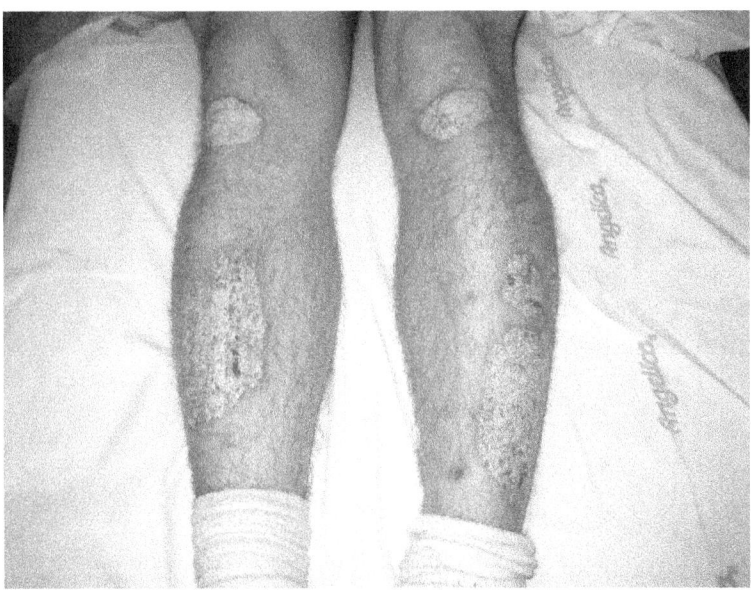

QUESTIONS

517. What is the likely diagnosis?
    a. Atopic Dermatitis
    b. Eczema
    c. Mycosis Fungoides
    d. Psoriasis
    e. Seborrheic Dermatitis

518. Which of the following signs is likely to be present?
    a. Auspitz Sign
    b. Cullen's Sign
    c. Darier's Sign
    d. Hutchinson's Sign
    e. Nikolsky's Sign

519. Which of the following medications is recommended as the first line treatment?
    a. Phototherapy
    b. Mildly Potent Steroid Ointment
    c. Oral Steroids
    d. Potent Steroid Ointment
    e. Topical Vitamin D Analog
    f. d and e

ANSWERS

517. d

518. a

519. f

VISUAL STIMULUS REVIEW

The image shows bilateral inflamed plaques that are covered with silvery white scales over the knees and extensor surfaces of the lower extremities.

REFERENCES

- Samarasekera E, Sawyer L, Parnham J, Smith CH; Guideline Development Group. Assessment and management of psoriasis: summary of NICE guidance. BMJ. 2012 Oct 24;345:e6712.

- Hsu LN, Armstrong AW. Psoriasis and autoimmune disorders: a review of the literature. J Am Acad Dermatol. 2012 Nov;67(5):1076-9.

CASE #153: SHORTNESS OF BREATH

CASE

A 20-year-old man is brought to the emergency department by EMS for a stab wound to his right chest. The patient is diaphoretic and in severe respiratory distress. His vital signs are heart rate 130/min, respiratory rate 50/min, blood pressure 70/30, and O_2Sat 87% on a non-rebreather face mask. The patient is awake and alert saying that he can't breathe. A chest X-ray is performed.

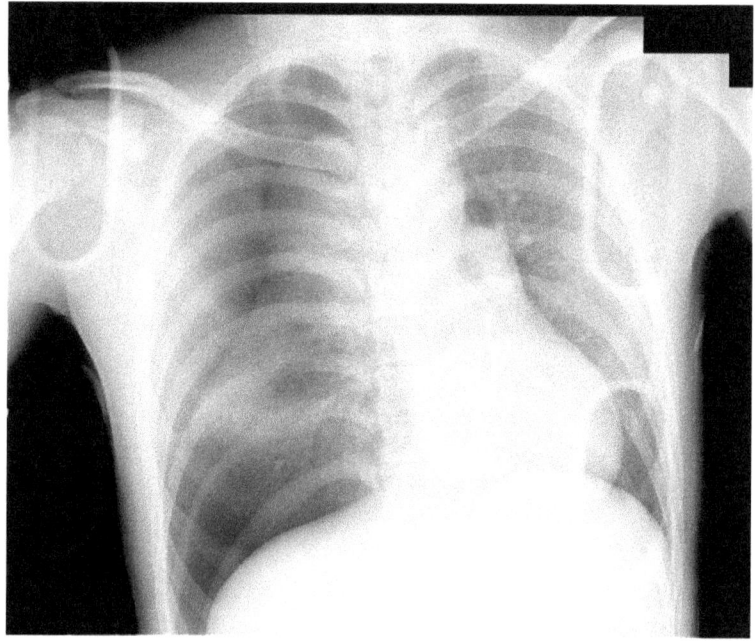

QUESTIONS

520. What is the likely diagnosis?
    a. Massive Hemothorax
    b. Pericardial Effusion
    c. Pericardial Tamponade
    d. Simple Pneumothorax
    e. Tension Pneumothorax

521. Which of the following is indicated for further evaluation of this patient at this time?
    a. Complete Blood Count
    b. CT Chest with Contrast
    c. Echocardiogram
    d. Inspiratory and Expiratory Chest Radiograms
    e. Repeat Chest Radiogram in Two Hours
    f. None of the above

522. What should be the next intervention in this patient?
    a. Endotracheal Intubation
    b. Noninvasive Ventilation Using BIPAP Device
    c. Noninvasive Ventilation Using CPAP Device
    d. Left-Sided Thoracotomy
    e. Pericardiocentesis
    f. Tube Thoracostomy

ANSWERS

520. e

521. f

522. f

VISUAL STIMULUS REVIEW

The chest radiogram shows large pneumothorax on the right with midline shift of the mediastinal structures to the left hemithorax.

REFERENCES

- Bernardin B, Troquet JM. Initial management and resuscitation of severe chest trauma. Emerg Med Clin North Am. 2012 May;30(2):377-400, viii-ix.

- Haynes D, Baumann MH. Management of pneumothorax. Semin Respir Crit Care Med. 2010 Dec;31(6):769-80.

CASE #154: SHORTNESS OF BREATH

CASE

A 72-year-old man is brought to the emergency department by EMS complaining of shortness of breath. He reports waking up at 3 a.m. in extreme dyspnea and drowning sensation. The patient appears in severe respiratory distress and is diaphoretic. His vital signs are temp of 98.7F (37C), heart rate 118/min, respiratory rate 38/min, blood pressure 220/140 mmHg, and O_2Sat of 86% on a non-rebreather face mask. On physical examination, the patient is awake and alert; he has bilateral rales on lung auscultation, tachycardic, and regular heart sounds with accentuated S3 as well as jugular vein distention on cardiovascular exam. A chest radiogram is obtained.

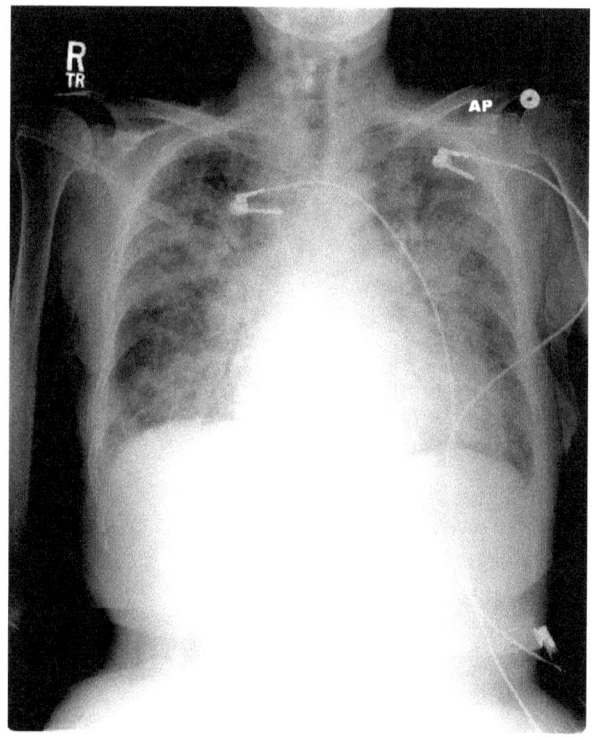

QUESTIONS

523. What is the likely diagnosis?
    a. Aspiration Pneumonitis
    b. Pneumonia
    c. Pneumothorax
    d. Pulmonary Edema
    e. Pulmonary Embolism

524. Which of the following is included in the first line management of this patient?
    a. Bilevel Positive Airway Pressure
    b. Continuous Positive Airway Pressure
    c. Nasal Canula

- d. Non-Rebreather Face Mask
- e. Rapid Sequence Intubation
- f. a or b

525. Which of the following medications is likely to improve the patient's condition most quickly?
    - a. Aspirin PO
    - b. Ceftriaxone IV
    - c. Furosemide IV
    - d. Heparin IV
    - e. Nitroglycerin IV

526. Presence of a loud aortic murmur over the apex or inferior sternal boarder suggests which of the following?
    - a. Aortic Regurgitation
    - b. Aortic Stenosis
    - c. Mitral Regurgitation
    - d. Tricuspid Regurgitation

ANSWERS

523. d

524. f

525. e

526. c

VISUAL STIMULUS REVIEW

The chest radiogram shows an enlarged cardiac silhouette, cephalization of the pulmonary vasculature, and bilateral alveolar infiltrates.

REFERENCES

- King M, Kingery J, Casey B. Diagnosis and evaluation of heart failure. Am Fam Physician. 2012 Jun 15;85(12):1161-8.

- Boldrini R, Fasano L, Nava S. Noninvasive mechanical ventilation. Curr Opin Crit Care. 2012 Feb;18(1):48-53.

- Frontin P, Bounes V, Houze-Cerfon CH, et al. Continuous positive airway pressure for cardiogenic pulmonary edema: a randomized study. Am J Emerg Med. Sep 2011;29(7):775-81.

CASE #155: RASH AND FEVER

CASE

A 23-year-old man presents to the emergency department for fever, rash, and abdominal pain that started two days ago. He reports dry cough, headaches, and sore throat. A couple hours ago he noticed a rash that quickly spread all over his body. His vital signs are temp 104.5F (40.2C), heart rate 130/min, respiratory rate 32/min, blood pressure 84/50 mmHg, and O_2Sat 94% on room air. On physical examination, the patient is confused and lethargic; his neck is supple, and he has a normal lung exam. His abdomen is soft and non-tender. His skin lesion increases in size and number during the first couple of hours of his evaluation.

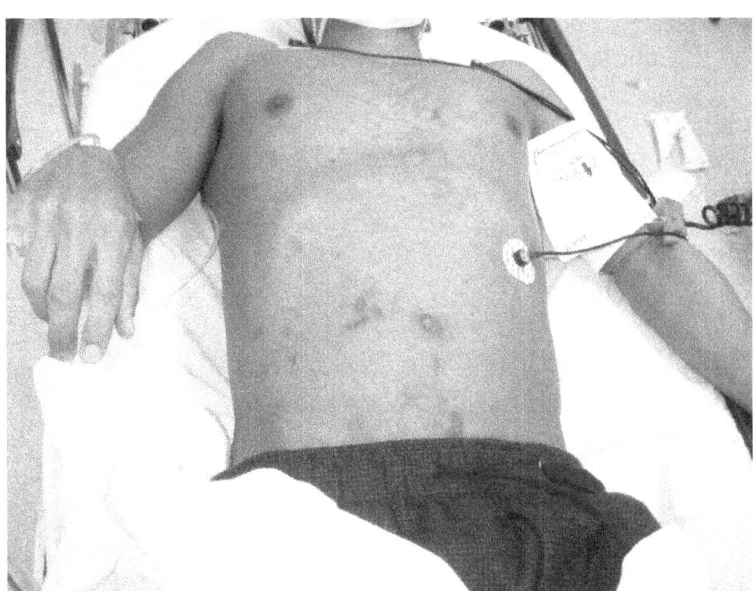

QUESTIONS

527. What is the likely diagnosis?
    a. Dengue Fever
    b. Endocarditis
    c. Influenza
    d. Meningococcemia
    e. Rocky Mountain Spotted Fever
528. What is the likely cause of this condition?
    a. Arbovirus
    b. Influenza Virus A
    c. Neisseria Meningitidis
    d. Rickettsia Rickettsii
    e. Staphylococcus Aureus
529. What is the most common reservoir of the causative agent of this condition?
    a. Bovine
    b. Canine
    c. Deer Ticks
    d. Humans
    e. Mosquitos
    f. Poultry
530. Which of the following is the antibiotic of first choice for use in this condition?
    a. Ceftriaxone IV
    b. Ciprofloxacin IV
    c. Clindamycin IV
    d. Gentamycin IV
    e. Oseltamivir PO
    f. Vancomycin IV

ANSWERS

527. d

528. c

529. d

530. a

VISUAL STIMULUS REVIEW

The image shows multiple petechial and purpuric lesions (Purpura Fulminans).

REFERENCES

- Pace D, Pollard AJ. Meningococcal disease: clinical presentation and sequelae. Vaccine. 2012 May 30;30 Suppl 2:B3-9.
- Prevention and control of meningococcal disease. MMWR Recomm Rep. Mar 22 2013;62:1-22.
- Rajapaksa S, Starr M. Meningococcal sepsis. Aust Fam Physician. 2010 May;39(5):276-8.

CASE #156: HEADACHE

CASE

A 46-year-old man is brought to the emergency department by EMS for a sudden onset severe headache that started an hour ago while lifting weights. He describes the headache as the worst headache in his life, and he has vomited twice since the onset. His vital signs are temp 98.7F (37C), heart rate 76/min, blood pressure 190/105 mmHg, and O_2Sat 99%. On physical examination, the patient is awake, alert, and holding his head. His cranial nerve exam shows abducens palsy on the left, but no other gross neurological deficit. A CT of the head is obtained.

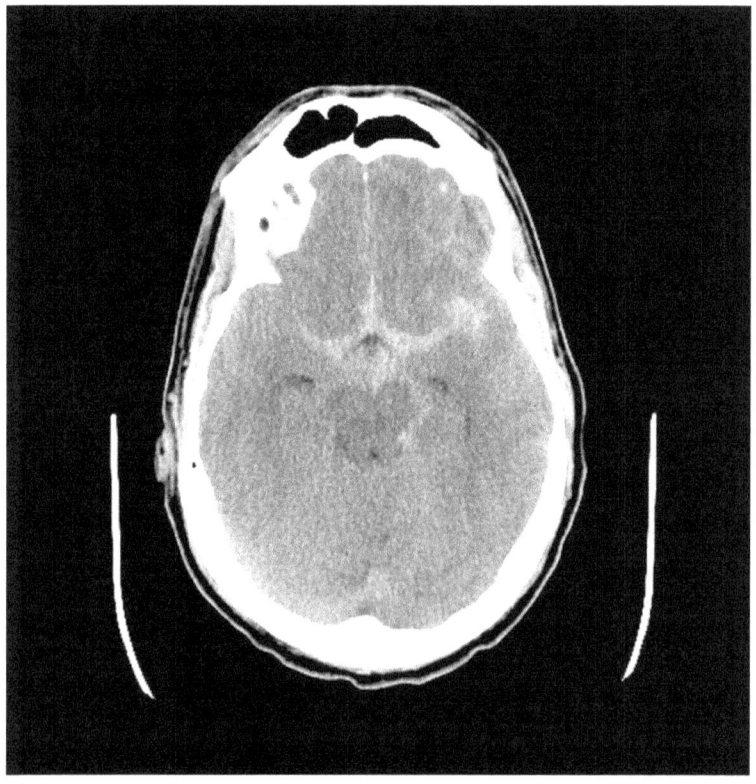

QUESTIONS

531. What is the likely diagnosis?
    a. Cavernous Sinus Thrombosis
    b. Epidural Hemorrhage
    c. Subarachnoid Hemorrhage
    d. Subdural Hemorrhage

532. What is the most likely cause of this condition?
    a. Berry Aneurism
    b. Brain Tumor
    c. Direct Trauma
    d. Infectious Thrombosis
    e. Mycotic Aneurism

533. Which of the following agents is likely to prevent short-term complications in patients with this condition?
    a. Aspirin PO
    b. Atenolol PO
    c. Metoprolol IV
    d. Nimodipine PO
    e. Tissue Plasminogen Activator IV

ANSWERS

531. c

532. a

533. d

VISUAL STIMULUS REVIEW

The CT image shows subarachnoid hemorrhage filling the basilar cisterns.

REFERENCES

- Mortimer AM, Bradley MD, Stoodley NG, Renowden SA. Thunderclap headache: diagnostic considerations and neuroimaging features. Clin Radiol. 2013 Mar;68(3):e101-13.

- Caceres JA, Goldstein JN. Intracranial hemorrhage. Emerg Med Clin North Am. 2012 Aug;30(3):771-94.

- Edlow JA, Samuels O, Smith WS, Weingart SD. Emergency neurological life support: subarachnoid hemorrhage. Neurocrit Care. 2012 Sep;17 Suppl 1:S47-53.

CASE #157: VOMITING

CASE

A 63-year-old man patient is brought to the emergency department for one day of abdominal pain, nausea, and vomiting. The patient reports that his last bowel movement was two days ago and that he hasn't been passing gas for the past 12 hours. The vital signs are temperature of 101.8F (38.8C), heart rate 108/min, blood pressure 120/60 mmHg, and O_2Sat 98% on room air. On physical examination, his abdomen is distended, soft, and diffusely tender to palpation with hypoactive bowel sounds. No hernias are palpated bilaterally.

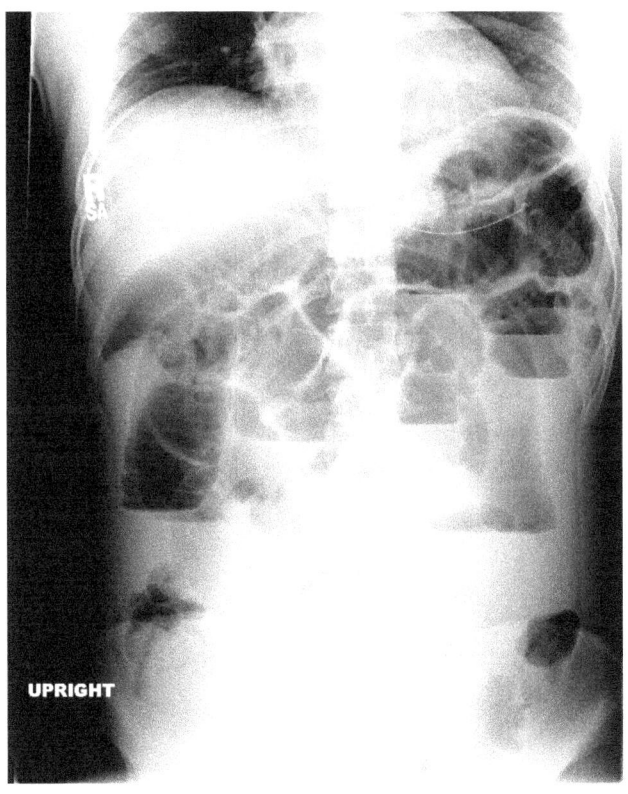

QUESTIONS

534. What is the likely diagnosis?

   a. Diverticulitis

   b. Ileus

   c. Large Bowel Obstruction

   d. Sigmoid Volvulus

   e. Small Bowel Obstruction

535. What is the likely cause of this condition?

   a. Food Bezoar

   b. Incarcerated Inguinal Hernia

   c. Inflammatory Bowel Disease

   d. Medication Side Effect

   e. Post-Operative Adhesions

536. Definitive management of this condition usually requires which of the following?

   a. Alvimopan PO

   b. Colonoscopy

   c. Intravenous Steroids

   d. Laparotomy

   e. Rectal Tube Decompression

ANSWERS

534. e

535. e

536. d

VISUAL STIMULUS REVIEW

The radiogram shows dilated small bowel loops with multiple air-fluid levels.

REFERENCES

- Mullan CP, Siewert B, Eisenberg RL. Small bowel obstruction. Am J Roentgenol. 2012 Feb;198(2):W105-17.

- Diaz JJ Jr, Bokhari F, Mowery NT et al. Guidelines for management of small bowel obstruction. J Trauma. 2008 Jun;64(6):1651-64.

- Moran BJ. Adhesion-related small bowel obstruction. Colorectal Dis. 2007 Oct;9 Suppl 2:39-44.

CASE #158: ITCHY RASH

CASE

A 21-year-old man, who has no past medical history and is not taking any medications, presents to his family doctor complaining of a worsening pruritic rash that started two weeks ago. He reports that the lesions itch more at night time as well as after he takes a shower.

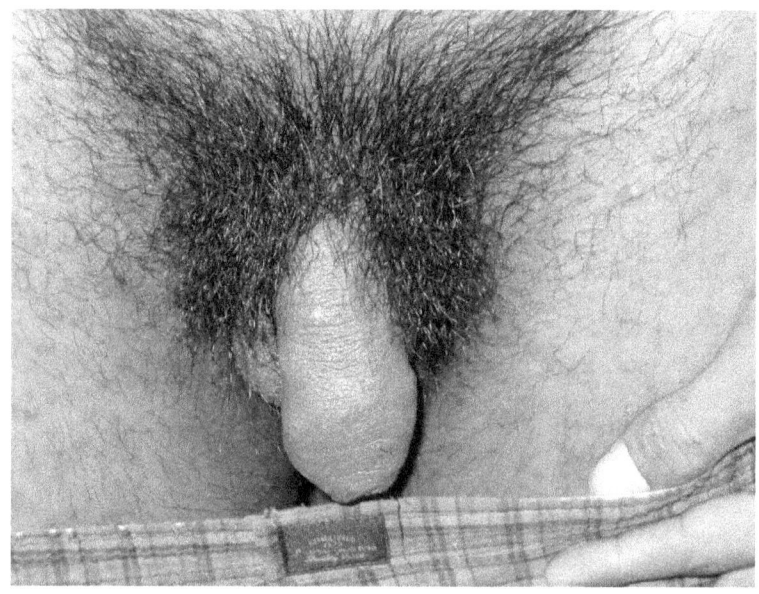

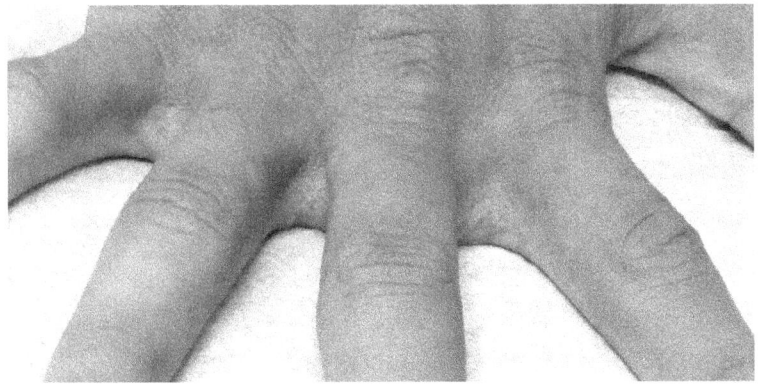

QUESTIONS

537. What is the likely diagnosis?

    a. Atopic Dermatitis

    b. Body Lice

    c. Eczema

    d. Pubic Lice

    e. Scabies

538. What is the mode of transmission of this condition?

    a. Autosomal Recessive

    b. Feline to Human

    c. Fomite to Human

    d. Human to Human

    e. b, c, and d

    f. c and d

539. Which of the following statements is correct?
    a. Barrier cream is a useful method to prevent future exacerbation of this condition.
    b. Close personal contacts should not be treated unless they share one household.
    c. Only symptomatic household members should be treated.
    d. Pruritus is expected to last for at least two weeks after successful treatment.
    e. This condition is often times a result of poor personal and household hygiene.

540. Severe forms of this condition that fail topical treatment may be treated with which of the following treatments?
    a. Doxycycline IV
    b. Ivermectin PO
    c. IVIG
    d. Methyl-Prednisolone IV
    e. Prednisone PO

ANSWERS

537. e

538. f

539. d

540. b

VISUAL STIMULUS REVIEW

The first image shows papules over the penis and the foreskin.

The second image shows small papules and burrows between the finger webs.

REFERENCES

- Gunning K, Pippitt K, Kiraly B, Sayler M. Pediculosis and scabies: treatment update. Am Fam Physician. 2012 Sep 15;86(6):535-41.
- Shmidt E, Levitt J. Dermatologic infestations. Int J Dermatol. 2012 Feb;51(2):131-41.
- Currie BJ, McCarthy JS. Permethrin and ivermectin for scabies. N Engl J Med. 2010 Feb 25;362(8):717-25.

CASE #159: LEG PAIN

CASE

A 47-year-old male presents to the emergency department complaining of severe left thigh pain worsening over the last 10 days. He has a history of HIV with a recent CD4 count of 700 cells/μl. He reports no recent or remote trauma and says that he already saw his doctor about a week prior and was diagnosed with a muscle strain. The patient is afebrile with a normal heart rate, blood pressure, and respiratory rate. Physical examination is remarkable for normal skin examination to bilateral lower legs. His left thigh is minimally swollen, when compared with the right thigh, and has localized severe tenderness to palpation over the proximal adductors. The skin temperature is the same when compared with the right thigh. The patient has normal painless passive internal and external rotation of both his hips.

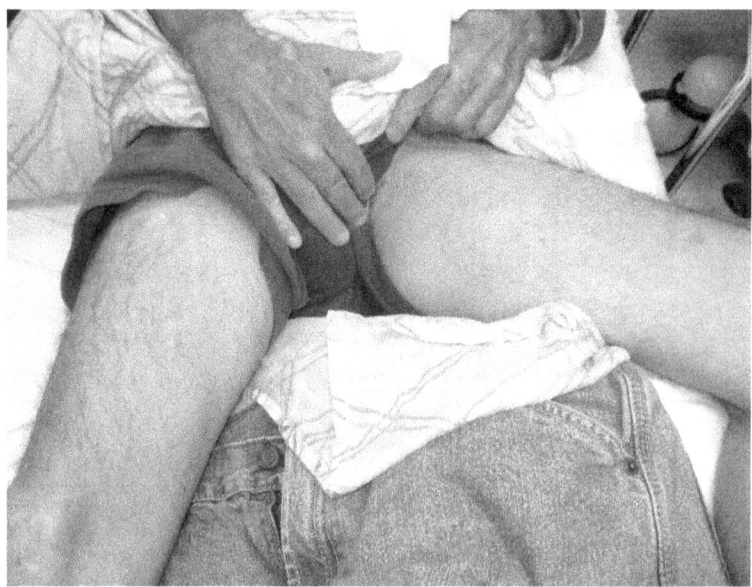

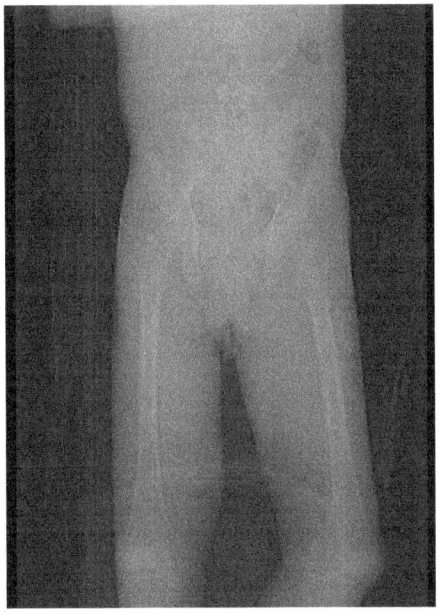

QUESTIONS

541. What is the likely diagnosis?
    a. Cellulitis
    b. Dermatomyositis
    c. Fibromyalgia
    d. Polymyositis
    e. Pyomyositis

542. What is the likely cause of this condition?
    a. Borrelia Burgdorferi
    b. Coxsackie Virus
    c. Cryptococcus Neoformans
    d. Staphylococcus Aureus
    e. Streptococcus pyogenes

543. Which of the following is the most sensitive test for evaluating this condition?
   a. CBC with Differential
   b. Erythrocyte Sedimentation Rate
   c. CT with IV Contrast
   d. MRI
   e. Nerve Conduction Study
   f. Serum CPK

ANSWERS

541. e

542. d

543. d

VISUAL STIMULUS REVIEW

The gross image shows a minimally swollen left thigh. The CT scout image shows soft tissue swelling to the medial left thigh when compared with the right.

REFERENCES

- Burdette SD et al. Staphylococcus aureus pyomyositis compared with non-Staphylococcus aureus pyomyositis. J Infect. 2012 Jan 13.
- Lo BM, Fickenscher BA. Primary pyomyositis caused by ca-MRSA. Int J Emerg Med. 2008 Dec;1(4):331-2.
- Lemonick DM. Non-tropical pyomyositis caused by methicillin-resistant Staphylococcus aureus: an unusual cause of bilateral leg pain. J Emerg Med. 2012 Mar;42(3):e55-62.
- Small LN, Ross JJ. Tropical and temperate pyomyositis. Infect Dis Clin North Am. 2005 Dec;19(4):981-9, x-xi.

CASE #160: JOINT PAIN

CASE

A 50-year-old woman presents to a new patient appointment with a family doctor complaining of two years of recurrent joint pain. The pain mostly involves her hands and wrists as well as her feet, and she can no longer use her hands or walk the way she used to. The reason for her current visit is progressive swelling and pain to her left wrist that no longer responds to ibuprofen and prevents her from sleeping at night. She reports that her wrist is never that painful or red. Her vital signs are within normal limits. Her left wrist is warm to palpation and exquisitely tender to movement in all directions.

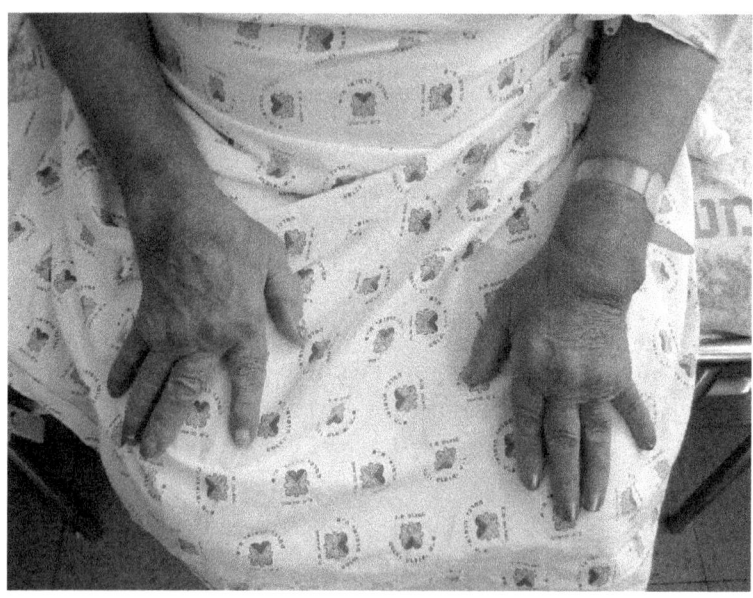

QUESTIONS

544. What is the likely diagnosis of this patient's chronic condition?

    a. Fibromyalgia

    b. Gout

    c. Osteoarthritis

    d. Rheumatoid Arthritis

    e. Septic Arthritis

545. Which of the following is commonly found in patients with this condition?

    a. Expanding Circular Rash

    b. Heberden Nodes

    c. Proximal Muscle Weakness

    d. Subcutaneus Nodules

    e. Tophaceous Deposits

546. Which of the following is indicated in order to dictate further management during this visit?

    a. Complete Blood Count with Differential

    b. ESR

    c. Joint Fluid Analysis

    d. None, Start Patient on Prednisone

    e. Rheumatoid Factor Titers

ANSWERS

544. d

545. d

546. c

VISUAL STIMULUS REVIEW

The image shows bilateral ulnar deviation of the fingers and swelling to the left wrist. The metacarpophalangeal joint also appears swollen.

REFERENCES

- Britsemmer K, Ursum J, Gerritsen M, van Tuyl L, van Schaardenburg D. Validation of the 2010 ACR/EULAR classification criteria for rheumatoid arthritis: slight improvement over the 1987 ACR criteria. Ann Rheum Dis. Aug 2011;70(8):1468-70.

- Aletaha D, Neogi T, Silman AJ, Funovits J, Felson DT, Bingham CO 3rd, et al. 2010 Rheumatoid arthritis classification criteria: an American College of Rheumatology/European League Against Rheumatism collaborative initiative. Arthritis Rheum. Sep 2010;62(9):2569-81.

CASE #161: PAINFUL RASH

CASE

A 25-year-old who has no past medical history woman presents to her family doctor complaining of a painful rash to her left thigh for two days. She reports a few days of tingling sensation to that area that evolved into severe, constant burning pain. She denies history of similar rash, dysuria, cough, nausea, vomiting, headache, or sore throat. Her vital signs are temp 103.5F (39.7C), heart rate 104/min, and blood pressure 130/76 mmHg.

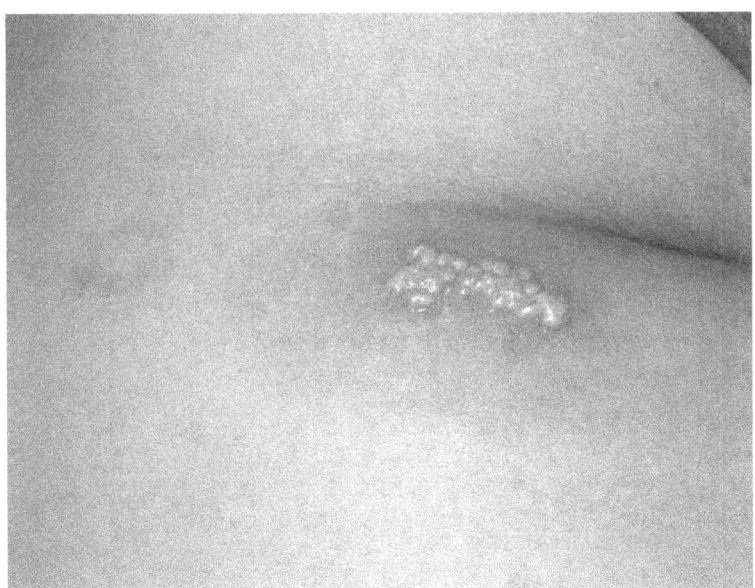

QUESTIONS

547. What is the likely diagnosis?
   a. Candidiasis
   b. Chancroid
   c. Pustular Cellulitis
   d. Herpes Simplex Lesion
   e. Shingles
   f. Syphilis

548. What is the likely cause of this condition?
   a. Candida Albicans
   b. Hemophilus Ducreyi
   c. Herpes Simplex Virus
   d. Methicillin Resistant Staphylococcus Aurous
   e. Varicella Zoster Virus
   f. Treponema Pallidum

549. Which of the following treatments is recommended in this condition?
   a. Acyclovir
   b. Ceftriaxone
   c. Clindamycin
   d. Fluconazole
   e. Penicillin
   f. Prednisone

ANSWERS

547. d

548. c

549. a

VISUAL STIMULUS REVIEW

The image shows clustered vesicles and pustules over an erythematous skin

REFERENCES

- Dawson AL, Dellavalle RP, Elston DM. Infectious skin diseases: a review and needs assessment. Dermatol Clin. 2012 Jan;30(1):141-51.

- Azwa A, Barton SE. Aspects of herpes simplex virus: a clinical review. J Fam Plann Reprod Health Care. 2009 Oct;35(4):237-42.

- Fatahzadeh M, Schwartz RA. Human herpes simplex virus infections: epidemiology, pathogenesis, symptomatology, diagnosis, and management. J Am Acad Dermatol. 2007 Nov;57(5):737-63.

CASE #162: PAINFUL FINGERS

CASE

A 40-year-old heavy-smoker male presents to a family doctor complaining of severe pain to his hands and feet for the past two years. The patient reports that walking or heavy hand use causes severe pain to his hands and feet. He reports ulcerations to his fingers and toes that progressed over the last six months to what his hands look like today. He denies skin rashes or joint pain. His vital signs are within normal limits.

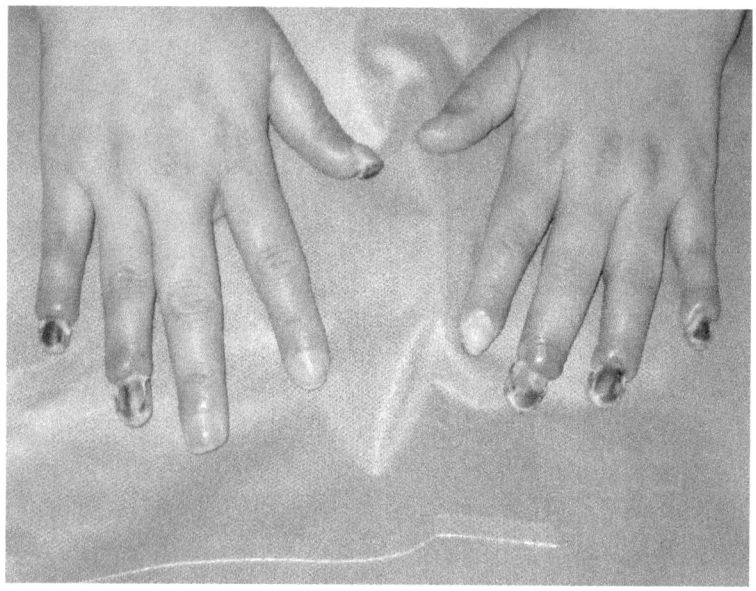

QUESTIONS

550. What is the likely diagnosis?
    a. Buerger Disease
    b. Giant Cell Arteritis
    c. Polyarteritis Nodosa
    d. Raynaud's Disease
    e. Scleroderma
    f. Systemic Lupus Erythematosus

551. Which of the following findings is expected in this patient?
    a. Elevated Anti-Double Stranded DNA Antibodies
    b. Elevated Rheumatoid Factor
    c. Malar Rash
    d. Segmental Occlusive Lesions of Digital and Plantar Arterioles.
    e. Tender Cord Over the Temporal Arteries

552. Which of the following treatments is effective in preventing disease progression?
    a. Angioplasty and Stenting
    b. High Dose Prednisone
    c. IVIG
    d. Nifedipine PO
    e. Smoking Cessation

ANSWERS

550. a

551. d

552. e

VISUAL STIMULUS REVIEW

The image shows bilateral fingertip dry gangrene.

REFERENCES

- Dargon PT, Landry GJ. Buerger's disease. Ann Vasc Surg. 2012 Aug;26(6):871-80.
- Piazza G, Creager MA. Thromboangiitis obliterans. Circulation. 2010 Apr 27;121(16):1858-61.
- Małecki R, Zdrojowy K, Adamiec R. Thromboangiitis obliterans in the 21st century--a new face of disease. Atherosclerosis. 2009 Oct;206(2):328-34.

CASE #163: CONSTIPATION

CASE

A 3-year-old girl is brought to her pediatrician's office for anal mass and constipation. The parents report that she has been straining in the bathroom for the last three months and that her stools are hard in consistency. This morning she complained of pain during defecation and a mass was present after her bowel movement. On exam the patient has normal vital signs and soft abdomen with normal bowel sounds.

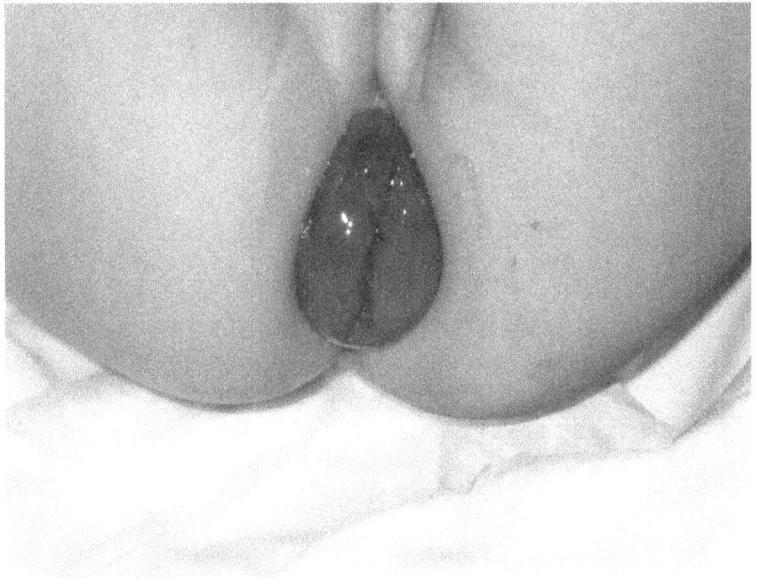

QUESTIONS

553. What is the likely diagnosis?
    a. External Hemorrhoids
    b. Internal Hemorrhoids

c. Rectal Prolapse
  d. Sigmoid Intussusception
  e. Ulcerative Colitis

554. What is the likely cause of this condition?
  a. Anal Hyperplasia
  b. Ascaris
  c. Chronic Constipation
  d. Hirschsprung Disease
  e. Rectal Polyps

555. What is the first line treatment of this condition?
  a. Hemorrhoidectomy
  b. Manual Reduction
  c. Rectopexy
  d. Steroid Ointment
  e. Stool Softeners
  f. b and e

556. What condition should be considered in a different patient of the same age who presents with the same physical findings but with a history of frequent respiratory infections as well as frequent malodorous, oily, and floating stools?
  a. Ascaris
  b. Cystic Fibrosis
  c. Clostridium Difficile Colitis
  d. Hirschsprung Disease
  e. Malnutrition

ANSWERS

553. c

554. c

555. f

556. b

VISUAL STIMULUS REVIEW

The image shows a rectal prolapse.

REFERENCES

- Melton GB, Kwaan MR. Rectal prolapse. Surg Clin North Am. 2013 Feb;93(1):187-98.

- Jones OM, Cunningham C, Lindsey I. The assessment and management of rectal prolapse, rectal intussusception, rectocoele, and enterocoele in adults. BMJ. 2011 Feb 1;342:c7099.

- Felt-Bersma RJ, Tiersma ES, Cuesta MA. Rectal prolapse, rectal intussusception, rectocele, solitary rectal ulcer syndrome, and enterocele. Gastroenterol Clin North Am. 2008 Sep;37(3):645-68.

CASE #164: WRIST PAIN

CASE

A 23-year-old man presents to the emergency department after a fall on his outstretched left hand complaining of wrist pain. He has no medical history and is taking no medications. On physical examination, he has tenderness to the radial aspect of his left wrist.

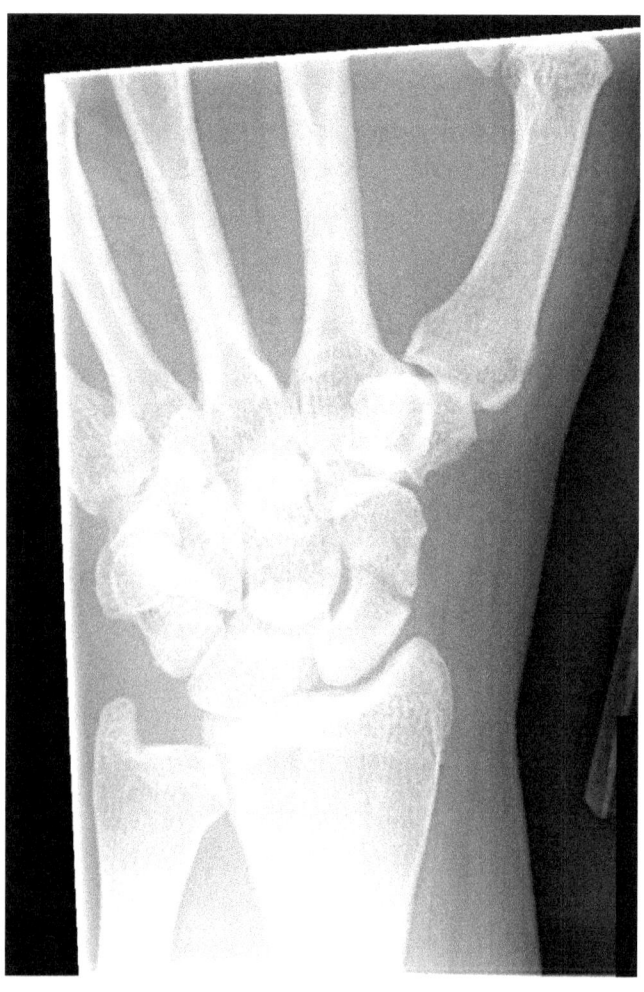

QUESTIONS

557. What is the likely diagnosis?

    a. Lunate Fracture
    b. Radial Fracture
    c. Scaphoid Fracture
    d. Trapezium Fracture
    e. Trapezoid Fracture

558. Which of the following conditions is a common complication of delayed diagnosis and treatment of this condition?

    a. Avascular Necrosis
    b. Chronic Pain
    c. Non-Union
    d. Osteoarthritis
    e. All of the above
    f. Only a and c

559. Which of the following findings is expected in this patient?

    a. Diminished Radial Artery Pulsation
    b. Markedly Reduced Wrist Range of Motion
    c. Snuffbox Tenderness
    d. Worsening Pain on Wrist Ulnar Deviation
    e. Worsening Pain on Distal Ulnar Palpation

ANSWERS

557. c

558. e

559. c

VISUAL STIMULUS REVIEW

The radiogram shows a complete scaphoid fracture at the waist.

REFERENCES

- Sendher R, Ladd AL. The scaphoid. Orthop Clin North Am. 2013 Jan;44(1):107-20.
- Alshryda S, Shah A, Odak S et al. Acute fractures of the scaphoid bone: Systematic review and meta-analysis. Surgeon. 2012 Aug;10(4):218-29.

CASE #165: ALTERED MENTAL STATUS

CASE

A 67-year-old chronic alcoholic male is brought to the emergency department by EMS. He was found unresponsive, lying down in the park with no signs of trauma. His vital signs are temp 97.5F (36.4), heart rate 45/min, blood pressure 190/100 mmHg, and O_2Sat 96% on room air. He is not responding to his name and is not following commands. He withdraws to painful stimuli on the right but has no movement on the left.

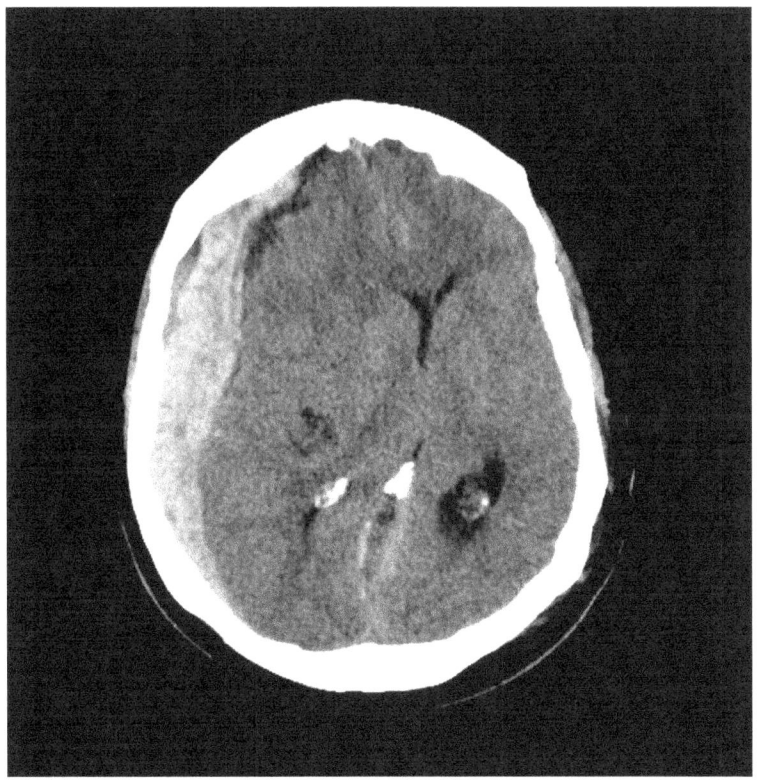

QUESTIONS

560. What is the likely diagnosis?

   a. Concussion

   b. Epidural Hemorrhage

   c. Glioblastoma Multiforme

   d. Subarachnoid Hemorrhage

   e. Subdural Hemorrhage

561. What is the likely cause of this condition in this patient?

   a. Arteriovenous Malformation

   b. Berry Aneurism

   c. Liver Failure

   d. Minor Head Trauma

   e. c and d

562. What finding is expected in this patient?

   a. Dilated and Nonreactive Right Pupil

   b. Extensor Plantar Reflex on the Right

   c. Respiratory Rate of 24/min

   d. Vertical Nystagmus

ANSWERS

560. e

561. e

562. a

VISUAL STIMULUS REVIEW

The CT image shows a right-sided subdural hematoma with a right to left midline shift.

REFERENCES

- Zammit C, Knight WA. Severe traumatic brain injury in adults. Emerg Med Pract. 2013 Mar;15(3):1-28.

- Harvey LA, Close JC. Traumatic brain injury in older adults: characteristics, causes and consequences. Injury. 2012 Nov;43(11):1821-6.

- Provenzale J. CT and MR imaging of acute cranial trauma. Emerg Radiol. 2007 Apr;14(1):1-12.

CASE #166: CHEST PAIN

CASE

A 64-year-old man is brought to the emergency department by EMS complaining of chest pain that started an hour ago. The patient reports a history of hypertension and hypercholesterolemia. He was in his usual health and sleeping when he woke up at 4 a.m. with chest pressure behind his sternum that radiated to his right arm accompanied by nausea and diaphoresis. He took an anti-acid as he thought that this was indigestion with no improvement. The vitals are temp 98.7F (37C), heart rate 64/min, blood pressure 90/50 mmHg, respiratory rate 14/hr, and O$_2$Sat 98% on room air. On exam he appears diaphoretic and ill-appearing and is holding his chest. His lung and heart exam is unremarkable.

QUESTIONS

563. What is the likely diagnosis?

   a. Angina Pectoris

   b. Aortic Dissection

   c. Early Repolarization ECG Pattern

   d. ST Elevation MI

   e. Takotsubo Cardiomyopathy

564. What is the location of the cardiac abnormality?

   a. Anterior Wall

   b. Global

   c. Inferior Wall

   d. Posterior Wall

   e. Septum

565. What is the first line treatment in this patient?

   a. Aspirin PO

   b. Lisinopril PO

   c. Nitroglycerin SL

   d. Streptokinase IV

566. Which of the following treatment is contraindicated in this patient?

   a. Aspirin PO

   b. Lisinopril PO

   c. Nitroglycerin SL

   d. Streptokinase IV

ANSWERS

563. d

564. c

565. a

566. c

VISUAL STIMULUS REVIEW

The ECG tracing shows ST segment elevation in lead II, III, aVF, V_5, and V_6.

REFERENCES

- Mistry NF, Vesely MR. Acute coronary syndromes: from the emergency department to the cardiac care unit. Cardiol Clin. 2012 Nov;30(4):617-27.

- Bates ER, Menees DS. Acute ST-elevation myocardial infarction.

- Yiadom MY. Emergency department treatment of acute coronary syndromes. Emerg Med Clin North Am. 2011 Nov;29(4):699-710.

CASE #167: RIGHT-SIDED WEAKNESS

CASE

A 54-year-old right-handed male is brought to the emergency department by EMS for right-sided weakness. He was in his usual health when he went to sleep 12 hours ago; upon awakening 45 minutes before arrival to the hospital, his wife noticed that he was not moving his right arm and leg and that he was slurring his words. The wife denies any past medical history or known trauma. Physical examination is remarkable for right-sided hemiplegia and aphasia. A non-contrast CT scan of the brain is ordered.

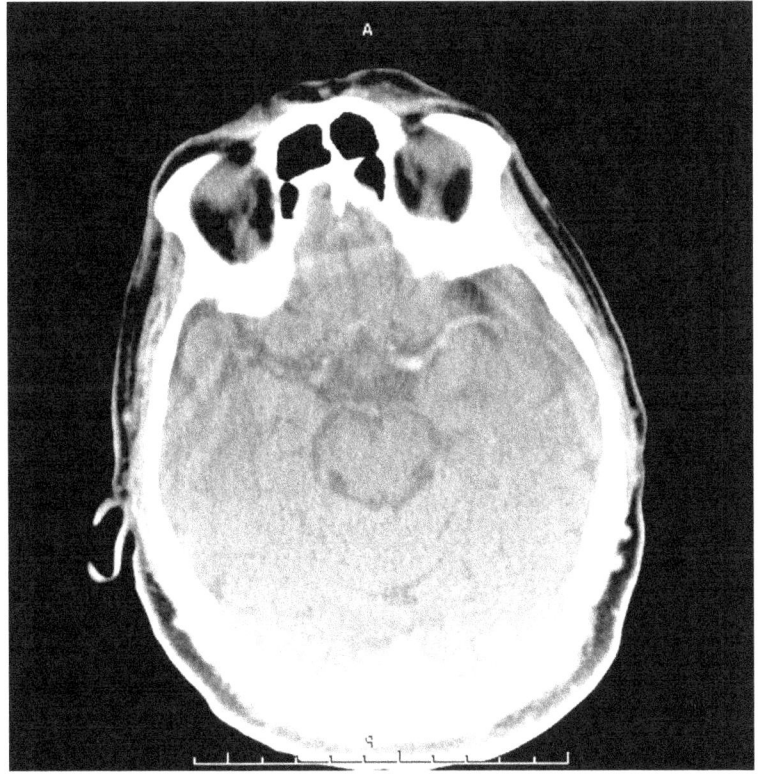

QUESTIONS

567. What is the likely diagnosis?

   a. Encephalitis

   b. Hemorrhagic Stroke

   c. Ischemic Stroke

   d. Todd's Paralysis

   e. Transient Ischemic Attack

568. Which of the following findings is expected in this patient?

   a. Left Facial Hypesthesia

   b. Left Gaze Preference

   c. Left Hemisensory Loss

   d. Left-Sided Neglect

   e. Left-Sided Extensor Plantar Reflex

569. Which of the following treatments is contraindicated in this patient?

   a. Aspirin

   b. Heparin

   c. Metoprolol

   d. Simvastatin

   e. Tissue Plasminogen Activator

ANSWERS

567. c

568. b

569. e

VISUAL STIMULUS REVIEW

The CT image shows a hyperdense middle cerebral artery sign that suggests the presence of an acute thrombus in the left MCA.

REFERENCES

- Nentwich LM, Veloz W. Neuroimaging in acute stroke. Emerg Med Clin North Am. 2012 Aug;30(3):659-80.
- Perry JM, McCabe KK. Recognition and initial management of acute ischemic stroke. Emerg Med Clin North Am. 2012 Aug;30(3):637-57.

CASE #168: VISION LOSS

CASE

A 67-year-old man presents to the emergency department complaining of headache and vision loss. He has a past medical history of diabetes and hypertension and is a smoker. The vital signs are temp 98.7F (37C), heart rate 70/min, and blood pressure 190/96 mmHg. On physical examination, the patient has a right-sided homonymous hemianopsia.

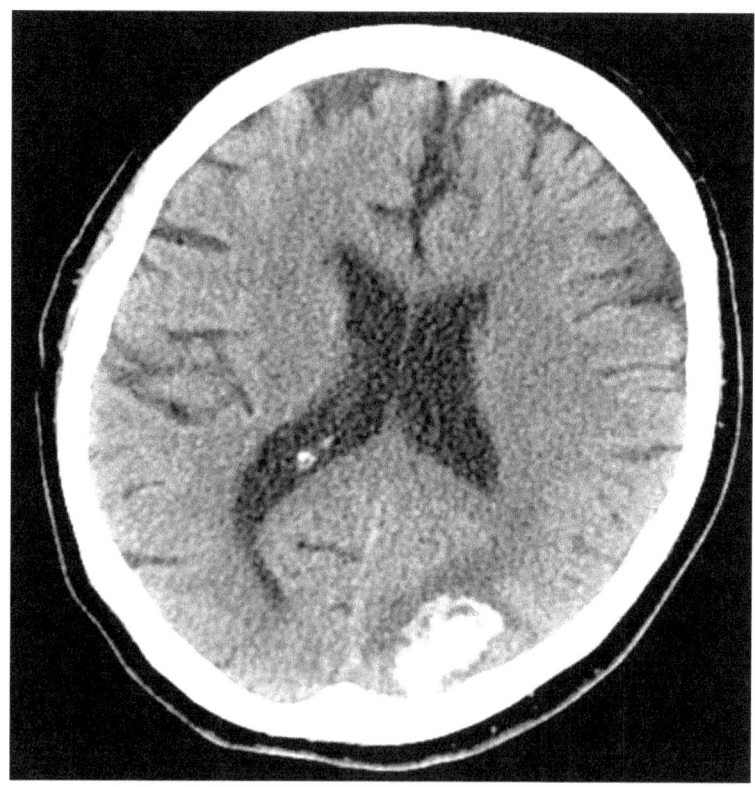

QUESTIONS

570. What is the likely diagnosis?

    a. Encephalitis

    b. Hemorrhagic Stroke

    c. Ischemic Stroke

    d. Transient Ischemic Attack

    e. Todd's Paralysis

571. Which of the following risk factors is the most common for this condition?

    a. Amyloidosis

    b. Diabetes Mellitus Type 2

    c. Hypercholesterolemia

    d. Hypertension

    e. Tobacco Use

572. Which of the following is an indication for immediate surgical intervention in this condition?

    a. Brainstem Compression

    b. Hydrocephalus

    c. Midline Shift

    d. Neurologic Deterioration

    e. All of the above

ANSWERS

570. b

571. d

572. e

VISUAL STIMULUS REVIEW

The CT image shows left occipital hemorrhage with surrounding edema.

REFERENCES

- Luu S, Lee AW, Daly A, Chen CS. Visual field defects after stroke--a practical guide for GPs. Aust Fam Physician. 2010 Jul;39(7):499-503.
- Caceres JA, Goldstein JN. Intracranial hemorrhage. Emerg Med Clin North Am. 2012 Aug;30(3):771-94.

CASE #169: SHORTNESS OF BREATH

CASE

A 52-year-old man presents to his family doctor complaining of progressive shortness of breath that developed over the last six months. The patient reports worsening dyspnea at rest and on exertion as well as hoarseness, nasal congestion, and sensation of head fullness. He reports that bending forward or lying down worsens his symptoms.

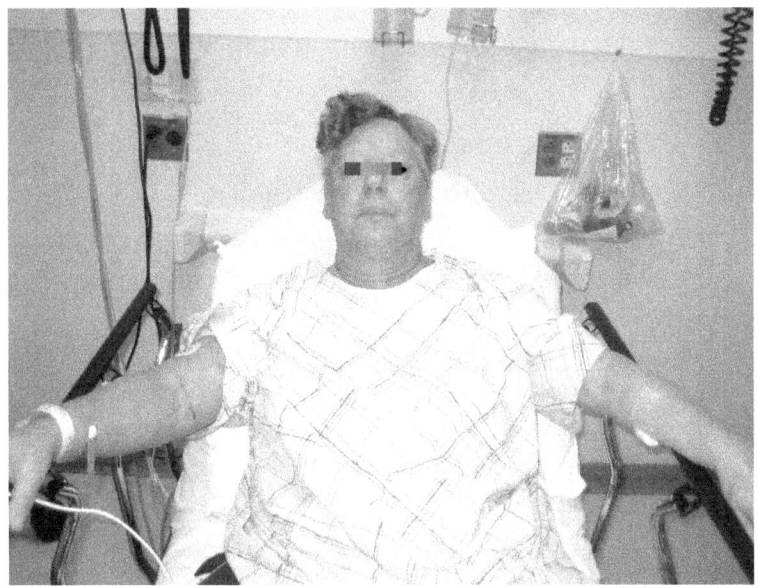

QUESTIONS

573. What is the likely diagnosis?
    a. Angioedema
    b. Axillary Vein Thrombosis
    c. Cardiac Tamponade
    d. Mediastinitis
    e. Superior Vena Cava Syndrome

574. What is the likely cause of this condition?
    a. Hypercoagulable State
    b. Lung Cancer
    c. Pericarditis
    d. Syphilis
    e. Tuberculosis
    f. Type I Allergic Reaction

575. Which of the following treatments often leads to symptomatic improvement in patients with this condition?
    a. Epinephrine IM
    b. IV Antibiotics
    c. Pericardiocentesis
    d. Radiotherapy
    e. Systemic Thrombolytics

ANSWERS

573. e
574. b
575. d

VISUAL STIMULUS REVIEW

The image shows facial and right upper extremity edema as well as plethora.

REFERENCES

- Armstrong BA, Perez CA, Simpson JR, et al. Role of irradiation in the management of superior vena cava syndrome. *Int J Radiat Oncol Biol Phys.* Apr 1987;13(4):531-9.
- Nieto AF, Doty DB. Superior vena cava obstruction: clinical syndrome, etiology, and treatment. *Curr Probl Cancer.* Sep 1986;10(9):441-84.
- Ahmann FR. A reassessment of the clinical implications of the superior vena caval syndrome. J Clin Oncol. Aug 1984;2(8):961-9.

CASE #170: COUGH

CASE

A 30-year-old homeless patient presents to a free clinic for evaluation of cough. He has no past medical history; he smokes one pack of cigarettes a day and occasionally uses IV heroin. He reports five weeks of cough, night sweats, fevers, and weight loss as well as occasional chest pain and blood mixed in his sputum. His vital signs are temperature 101.3F, heart rate 98/min, blood pressure 120/70 mmHg, respiratory rate 20/min, and O_2Sat 95% on room air. On physical exam, he has rales over the right and left upper fields.

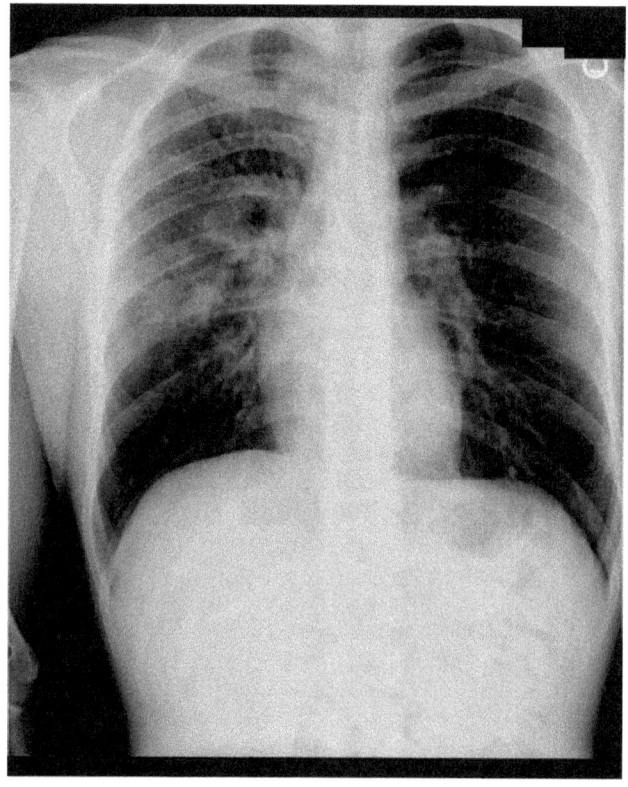

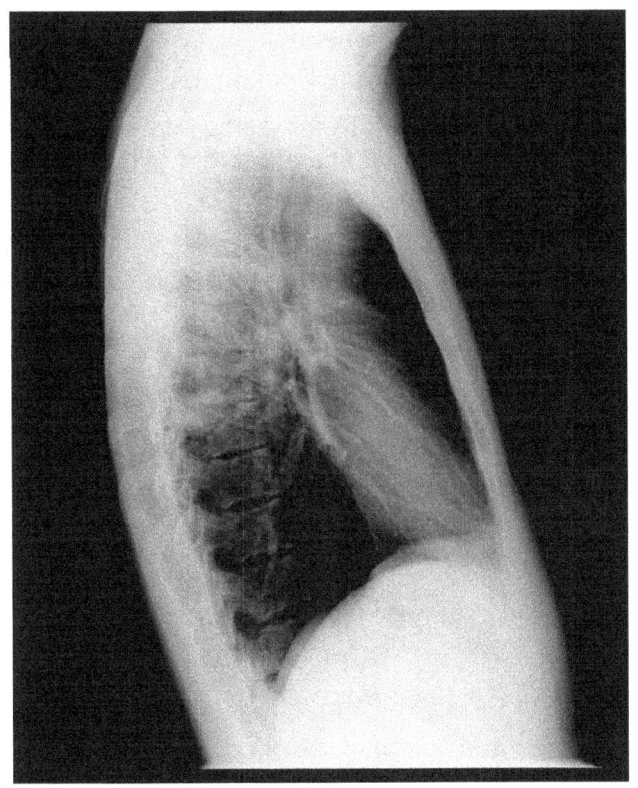

QUESTIONS

576. What is the likely diagnosis?
    a. Active Pulmonary TB
    b. Bronchitis, Bacterial
    c. Bronchitis, Fungal
    d. Bronchitis, Viral
    e. Pneumonia

577. What is the likely cause of this condition?
    a. Aspergillosis
    b. Parainfluenza Virus
    c. Mycobacterium Tuberculosis

d. Mycoplasma

   e. Streptococcus Pneumonia

578. Which of the following medications is usually included in the first line treatment of this condition?

   a. Amphotericin IV

   b. Azithromycin PO

   c. Isoniazid PO

   d. Rifampin PO

   e. A and b

   f. c and d

579. Which of the following is an expected complication of an overdose on an agent that is typically used for treatment of this condition?

   a. Acute Renal Failure

   b. Altered Mental Status

   c. Hearing Loss

   d. Methemoglobinemia

   e. Neuropathy

   f. Seizure

580. Which of the following is indicated for the treatment of the complication mentioned in the previous question?

   a. Diazepam IV

   b. Hemodialysis

   c. Methylene Blue

   d. Pyridoxine IV

   e. Vitamin B12 IV

ANSWERS

576. a

577. c

578. e

579. f

580. d

VISUAL STIMULUS REVIEW

The image shows a posterior segment right upper-lobe density consistent with active tuberculosis.

REFERENCES

- Zumla A, Raviglione M, Hafner R, von Reyn CF. Tuberculosis. N Engl J Med. 2013 Feb 21;368(8):745-55.
- CDC. Recommendations for use of an isoniazid-rifapentine regimen with direct observation to treat latent Mycobacterium tuberculosis infection. MMWR. 2011;60:1650-1653.

CASE #171: PAINFUL RASH

CASE

A previously healthy five-year-old boy is brought to the emergency department for a painful rash. His parents report three days of fever, cough, and runny nose as well as fine rash mostly over his face, torso, and extremities. Overnight, the rash progressed and turned into painful lesions. The vital signs are temp 103.4F (39.6C), heart rate 130/min, blood pressure 80/50 mmHg, respiratory rate 24/min, and O_2Sat 97% on room air. Oral exam shows extensive hemorrhagic erosions of the oral mucosa and hemorrhagic crusting of the lips. Skin exam shows involvement of at least 40% of his total body surface area.

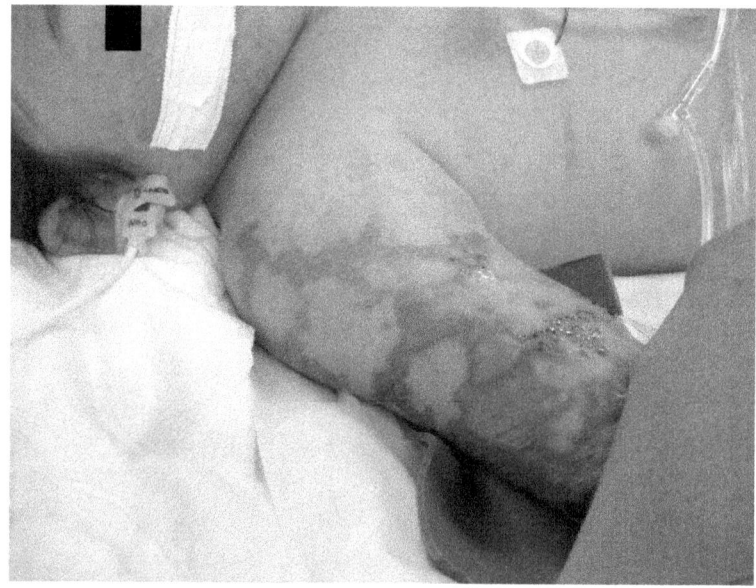

QUESTIONS

581. What is the likely diagnosis?
    a. Exfoliative Dermatitis
    b. Pemphigus Vulgaris
    c. Stevens Johnson Syndrome
    d. Toxic Epidermal Necrolysis
    e. Toxic Shock Syndrome

582. Use of which of the following has been associated with this condition?
    a. Ampicillin
    b. Ibuprofen
    c. Phenobarbital
    d. Phenytoin
    e. All of the above

583. Which of the following treatment is key in improving prognosis in this condition?
    a. Ceftriaxone IV
    b. Hemodialysis
    c. Methylprednisolone IV
    d. IVIG
    e. Plasmapheresis
    f. Supportive Care

ANSWERS

581. d

582. e

583. f

VISUAL STIMULUS REVIEW

The image shows some macular rash with diffuse blistering and hemorrhagic bullae.

REFERENCES

- Fernando SL. The management of toxic epidermal necrolysis. Australas J Dermatol. 2012 Aug;53(3):165-71.

- Downey A, Jackson C, Harun N, Cooper A. Toxic epidermal necrolysis: review of pathogenesis and management. J Am Acad Dermatol. 2012 Jun;66(6):995-1003.

CASE #172:   TESTICULAR PAIN

CASE

A 13-year-old boy is brought to the emergency department for sudden onset left testicular pain, nausea, and vomiting about an hour ago. He is in severe distress with a tender left scrotum that is also swollen and erythematous. A scrotal ultrasound is performed.

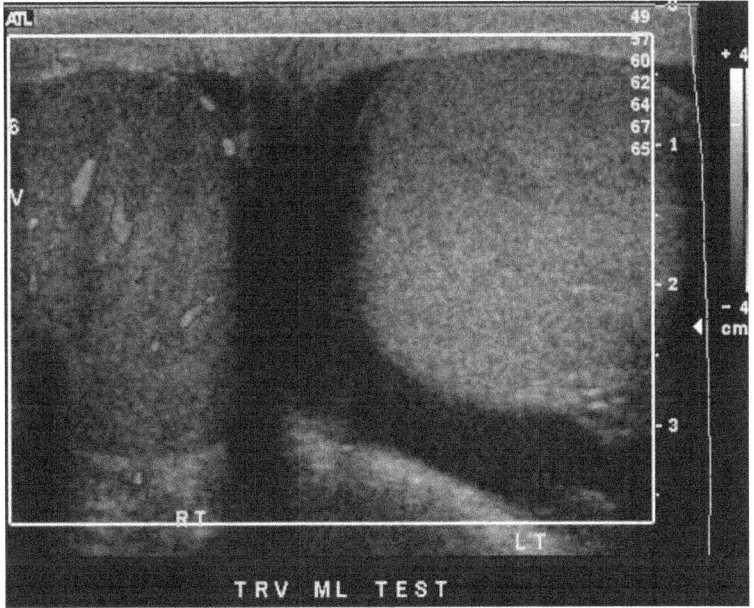

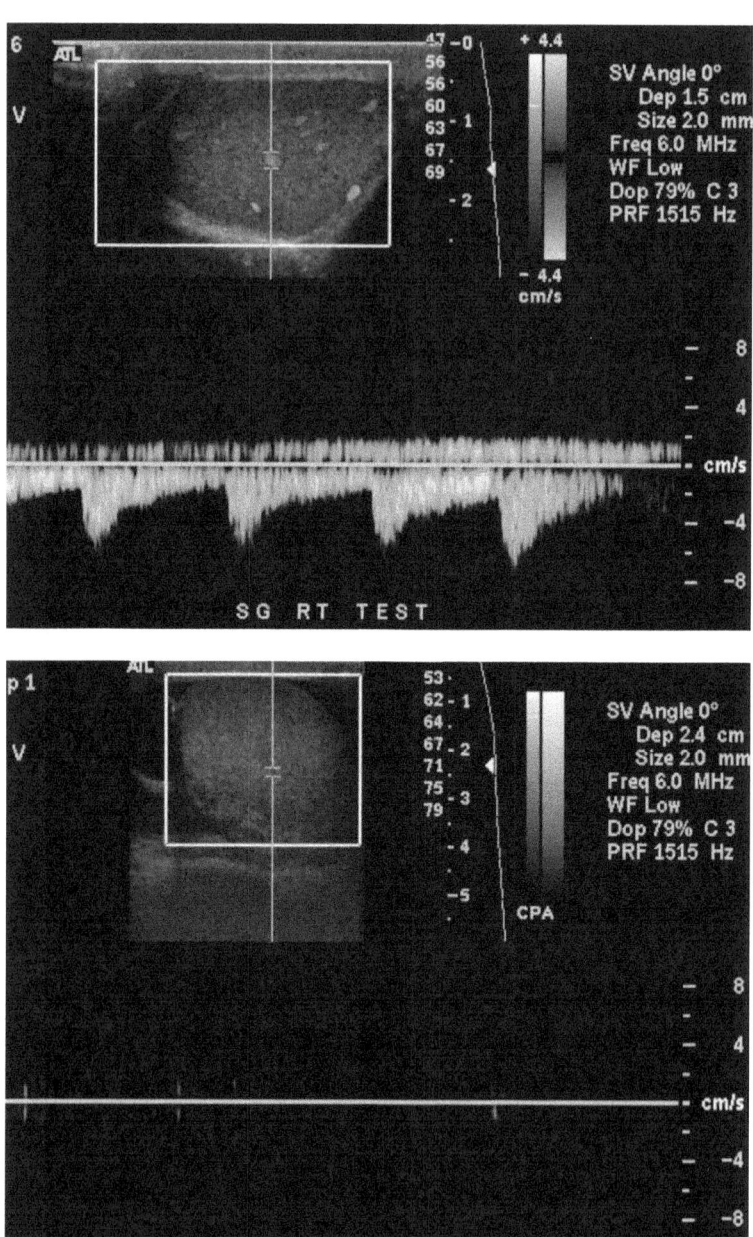

QUESTIONS

584. What is the likely diagnosis?
    a. Acute Appendicitis
    b. Idiopathic Scrotal Edema
    c. Incarcerated Inguinal Hernia
    d. Testicular Torsion
    e. Torsion of the Testicular Appendix

585. What is the likely cause of this condition?
    a. Bell Clapper Deformity
    b. Congenital Abdominal Wall Defect
    c. Cryptorchidism
    d. Direct Trauma
    e. Hot Ambient Temperature

586. Which of the following is most sensitive for the diagnosis of this condition?
    a. Absence of Cremasteric Reflex
    b. Radioisotope Scanning
    c. Surgical Exploration
    d. Testicular Doppler
    e. Testicular Ultrasound

ANSWERS

584. d

585. a

586. c

VISUAL STIMULUS REVIEW

The ultrasound images show no blood flow in the left testicle with some surrounding fluid.

REFERENCES

- Davis JE, Silverman M. Scrotal emergencies. Emerg Med Clin North Am. 2011 Aug;29(3):469-84.
- Ringdahl E, Teague L. Testicular torsion. Am Fam Physician. 2006 Nov 15;74(10):1739-43.

CASE #173: SORE THROAT

CASE

A 63-year-old man presents to his family doctor complaining of sore throat for three months. He has no past medical history but has been smoking a pack of cigarettes a day for the last 45 years. His sore throat started three months ago and was treated with oral amoxicillin for 10 days with no improvement. He denies any dysphagia, hoarseness, or trismus and reports that the pain mostly involves the right side of his throat. His vital signs are within normal limits. A CT scan is obtained.

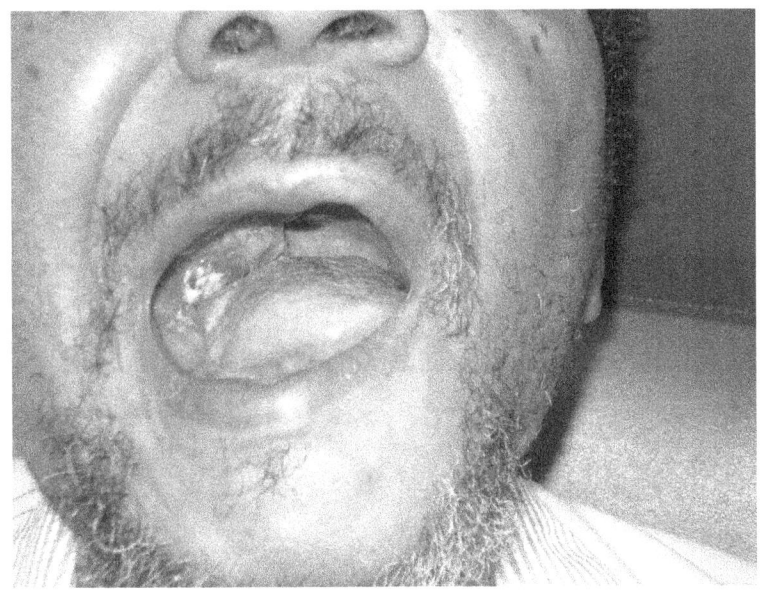

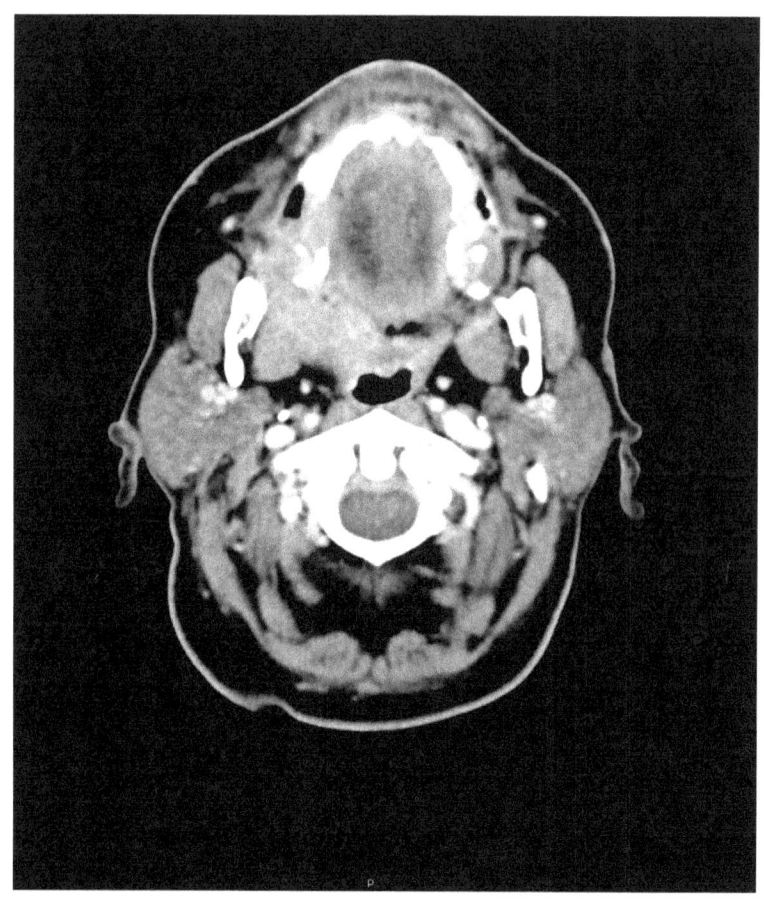

QUESTIONS

587. What is the likely diagnosis?
- a. Chronic Tonsillitis
- b. Infectious Mononucleosis
- c. Lymphoma
- d. Oral Cancer
- e. Peritonsillar Abscess
- f. Retropharyngeal Abscess

588. What is the likely cause of this condition?
   a. Actinomyces
   b. Epstein Bar Virus
   c. Human Papilloma Virus
   d. Squamous Cell Carcinoma
   e. Staphylococcus Aureus
   f. Streptococcus Group A

589. What is the typical anatomical origin of this condition?
   a. Frenulum
   b. Lymph Node
   c. Posterior Lateral Tongue
   d. Tonsils
   e. Uvula

590. Which of the following is a known risk factor for this condition?
   a. Alcohol Use
   b. Betel Consumption
   c. Cigarette Smoking
   d. Poor Dentition
   e. All of the above

ANSWERS

587. d

588. d

589. c

590. e

VISUAL STIMULUS REVIEW

The gross image shows a white and red soft tissue mass to the right of the tongue, involving the right tonsillar fossa as well as the soft and hard palates.

The CT image shows a soft tissue density that seems to origin from the right base of tongue to involve the right tonsil and extend into the soft and hard palates. The CT also shows a necrotic right submandibular lymph node.

REFERENCES

- Hunter KD, Yeoman CM. An update on the clinical pathology of oral precancer and cancer. Dent Update. 2013 Mar;40(2):120-2, 125-6.

- Carlson ER, Ghali GE, Herb-Brower KE. Diagnosis and management of pathological conditions. J Oral Maxillofac Surg. 2012 Nov;70(11 Suppl 3):e232-71.

CASE #174: WHITE TONGUE

CASE

A 20-year-old woman presents to her family doctor complaining of white coating to her tongue that developed over the last week. She has no past medical history but did develop poison ivy dermatitis a couple weeks prior and just finished a two-week course of prednisone. She has no cough and no difficulty swallowing solids or liquids. Her vital signs are within normal limits. On physical examination, the white coating was difficult to scrape off using a tongue blade.

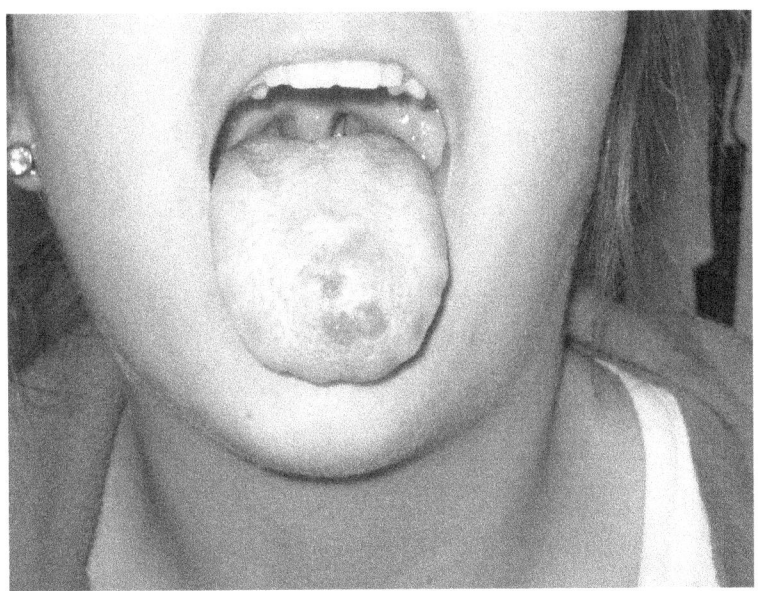

QUESTIONS

591. What is the likely diagnosis?
   a. Aphthous Ulcers
   b. Diphtheria

- c. Herpangina
- d. Leukoplakia
- e. Syphilis
- f. Thrush

592. What is the likely cause of this condition?
- a. Candida Albicans
- b. Corynebacterium
- c. Coxsackie Virus
- d. Epstein Bar Virus
- e. Herpes Simplex Virus
- f. Treponema Pallidum

593. Which of the following is a known risk factor for this condition?
- a. Antibiotic Use
- b. Diabetes Mellitus
- c. HIV
- d. Steroid Use
- e. Xerostomia
- f. All of the above

594. What is the first line of therapy for this condition?
- a. Acyclovir PO
- b. Doxycycline PO
- c. Nystatin Suspension Swish and Swallow
- d. Penicillin G IM
- e. Tongue Brushing
- f. c and e

ANSWERS

591. f

592. a

593. f

594. f

VISUAL STIMULUS REVIEW

The image shows white coating (plaque) to the tongue. The scraped areas demonstrate an inflamed base.

REFERENCES

- Rautemaa R, Ramage G. Oral candidosis--clinical challenges of a biofilm disease. Crit Rev Microbiol. 2011 Nov;37(4):328-36.
- Giannini PJ, Shetty KV. Diagnosis and management of oral candidiasis. Otolaryngol Clin North Am. 2011 Feb;44(1):231-40.

CASE #175: NECK PAIN

CASE

A 42-year-old woman presents to her family doctor complaining of anterior neck pain for three days. She has no medical history and is taking no medications. She reports progressive fever, chills, and anterior lower neck pain that worsens with head extension. Her vital signs are temp 103.2F (39.5C), heart rate 108/min, blood pressure 130/80 mmHg, respiratory rate 18/min, and O_2Sat 99% on room air. On physical exam, she has bilateral tenderness to palpation over her lower anterior neck.

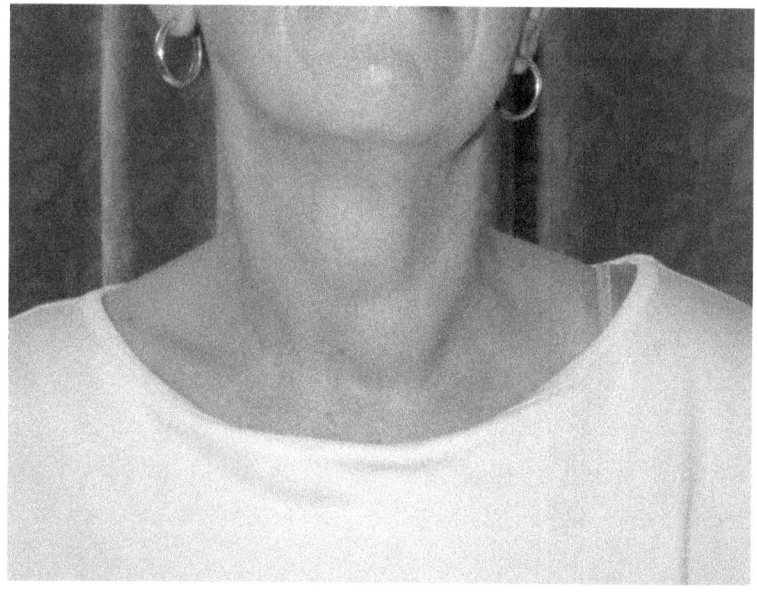

QUESTIONS

595. What is the likely diagnosis?
    a. Acute Thyroiditis
    b. Grave's Disease

c. Neck Cellulitis
   d. Photosensitivity
   e. Subacute Thyroiditis

596. What is the likely cause of this condition?
   a. Autoantibodies
   b. Chlamydia Trachomatis
   c. Influenza
   d. Mumps
   e. Staphylococcus Aureus

597. Which of the following findings is expected in this patient?
   a. Decreased TSH
   b. Elevated Amylase
   c. Elevated Antithyroid Peroxidase
   d. Elevated TSH
   e. Normal Thyroid Function Tests

598. Which of the following is indicated as part of the first line treatment of this condition?
   a. Antibiotics
   b. Prednisone
   c. Propranolol
   d. PTU
   e. Thyroidectomy
   f. Thyroxine

ANSWERS

595. a

596. e

597. e

598. a

VISUAL STIMULUS REVIEW

The image shows an enlarged and erythematous thyroid gland (left lobe > right) with some overlying erythema.

REFERENCES

- Paes JE, Burman KD, Cohen J et al. Acute bacterial suppurative thyroiditis: a clinical review and expert opinion. Thyroid. 2010 Mar;20(3):247-55.
- Pearce EN, Farwell AP, Braverman LE. Thyroiditis. N Engl J Med. Jun 26 2003;348(26):2646-55.

CASE #176:   ITCHY RASH

CASE

A 34-year-old man presents to his family doctor complaining of pruritic rash to his legs that started about six weeks ago. He denies any history of travel or exposure to animals. He describes that the lesions started as small red areas that progressed and grew in size. His vital signs are normal.

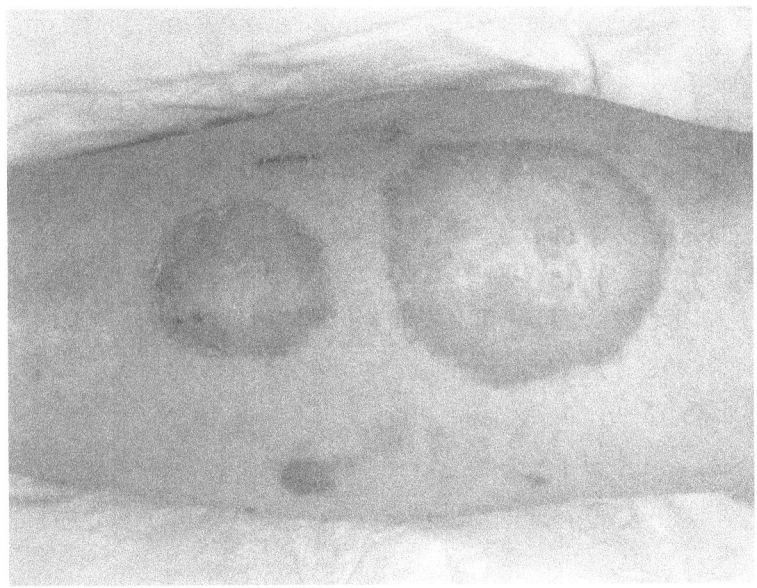

QUESTIONS

599. What is the likely diagnosis?
   a. Atopic Dermatitis
   b. Impetigo
   c. Psoriasis
   d. Tinea Corporis
   e. Swimmer's Itch
   f. Syphilis

600. What is the most common cause of this condition?
   a. Candida Albicans
   b. Epidermophyton Floccosum
   c. Microsporum Canis
   d. Schistosoma Mansoni
   e. Trichophyton Rubrum

601. What is the first line treatment for this condition?
   a. Oral Antibiotics
   b. Oral Antifungal
   c. Penicillin G
   d. Topical Antibiotic
   e. Topical Antifungal

ANSWERS

599. d

600. e

601. e

VISUAL STIMULUS REVIEW

The image show erythematous patches and plaques with fine scales. Some of the lesions show central clearing with a more intense erythema to the expanding border.

REFERENCES

- Moriarty B, Hay R, Morris-Jones R. The diagnosis and management of tinea. BMJ. 2012 Jul 10;345:e4380.
- Andrews MD, Burns M. Common tinea infections in children. Am Fam Physician. 2008 May 15;77(10):1415-20.

CASE #177: RASH

CASE

A previously healthy 30-year-old man presents to his family doctor complaining of a rash that started about a month ago. He reports that his wife noticed areas to the back of his neck that don't seem to tan as much. Over the last week the areas itch after he takes a shower.

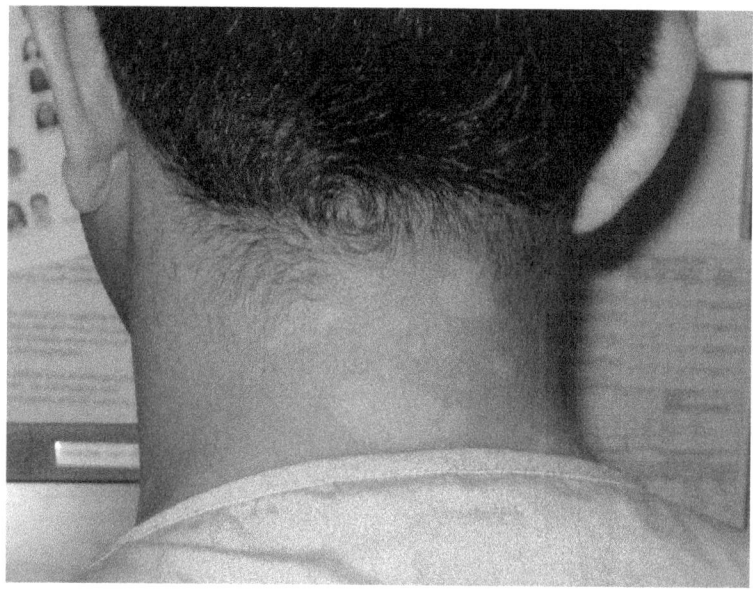

QUESTIONS

602. What is the likely diagnosis?
- a. Erythrasma
- b. Seborrheic Dermatitis
- c. Tinea Corporis
- d. Tinea Versicolor
- e. Vitiligo

603. What is the likely cause of this condition?
- a. Autoantibodies
- b. Candida Albicans
- c. Corynebacterium Minutissimum
- d. Malassezia Furfur
- e. Trichophyton Rubrum

604. What is the first line therapy of this condition?
- a. Betamethasone Ointment
- b. Fusidic Acid
- c. Prednisone PO
- d. Selenium Sulfide
- e. Terbinafine Cream

ANSWERS

602. d

603. d

604. d

VISUAL STIMULUS REVIEW

The image shows numerous hypopigmented macules with larger areas of macules that coalesce into irregularly shaped hypopigmented patches.

REFERENCES

- Hay RJ. Malassezia, dandruff and seborrhoeic dermatitis: an overview. Br J Dermatol. 2011 Oct;165 Suppl 2:2-8.

- Hu SW, Bigby M. Pityriasis versicolor: a systematic review of interventions. Arch Dermatol. 2010 Oct;146(10):1132-40.

- Bonifaz A, Gómez-Daza F, Paredes V, Ponce RM. Tinea versicolor, tinea nigra, white piedra, and black piedra. Clin Dermatol. 2010 Mar 4;28(2):140-5.

CASE #178: SORE THROAT

CASE

A previously healthy 19-year-old girl presents to her family doctor complaining of sore throat and odynophagia for the last two days. She reports sudden onset of sore throat, fever, and chills and denies cough, coryza, dysuria, vaginal discharge, or being sexually active. Her vital signs are temp 102.5F (39.1C), heart rate 100/min, and blood pressure 110/60 mmHg. Her neck is supple, her lung sounds are clear, and there are no murmurs on heart sounds auscultation.

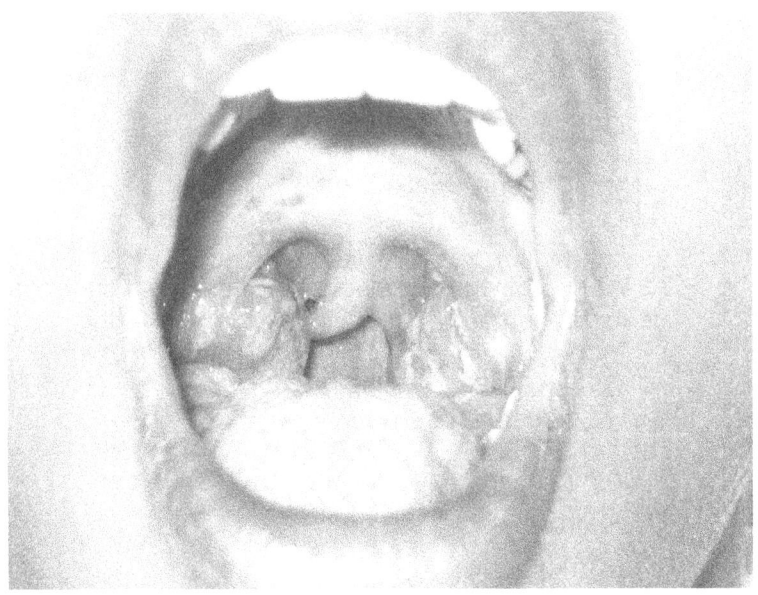

QUESTIONS

605. What is the likely diagnosis?

    a. Diphtheria

    b. Epiglottitis

c. Mononucleosis

d. Peritonsillar Abscess

e. Tonsillitis

606. What is the likely cause of this condition?

   a. Bartonella

   b. Cytomegalovirus

   c. Epstein Bar Virus

   d. Hemophilus Influenza

   e. Streptococcus Pyogenes

607. Which of the following is part of the first line treatment for this condition?

   a. Ceftriaxone IM

   b. Penicillin G IM

   c. Penicillin VK PO

   d. Prednisone PO

   e. b or c

608. Which of the following is the most common complication of this condition?

   a. Abscess Formation

   b. Disseminated Septic Arthritis

   c. Glomerulonephritis

   d. Hepatitis

   e. Rheumatic Heart Disease

   f. Splenic Rupture

ANSWERS

605. e

606. e

607. e

608. a

VISUAL STIMULUS REVIEW

The image shows erythematous and enlarged tonsils that are covered with white exudate. The image also shows soft palate petechiae, mostly to the right side. The uvula is midline and normal size.

REFERENCES

- Kociolek LK, Shulman ST. In the clinic. Pharyngitis. Ann Intern Med. 2012 Sep 4;157(5):ITC3-1 - ITC3-16.
- Tagliareni JM, Clarkson EI. Tonsillitis, peritonsillar and lateral pharyngeal abscesses. Oral Maxillofac Surg Clin North Am. 2012 May;24(2):197-204.
- Wessels MR. Clinical practice. Streptococcal pharyngitis. N Engl J Med. 2011 Feb 17;364(7):648-55.

CASE #179: CONFUSION

CASE

A 43-year-old man is brought to the emergency department for altered mental status and right-sided weakness the developed over the past week. The patient has no known past medical history, and, per his neighbors who called 911 and joined him at the hospital, he has been confused and disoriented over the past week and complained of right arm weakness. They tried to take him to the hospital a couple of days ago, but he refused. On exam, the patient is lethargic, opens his eyes to his name, and follows command in four extremities. He has a pronator drift on the right. He does have meningismus but is not febrile. A CT scan of his brain is ordered followed by an MRI.

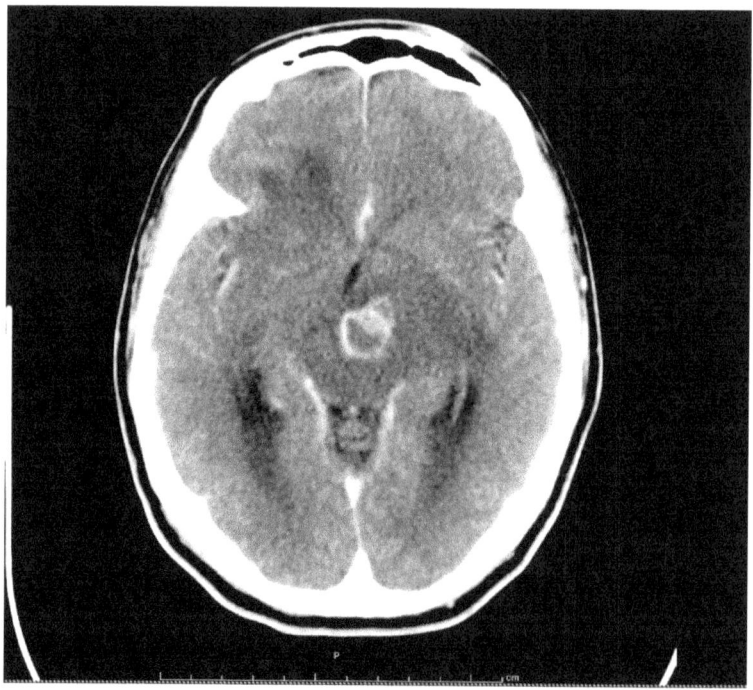

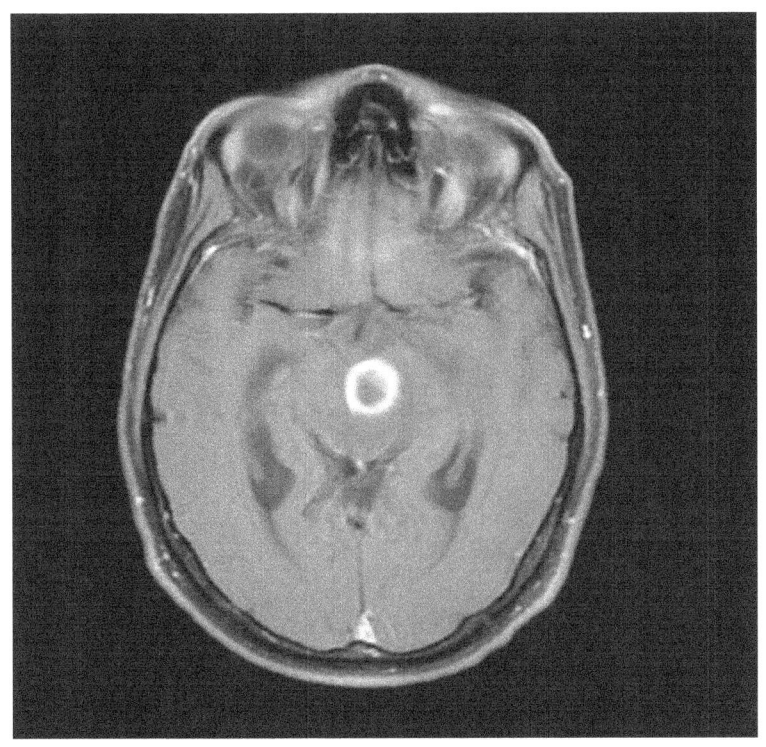

QUESTIONS

609. What is the likely diagnosis?
    a. Bacterial Meningitis
    b. Brain Abscess
    c. Herpes Encephalitis
    d. Neuro Cysticercosis
    e. Toxoplasmosis

610. What is the likely cause of this condition?
    a. Cysticercosis
    b. Neisseria Meningitidis

c. Herpes Simplex Virus
   d. Streptococcus Pneumonia
   e. Toxoplasma Gondii
611. What is the most common host of this condition?
   a. Birds
   b. Cats
   c. Cattle
   d. Dogs
   e. Pigs
612. Which of the following is a likely comorbidity that exists in this patient?
   a. AIDS
   b. Anemia
   c. C3 Deficiency
   d. Chronic Renal Failure
   e. Diabetes Mellitus
613. Which of the following medications is effective in treatment of this condition?
   a. Acyclovir
   b. Albendazole
   c. Ceftriaxone
   d. Pyrimethamine
   e. Vancomycin

ANSWERS

609. e

610. e

611. b

612. a

613. d

VISUAL STIMULUS REVIEW

The CT and MRI images show a ring enhancing lesion with surrounding edema.

REFERENCES

- Weiss LM, Dubey JP. Toxoplasmosis: A history of clinical observations. Int J Parasitol. 2009 Jul 1;39(8):895-901.

- Montoya JG, Liesenfeld O. Toxoplasmosis. Lancet. Jun 12 2004;363(9425):1965-76.

- Hill D, Dubey JP. Toxoplasma gondii: transmission, diagnosis and prevention. Clin Microbiol Infect. 2002 Oct;8(10):634-40.

CASE #180: RASH AND FEVER

CASE

A 35-year-old woman is brought to emergency department by EMS. She is two-weeks postpartum and has been in good health until two days ago when she developed generalized weakness, fatigue, and a fine rash to her bilateral legs. Her husband noticed about an hour ago that she became confused and that the rash progressed. Her vital signs are temp 102.5F (39.1C), heart rate 110/min, blood pressure 117/60 mmHg, respiratory rate 20/min, and O_2Sat 98%. On physical exam she is lethargic, not answering questions, and not following commands. The rash to her legs and torso is not palpable and does not blanch. The feet and palms are not involved.

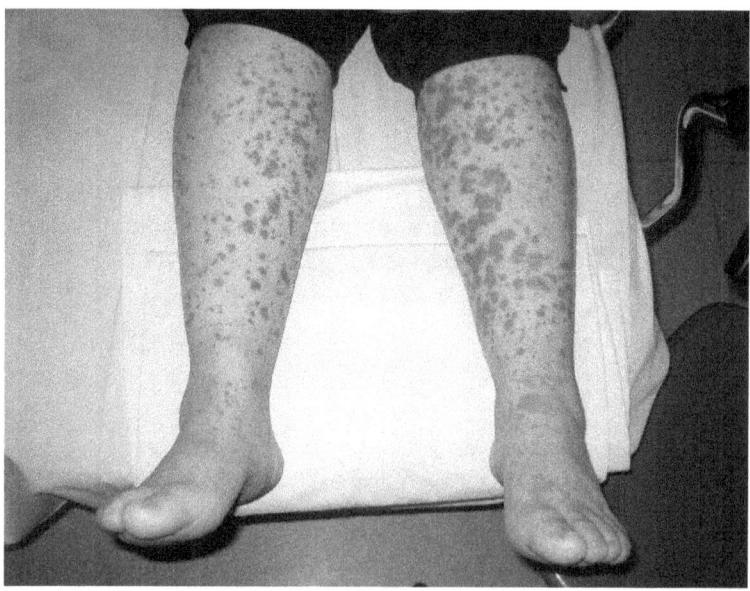

QUESTIONS

614. What is the likely diagnosis?
    a. Disseminated Intravascular Coagulation
    b. Hemolytic Uremic Syndrome
    c. Henoch Schönlein Purpura
    d. Immune Thrombocytopenia Purpura
    e. Thrombotic Thrombocytopenia Purpura

615. Which of the following is an expected finding in this condition?
    a. Basophilic Stippling
    b. Howell-Jolly Bodies
    c. Rouleaux Formation
    d. Schistocytes
    e. Stomatocytes

616. Which of the following is an expected finding in this condition?
    a. Elevated PT/INR
    b. Low Fibrinogen
    c. Low Platelet Count
    d. Markedly Elevated D-dimers

617. Which of the following is the treatment of choice for this condition?
    a. IVIG
    b. Methylprednisolone IV
    c. Plasma Exchange
    d. Plasmapheresis
    e. Prednisone PO
    f. a and e

ANSWERS

614. e

615. d

616. c

617. c

VISUAL STIMULUS REVIEW

The image shows diffuse petechiae and purpura to the lower extremities.

REFERENCES

- George JN, Al-Nouri ZL. Diagnostic and therapeutic challenges in the thrombotic thrombocytopenic purpura and hemolytic uremic syndromes. Hematology Am Soc Hematol Educ Program. 2012;2012:604-9.

- Kessler CS, Khan BA, Lai-Miller K. Thrombotic thrombocytopenic purpura: a hematological emergency. J Emerg Med. 2012 Sep;43(3):538-44.

CASE #181: DYSURIA

CASE

A previously healthy 20-year-old man presents to his family doctor complaining of painful urination. He reports five days of dysuria mostly localized to the meatus and worst during the first morning void. He also reports yellow stains on his underpants. His vitals are normal, and so are his testicular and prostate exams.

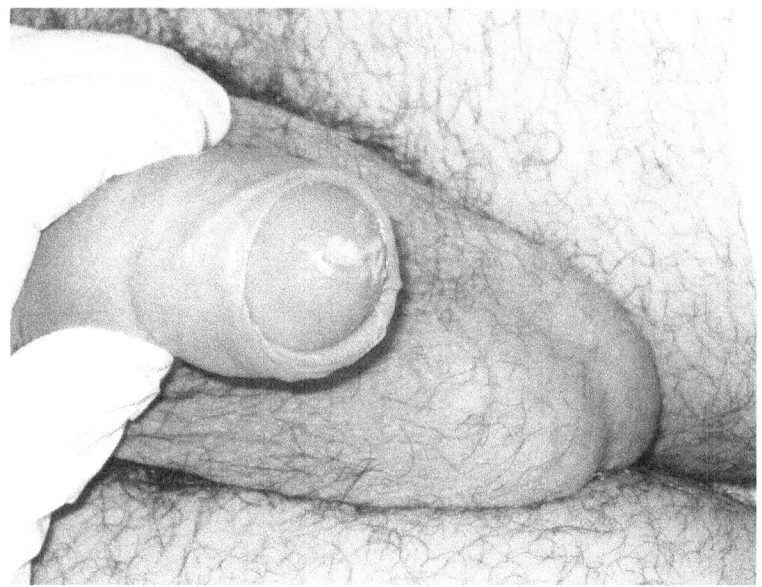

QUESTIONS

618. What is the likely diagnosis?

    a. Balanitis

    b. Cystitis

    c. Prostatitis

    d. Syphilis

    e. Urethritis

619. Which of the following organism is likely to be resistant to Levofloxacin?

    a. Chlamydia Trachomatis

    b. Escherichia Colli

    c. Mycoplasma Hominis

    d. Neisseria Gonorrhea

    e. Ureaplasma Urealyticum

620. Which of the following is correct in regards to patients with this condition?

    a. Patients with positive gram stain should be treated with Ceftriaxone.

    b. Patients with negative gram stain should be treated with Azithromycin.

    c. All patients should be treated with Ceftriaxone.

    d. All patients should be treated with Azithromycin or Doxycycline.

    e. c and d

ANSWERS

618. e

619. d

620. e

VISUAL STIMULUS REVIEW

The image shows purulent urethral discharge.

REFERENCES

- Centers for Disease Control and Prevention. Sexually Transmitted Diseases Treatment Guidelines, 2010. MMWR 2010;59(No. RR-12):1-110.
- Brill JR. Sexually transmitted infections in men. Prim Care. 2010 Sep;37(3):509-25.

ABOUT THE AUTHOR

Dr. Gil Shlamovitz is a practicing Emergency Physician at the Ben Taub General Hospital in Houston, TX, and the Director of Medical Informatics for the section of Emergency Medicine at Baylor College of Medicine. He earned his Doctor of Medicine degree from the Sackler School of Medicine in Tel-Aviv University and completed his residency training in Emergency Medicine at the UCLA / Olive-View-UCLA integrated residency program in Los-Angeles, CA. Gil is a frequently invited guest speaker both nationally and abroad in the subject of visual diagnosis and has been a regular speaker at the annual Scientific Assembly of the American College of Emergency Physicians since 2010. He is also an established medical researcher and author with a publications record of more than 14 articles in peer reviewed journals, and 17 book chapters in Medscape® Reference by WebMD. Gil also serves as CME and medical editor for Medscape® and a peer reviewer for the "Emergency Medicine Update" monthly e-publication and is the author and chief editor of the Visual Diagnosis Series® - http://www.visualdxseries.com.

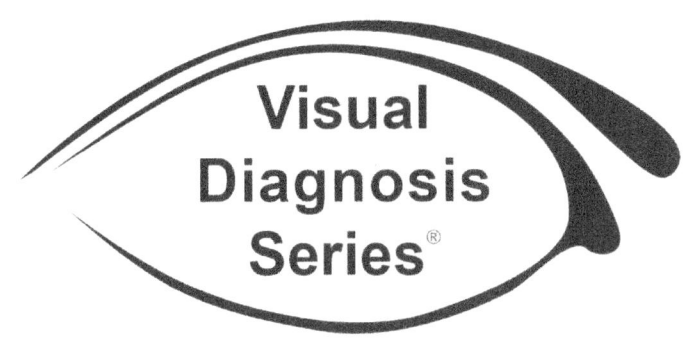

www.visualdxseries.com

www.ingramcontent.com/pod-product-compliance
Lightning Source LLC
Chambersburg PA
CBHW051620170526
45167CB00001B/3